The Role of Genetic Testing in Surgical Oncology

Editor

THOMAS K. WEBER

SURGICAL ONCOLOGY CLINICS OF NORTH AMERICA

www.surgonc.theclinics.com

Consulting Editor
NICHOLAS J. PETRELLI

October 2015 • Volume 24 • Number 4

ELSEVIER

1600 John F. Kennedy Boulevard ● Suite 1800 ● Philadelphia, Pennsylvania, 19103-2899

http://www.theclinics.com

SURGICAL ONCOLOGY CLINICS OF NORTH AMERICA Volume 24, Number 4
October 2015 ISSN 1055-3207, ISBN-13: 978-0-323-40108-1

Editor: John Vassallo
Developmental Editor: Meredith Clinton

Surgical Oncology Clinics of North America (ISSN 1055-3207) is published quarterly by Elsevier Inc., 360 Park Avenue South, New York, NY 10010-1710. Months of publication are January, April, July, and October. Business and Editorial Offices: 1600 John F. Kennedy Blvd., Ste. 1800, Philadelphia, PA 19103-2899. Customer Service Office: 3251 Riverport Lane, Maryland Heights, MO 63043. Periodicals postage paid at New York, NY and additional mailing offices. Subscription prices are $290.00 per year (US individuals), $421.00 (US institutions) $140.00 (US student/resident), $330.00 (Canadian individuals), $533.00 (Canadian institutions), $205.00 (Canadian student/resident), $410.00 (foreign individuals), $533.00 (foreign institutions), and $205.00 (foreign student/resident). Foreign air speed delivery is included in all *Clinics* subscription prices. All prices are subject to change without notice. **POSTMASTER**: Send address changes to *Surgical Oncology Clinics of North America*, Elsevier Health Science Division, Subscription Customer Service, 3251 Riverport Lane, Maryland Heights, MO 63043. **Customer Service: 1-800-654-2452 (US and Canada). 314-447-8871 (outside US and Canada). Fax: 314-447-8029. E-mail: journalscustomerservice-usa@elsevier.com (for print support); journalsonline support-usa@elsevier.com (for online support).**

Reprints. For copies of 100 or more, of articles in this publication, please contact the Commercial Reprints Department, Elsevier Inc., 360 Park Avenue South, New York, New York 10010-1710. Tel. 212-633-3874; Fax: 212-633-3820; E-mail: reprints@elsevier.com.

Surgical Oncology Clinics of North America is covered in *MEDLINE/PubMed (Index Medicus)* and *EMBASE/ Excerpta Medica, Current Contents/Clinical Medicine, and ISI/BIOMED.*

Contributors

CONSULTING EDITOR

NICHOLAS J. PETRELLI, MD, FACS
Bank of America Endowed Medical Director, Helen F. Graham Cancer Center and Research Institute, Christiana Care Health System, Newark, Delaware; Professor of Surgery, Thomas Jefferson University, Philadelphia, Pennsylvania

EDITOR

THOMAS K. WEBER, MD
Professor of Surgery, State University of New York Health Sciences Center at Downstate, Brooklyn, New York

AUTHORS

JOHN BURN, MD
Professor of Clinical Genetics, Institute of Genetic Medicine, International Centre for Life, Newcastle University, Newcastle upon Tyne, United Kingdom

RANDALL W. BURT, MD
Emeritus Professor of Medicine, Department of Internal Medicine, Huntsman Cancer Institute, The University of Utah, Salt Lake City, Utah

ZOHRA ALI-KHAN CATTS, MS, LGC
Director, Cancer Genetic Counseling, Christiana Care Health System, Helen F. Graham Cancer Center and Research Institute, Newark, Delaware

HUGH COLVIN, MB, Bchir, MRCS
Department of Gastroenterological Surgery, Osaka University Graduate School of Medicine, Suita, Osaka, Japan

ASHTON A. CONNOR, MD
Division of General Surgery, Department of Surgery, Faculty of Medicine, University of Toronto, Toronto, Ontario, Canada

STEVEN GALLINGER, MD, MSc
Professor, Division of General Surgery, Department of Surgery, Faculty of Medicine, University of Toronto, Toronto, Ontario, Canada

AMANDA GAMMON, MS
High Risk Cancer Research, Huntsman Cancer Institute, The University of Utah, Salt Lake City, Utah

MARC S. GREENBLATT, MD
Professor of Medicine, University of Vermont College of Medicine, Burlington, Vermont

HEATHER HAMPEL, MS, LGC
Professor, Department of Internal Medicine; Associate Director, Division of Human Genetics, Associate Director of Biospecimen Research, The Ohio State University Comprehensive Cancer Center, Columbus, Ohio

KORY JASPERSON, MS
Certified Genetic Counselor, Department of Internal Medicine, Huntsman Cancer Institute, The University of Utah, Salt Lake City, Utah

ROBERT T. JENSEN, MD
Chief, Cell Biology Section, Digestive Diseases Branch, National Institute of Arthritis, Diabetes, Digestive and Kidney Disease, National Institutes of Health, Bethesda, Maryland

GEOFFREY KRAMPITZ, MD
Professor, Department of Surgery, Stanford University School of Medicine, Stanford, California

MASAKI MORI, MD, PhD, FACS
Professor, Department of Gastroenterological Surgery, Osaka University Graduate School of Medicine, Suita, Osaka, Japan

DEBORAH W. NEKLASON, PhD
Department of Internal Medicine, High Risk Cancer Research, Huntsman Cancer Institute, The University of Utah, Salt Lake City, Utah

JEFFREY A. NORTON, MD
Department of Surgery, Stanford University School of Medicine, Stanford, California

OMAR M. RASHID, MD, JD
Department of Cutaneous Oncology, Graduate Medical Education, Moffitt Cancer Center, Tampa; Bienes Comprehensive Cancer Center, Holy Cross Hospital, Fort Lauderdale, Florida

MAREN T. SCHEUNER, MD, MPH
Professor, Department of Medicine, David Geffen School of Medicine at UCLA; Chief, Medical Genetics, VA Greater Los Angeles Healthcare System, Los Angeles, California

VICKIE L. VENNE, MS
Senior Genetic Counselor, Genomic Medicine Service, Salt Lake City, Utah

NORIKO WADA, MD
Department of Gastroenterological Surgery, Osaka University Graduate School of Medicine, Suita, Osaka, Japan

JEFFREY N. WEITZEL, MD
Professor of Oncology and Population Sciences, Chief, Division of Clinical Cancer Genetics, City of Hope Comprehensive Cancer Center, Duarte, California

KEN YAMAMOTO, MD, PhD
Professor, Department of Medical Chemistry, Kurume University School of Medicine, Kurume, Fukuoka, Japan

JONATHAN S. ZAGER, MD, FACS
Director of Regional Therapies, Department of Cutaneous Oncology, Chair, Graduate Medical Education; Senior Member, Moffitt Cancer Center; Professor of Surgery, University of South Florida School of Medicine, Tampa, Florida

Contents

> Alison's story illustrates the disastrous consequences of not securing an accurate family history when evaluating a patient for solid tumor malignancy; this is even more acute when the patient is diagnosed at a young age, or has other close relatives affected by the disease. Rapidly advancing genomic technologies directly challenge traditional management practices of referring all patients who may require genetic testing to a genetic counselor or clinical genetics service because next-generation targeted molecular therapies may be indicated based on genomic DNA analysis, and may be required urgently to treat life-threatening advanced disease, at times, before genetic counseling.

> Family health history is one of the least expensive, most useful, and most underused methods available to conduct assessments of the genetic aspect of a condition or to target the need for a genetic evaluation. This article introduces to the surgical oncologist the reason and process of collecting family history information. As medical records shift from paper to electronic formats, pedigree drawings are not readily available within the electronic health records. International efforts are underway to develop searchable, updatable, and interoperable formats that can collect family history information to inform clinical decision support for genetic risk assessment.

> The role of the cancer genetic counselor in the management of patients with cancer is discussed in this article. This includes explaining what a genetic counselor is trained to do and how they are credentialed and licensed. In addition, the article explains who to refer for cancer genetic counseling. Once referred, the article describes what actually happens in a pretest and posttest cancer genetic counseling session, use of a cancer genetic registry, and how it can help in practice is discussed. Finally,

several mechanisms for identifying a cancer genetic counselor at one's institution are outlined.

In the past decade, laws have been passed to provide legal protections against genetic discrimination. Many members of the public, and medical providers, are unaware of the legislation, and concerns about genetic privacy can prevent delivery of optimal medical care. Patient health information, including genetic testing and family history, is protected under the Health Insurance Portability and Accountability Act and the Genetic Information Nondiscrimination Act. Additional protections are granted through the Americans with Disabilities Act, state laws, and the Affordable Care Act. Communicating a genetic test result back to a patient is important for medical management decisions and family members.

The hereditary colorectal cancer syndromes comprise a heterogeneous group of conditions with varying cancer risks, gastrointestinal polyp types, nonmalignant findings, and inheritance patterns. Although each one is unique in its own right, these syndromes often have overlapping features, making diagnoses difficult in select cases. Obtaining accurate polyp history (histologic type, number, location, and age of onset), cancer history (location, type, and age of onset), and other nonmalignant features is imperative in determining the likely disease diagnosis and thereby the appropriate genetic tests for precise diagnosis in a timely fashion. This process often necessitates collaboration among surgical oncology team members and genetic counselors.

This article summarizes the impact of germline predisposition to breast cancer on the surgical management of breast cancer and breast cancer risk. Surgical implications of germline predisposition to breast cancer are now more nuanced due to the application of increasingly more complicated next-generation sequencing-based tests. The rapid pace of change will continue to challenge paradigms for genetic cancer risk assessment, which can influence the medical and surgical management of breast cancer risk as well as strategies for screening and for risk reduction.

Despite decades of scientific and clinical research, pancreatic ductal adenocarcinoma (PDAC) remains a lethal malignancy. The clinical and pathologic features of PDAC, specifically the known environmental and genetic risk factors, are reviewed here with special emphasis on the hereditary pancreatic cancer (HPC) syndromes. For these latter conditions, strategies are described for their identification, for primary and secondary prevention in unaffected carriers, and for disease management in affected carriers. Nascent steps have been made toward personalized medicine based on the rational use of screening, tumor subtyping, and targeted therapies; these have been guided by growing knowledge of HPC syndromes in PDAC.

Hugh Colvin, Ken Yamamoto, Noriko Wada, and Masaki Mori

Hereditary gastric cancer syndromes are a rare but distinct cause of gastric cancers. The genetic mutations underlying most affected families are unknown. Mutations of CDH1 occur in some patients affected by hereditary diffuse gastric cancer, and is the only practical marker for guiding management. Carriers of CDH1 mutations are at risk for a highly penetrant, aggressive and early-onset diffuse-type gastric cancer, and these individuals are usually offered prophylactic total gastrectomy. Further research is required to identify other genetic mutations responsible for these syndromes to improve our understanding of the underlying disease mechanisms and optimize the clinical management of affected individuals.

Omar M. Rashid and Jonathan S. Zager

Melanoma is increasing in incidence and represents an aggressive type of cancer. Efforts have focused on identifying genetic factors in melanoma carcinogenesis to guide prevention, screening, early detection, and targeted therapy. This article reviews the hereditary risk factors associated with melanoma and the known molecular pathways and genetic mutations associated with this disease. This article also explores the controversies associated with genetic testing and the latest advances in identifying genetic targets in melanoma, which offer promise for future application in the multidisciplinary management of melanoma.

Jeffrey A. Norton, Geoffrey Krampitz, and Robert T. Jensen

Early diagnosis of multiple endocrine neoplasia (MEN) syndromes is critical for optimal clinical outcomes; before the MEN syndromes can be diagnosed, they must be suspected. Genetic testing for germline alterations in both the MEN type 1 (MEN1) gene and RET proto-oncogene is crucial to identifying those at risk in affected kindreds and directing timely surveillance and surgical therapy to those at greatest risk of potentially life-threatening neoplasia. Pancreatic, thymic, and bronchial neuroendocrine tumors are the leading cause of death in patients with MEN1 and should be aggressively considered by at least biannual computed tomography imaging.

Marc S. Greenblatt

Clinical genetic testing for cancer predisposition syndromes often identifies DNA changes whose effects cannot be interpreted easily. These changes, often referred to as variants of uncertain significance (VUS), are not useful for clinical management. In contrast with clearly pathogenic mutations, VUS do not firmly diagnose a specific syndrome at the molecular level and cannot be used to identify with certainty which relatives are mutation carriers and which relatives are free of the syndrome. This article discusses the approach to evaluating VUS and how clinicians can play a key role in advancing the field to benefit all patients.

SURGICAL ONCOLOGY
CLINICS OF NORTH AMERICA

RELATED INTEREST

Surgical Clinics of North America, October 2015 (Vol. 95, Issue 5)
Cancer Screening and Genetics
Christopher L. Wolfgang, *Editor*
Available at: http://www.surgical.theclinics.com/

THE CLINICS ARE AVAILABLE ONLINE!
Access your subscription at:
www.theclinics.com

Foreword

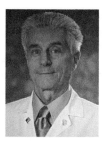

Nicholas J. Petrelli, MD, FACS
Consulting Editor

This issue of the *Surgical Oncology Clinics of North America* is devoted to genetic testing and its surgical oncology implications. The guest editor is Thomas K. Weber, MD, Professor of Surgery, State University of New York at Downstate, Brooklyn, New York. Dr Weber is also Chief of Surgery at the Department of Veterans Affairs, New York Harbor Healthcare System, Brooklyn Campus. Dr Weber is an American Cancer Society research scholar and an NIH-funded scientific investigator, has published extensively on hereditary colorectal cancer, and is a frequent invited speaker on that subject at national and international meetings.

We are presently in a medical era where advances in molecular biology and genetics have logarithmically improved our knowledge of how cells can change during a person's lifetime to evolve into cancer. It is important to realize that genetic testing can be useful for people with different types of cancer that are common in families, but genetic testing is not recommended for everyone. This issue of the *Surgical Oncology Clinics of North America* will help readers to understand what genetic testing is and how it can be used in cancer.

An excellent article by Drs Venne and Scheuner entitled, "Securing and Documenting Cancer Family History in the Age of the Electronic Medical Record," utilizes a case history of a 33-year-old woman with no cancer history referred for a surgical consultation after requesting prophylactic mastectomy because of her strong family history of breast cancer. Another article, by Drs Gammon and Neklason entitled, "Confidentiality and the Risk of Genetic Discrimination, What Surgeons Need to Know," centers on issues related to health insurance and job status.

Aside from the topics above, there are also articles that discuss in detail the role of genetic testing in specific cancers. For example, Drs Rashid and Zager discuss genetic testing in the management of melanoma, and Drs Jasperson and Burt discuss the genetics of colorectal cancer.

Like our individual fingerprints, each person's cancer has a unique combination of genetic alterations. Importantly, some of these genetic mutations may be the result of cancer rather than the cause. As our knowledge continues to grow in the field of genetics and proteomics, we will continue to offer patients the ultimate in cancer

Surg Oncol Clin N Am 24 (2015) xi–xii
http://dx.doi.org/10.1016/j.soc.2015.07.002
1055-3207/15/$ – see front matter © 2015 Published by Elsevier Inc.

surgonc.theclinics.com

prevention led by the experts that Dr Weber has brought together in this special issue of the *Surgical Oncology Clinics of North America*.

Nicholas J. Petrelli, MD, FACS
Bank of America Endowed Medical Director
Helen F Graham Cancer Center & Research Institute
Christiana Care Health Systems
4701 Ogletown Stanton Road, Suite 1233
Newark, DE 19713, USA

Professor of Surgery
Thomas Jefferson University

E-mail address:
npetrelli@christianacare.org

Preface

Surgical Oncology in the Age of Genomic Medicine

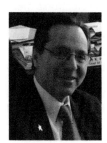

Thomas K. Weber, MD
Editor

Practicing Surgical Oncology in the age of genomic medicine is an exhilarating challenge. A quarter century after the launch of the Human Genome Project, the impact of the information it has delivered on clinical practice continues to expand exponentially. And yet, for many practicing surgical oncologists, the benefits of cancer genomics in everyday practice often seem remote if not frankly problematic on many counts, including basic logistics and medical-legal issues.

In this issue of *Surgical Oncology Clinics of North America*, we provide the practicing surgical oncologist with an impressive array of articles, each designed to deliver state-of-the-art cancer genetics information that is clinically relevant and readily usable in everyday practice. We cover all of the principle solid tumor malignancy syndromes on which surgical oncologists are most frequently consulted. Every article is written by world-class experts, each of whom is an active clinician practicing at internationally renowned academic medical centers. Our goal is to provide you with the definitive information, evidence-based guidelines, and exhaustive references you need to navigate twenty-first century cancer genetics and provide the best possible care to your patients. Our issue is filled with easy-to-read and easy-to-use tables of clinical practice guidelines, online resources, and exhaustive references.

We begin the issue with John Burn's testament to the vital importance of that simple question: "Have you or anyone else in your family ever had cancer?" We regularly remind our medical students, residents, and fellows that you do not need to know an intron from an exon to save a life. We remind them that recording family health

Surg Oncol Clin N Am 24 (2015) xiii–xv
http://dx.doi.org/10.1016/j.soc.2015.07.001
1055-3207/15/$ – see front matter © 2015 Published by Elsevier Inc.
surgonc.theclinics.com

history is the standard of care for a comprehensive history and physical examination (H&P). We remind them because we know the vast majority of recorded H&Ps have absent or deficient cancer family history information. Recent literature confirms that even among oncology practices, 70% of H&Ps are incomplete with regard to cancer family history, including critical age at diagnosis information.[1] The article by Vickie L. Venne and Maren T. Scheuner reviews the barriers and provides the tools necessary to secure accurate cancer family history information in the age of the electronic medical record. Zohra Ali-Kahn Catts with Heather Hampel and Amanda Gammon with Deborah W. Neklason review the dramatic extent to which genetic counselors can assist surgical oncologists and their patients. Importantly for all concerned, the underappreciated, surprisingly supportive legal framework protecting genetic information confidentiality is also reviewed.

In the next article, we begin our in-depth review of solid tumor genetics with a detailed summary of the clinical features, management, and genetic principles of each of the *eleven* currently known hereditary CRC syndromes. We bet you can't name them all—but you'll know how to manage each and every one of them after studying Kory Jasperson and Randall W. Burt's impressive work. Recertifying exams and daily clinical practice are full of tough questions regarding hereditary and familial breast cancer. In the next article, Jeffrey N. Weitzel takes us through what we need to know about hereditary breast and ovarian cancer syndrome as well as the *seven* other genetic syndromes associated with increased risk of invasive breast cancer. The advantages and limitations of newly available gene panels are also discussed.

In the articles by Ashton A. Connor with Steven Gallinger and Hugh Colvin with Ken Yamamoto, Noriko Wada, and Masaki Mori, we are taken through the most up-to-date information available on hereditary pancreatic and gastric cancer, respectively. Both of these articles outline clearly the multiple heritable syndromes that confer pancreatic and gastric cancer susceptibility. Each syndrome requires specific surveillance strategies and surgical care, including prophylactic surgery in some cases; all of which is reviewed.

In the article by Omar M. Rashid and Jonathan S. Zager, we are provided a thorough review of the impact of advances in germline as well as somatic genetics on the standard of care of malignant melanoma. This includes both new and soon to be released genomic-based targeted molecular therapies. In the article by Jeffrey A. Norton, Geoffrey Krampitz, and Robert T. Jensen, a thorough compendium of clinically relevant genetics and the clinical management of multiple endocrine neoplasia (MEN) are presented. It is an impressive body of work.

We close with an article by Marc S. Greenblatt, which is a sobering but extremely useful review of "what to do when genetic test results are not definitive": the significance and management of DNA sequence variants of unknown clinical significance, so-called VUS, are major issues in clinical cancer genetics and issues that we need to know how to navigate with our patients.

In what is perhaps the most poignant comment of this issue, Professor Jeffrey A. Norton observes in the early pages of his article: "Before MEN-1 can be diagnosed it must be *suspected*." Louis Pasteur reminded us in 1854 that "chance favors the prepared mind." At the end of the clinical day, it is indeed our responsibility to ask the cancer family history question described above. It is up to us to be prepared, to ask the key questions, to *suspect* those syndromes that pose the gravest risk to those who entrust their care to us, and then, based on the best objective information we have, act in the very best interest of our patients and their families. We trust this issue will assist you in those efforts. It is our sincere hope that it will help to "prepare the mind" to deliver optimal cancer prevention and care.

Thomas K. Weber, MD
Professor of Surgery
State University of New York Health Sciences Center at Downstate
Suite 112, 800 Poly Place
Brooklyn, NY 11209, USA

E-mail address:
thomaskweber@gmail.com

REFERENCE

1. Wood ME, Kadlubek P, Pham TH, et al. Quality of cancer family history and referral for genetic counseling and testing among oncology practices: a pilot test of quality measures as part of the American Society of Clinical Oncology Quality Oncology Practice Initiative. J Clin Oncol 2014;32(8):824–9.

Alison's Story—A Cautionary Tale in the Age of Genomic Medicine

John Burn, MD

KEYWORDS

- Breast cancer - Family history - Targeted molecular therapy - Genetic testing

KEY POINTS

- Documentation of patient family history is essential for all patients with cancer and especially critical for those diagnosed at an early age (younger than 50 years).
- Patients with early-age-onset cancer should be referred to clinical genetics services for consideration of genetic testing.
- The advent of targeted molecular therapies, the indications for which are based on germline genetic information, increases the rationale for immediate germline DNA analysis, independent of genetic counseling services.
- These services may not be available in a timely manner or, in many parts of the world, not available at all.

It was a routine clinic in 2008, 2 hours' drive from base and covering for a colleague. Alison's enthusiasm dispelled weary thoughts. A science teacher at a local high school, her desire to understand shone through, encouraging eyes hanging on each question. An only child of older parents, she had lost contact with her relatives but recalled as a teenager commenting on the number of women who had died of breast or womb cancer in her family tree. Older wiser heads had assured her that such cancers did not run in families. Then at age 34 years, she had a developed breast cancer herself and undergone curative mastectomy, but again, discussion of a possible inherited cause prompted no reaction or referral.

Now, at 50 years, Alison had finally found her way to our door. At the time, we were encouraged to validate family histories before ordering BRCA testing, but I knew it would be challenging and, noting my reliance on her excellent history, I ordered the test and told her I would see her in a few months once her sample had progressed up the long queue.

The author has nothing to disclose.
Institute of Genetic Medicine, International Centre for Life, Newcastle University, Central Parkway, Newcastle upon Tyne NE1 3BZ, UK
E-mail address: john.burn@newcastle.ac.uk

Surg Oncol Clin N Am 24 (2015) 635–637
http://dx.doi.org/10.1016/j.soc.2015.06.010
1055-3207/15/$ – see front matter © 2015 Elsevier Inc. All rights reserved.
surgonc.theclinics.com

Six months elapsed before Alison's name returned to my desk, not attached to a result, but as a message that she had been admitted to her local hospital having suffered a stroke. She had refused to cooperate, despite her dysphasia, unless they performed an ultrasound examination of her pelvis. She later told me that she guessed the diagnosis as she had begun to have menstrual bleeding again and she could see the obvious masses as soon as the ultrasound probe captured her pelvic image. The cranial computed tomographic scan confirmed the metastasis.

I invited her to our department to discuss the pathogenic splice variant in BRCA2 we had discovered, and she focused on the value that would have to her family. She agreed to record an interview and meet with our senior medical students. Despite struggling with her words, she was able to marvel at her excellent response to chemotherapy and express her gratitude for our efforts. This interview can be seen using the following link: http://youtu.be/SMLO-anbycQ.

Three more months passed, and I heard that Alison had died. I met her children who recounted her positive demeanor to the end. Her smiling face stayed with me. Should I have asked for a gynecological examination while awaiting her BRCA result? Clinical utility of ovarian ultrasound imaging is not established. It was probably already too late. Should it have taken her so long to even reach the discussion about genetic testing? The ignorance of her clinical team at the time of her mastectomy was defensible, but did anyone reconsider the possibility on her multiple subsequent mammogram visits? Clearly not.

As I write, my head is full of details about olaparib, newly licensed for treatment of relapsed BRCA mutated ovarian cancer, a 20-year journey since I first heard my colleagues in Medicinal Chemistry in Newcastle describe their newly invented PARP (pharmacologic inhibitors of the enzyme poly ADP ribose polymerase) inhibitors. The development of these new agents provides added incentive to proceed with genetic testing as early as possible so as to provide patients with the relevant BRCA mutations with effective targeted molecular therapies. This new time pressure to treat, based on genomic DNA information, calls into question traditional genetic counseling strategies that take excessive time, even in the most advanced academic medical center settings, and are simply not available across most of the world.

All health systems are under financial pressure, so we have to keep an eye on the financial bottom line but the case for first-line deployment of diagnostic gene testing in patients with solid tumors is steadily growing in strength. There will be casualties; some people with cancer would rather not know that their tumor is the result of an inherited genetic change, but the availability of targeted effective therapies and access to surveillance for their close family means these individuals are few.

Those who demand that germline testing must remain locked away behind a gateway guarded by the handful of genetic counselors and clinical geneticists available in developed countries must recognize the futility of this restraint. The latest analysis in the United Kingdom reveals that half of all people born since 1960 will develop a cancer during their life time. All cancer results from disruption of genetic control of cell function. Soon, all multimodal therapeutic interventions for cancer will be influenced by the genetic profile of the tumor. No doubt the dyes invented in the nineteenth century coupled with microscopy invented a century earlier will continue to play a central role, but, like the histopathologists before them, today's geneticists cannot remain the sole guardians of the tools of molecular biology, demanding expert consideration before DNA testing is offered and performed. But equally, expansion into rapid diagnostics means every clinician must acquire a core knowledge of genomics and respect their own limitations and the value of those who have specialist knowledge of genetic medicine.

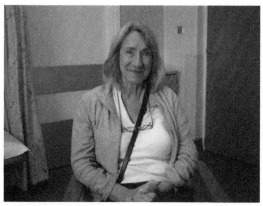

Fig. 1. Alison in brief remission after chemotherapy for her cerebral metastasis from undiagnosed BRCA2 deficient ovarian cancer.

The cost of whole-genome sequencing has reduced in less than 2 decades from 100 million dollars per genome to $1000 and will reduce further. Full disclosure, I must declare an interest as chairman and part owner of a young biotech company that will soon have on offer technology that can extract DNA in 2 minutes and perform selected genotyping automatically on the product in less than 20 minutes for $20. However, ours is only one of a dozen or more point-of-care technologies heading for the market or already there. The landscape on which genetics and molecular biology directly affect the care of patients with cancer and their families is rapidly changing. Soon, failure to test the somatic DNA of a tumor as well as the patient's germline DNA will generate the same incredulity that would meet a doctor performing a blood transfusion without first testing the patient's blood group. And perhaps even sooner, failure to take a diligent family history and offer genetic testing to a young 34-year-old science teacher with breast cancer will be considered medical malpractice. For the sake of all those Alisons out there, I hope the day is not far off **(Fig. 1)**.

Securing and Documenting Cancer Family History in the Age of the Electronic Medical Record

 CrossMark

Vickie L. Venne, MS[a],*, Maren T. Scheuner, MD, MPH[b,c]

KEYWORDS

- Family health history • Pedigree • Genetic risk assessment
- Electronic medical records

KEY POINTS

- Family health history (FHHx) is one of the least expensive, most useful, and most under-used methods to assess genetic risk and target the need for a genetic evaluation.
- In an era of increasingly comprehensive genetic testing, family history is still vital to the interpretation of many genetic test results.
- FHHx information sufficient to assess the need for a genetic consultation can be obtained reasonably quickly.
- Documenting family history electronically may inform clinical decisions regarding a diagnosis, screening, and prevention, as well as identify the need for referral for genetic evaluation, which might include genetic testing.

Case example: Maria is a healthy 33-year-old woman with no cancer history referred for a surgical consultation after requesting prophylactic mastectomy because of her strong family history of breast cancer.

Most individuals are aware when a health condition, whether it is cancer, cardiovascular disease, asthma, obesity, or a mental health disorder, runs in a family. What most individuals do not do is distinguish among the various factors, be they environmental, lifestyle, or genetic, that can impact the development and management of those conditions. Collecting and documenting an FHHx is one of the least

Ms V.L. Venne and Dr M.T. Scheuner are both employed by the Department of Veterans Affairs. The views expressed within are solely those of the authors, and do not necessarily represent the views of the Department of Veterans Affairs or the US government.

[a] Genomic Medicine Service, SLC VA Medical Center, 500 Foothill Drive, Salt Lake City, UT 84148, USA; [b] Department of Medicine, David Geffen School of Medicine at UCLA, 10833 Le Conte Ave, Los Angeles, CA 90095, USA; [c] Medical Genetics, VA Greater Los Angeles Healthcare System, 11301 Wilshire Boulevard, Los Angeles, CA 90073, USA
* Corresponding author.
E-mail address: vickie.venne@va.gov

expensive, most useful, and most underused methods to target the need for a genetic evaluation for risk assessment. FHHx is valuable when making a differential diagnosis or identifying surveillance and prevention options. Especially in an era when genetic testing is moving from single gene analysis to multigene panels and exome/genome sequencing, an FHHx may become even more vital in interpreting those laboratory results. Even for families without an identifiable genetic mutation, the FHHx can be important in changing surveillance, such as the first-degree relatives of a 47-year-old individual with colon cancer who are now candidates for earlier colon screening.

FHHx has long been recognized as an important component in prediction, prevention, and management of common, complex diseases, including cancers.[1] Half of all families have a positive FHHx for one or more common chronic diseases. Depending on the condition, a positive FHHx increases a person's chance of developing a particular disease from 2 to 10 times.[2] Consequently, FHHx has always been part of a comprehensive medical intake, because it represents the complex interaction of genes, environment, and other lifestyle risk factors for diseases shared among relatives.

However, several barriers have been identified that hinder the collection of an FHHx, not only at the provider level but also with patients and health care systems in general.[3–6] It takes time, it is not clear to most clinicians as to which questions are the most useful, and even when asked, patients are not always aware of the health nuances that are relevant to a genetic assessment.[2,7–9]

At present, a significant health care system barrier to the use of documented FHHx is the lack of consistent structured data elements.[10] Examples of structured data elements include gender, age, age at death and cause, diagnosis, age at diagnosis, and sometimes screening behaviors or treatment options. Without these data elements that can be queried by the electronic health record (EHR) system, clinical decision support (CDS) that assesses the FHHx data to assist with risk assessment or referral for genetic evaluation is not possible. Given the importance of FHHx for effective screening and prevention, several federal agencies, including the Centers for Disease Control and Prevention and the National Institutes of Health (NIH), have emphasized the importance of research and development of FHHx tools.[11] At present, many teams are exploring methods of incorporating FHHx into EHRs using structured data and interoperable formats.

This article reviews the process of collecting an initial family history within the EHR and updating it during subsequent clinic visits. This process can be facilitated if the information is collected, stored, accessed, and updated in a designated section of the EHR, and the data could be more valuable to the clinician if tied to CDS. With complete family history information documented in the medical record, the surgeon can then assess if the patient is a candidate for a comprehensive genetic evaluation or if alternative or enhanced screening, medication, or surgical options should be considered.

REASONS FOR COLLECTING AND DOCUMENTING A CANCER FAMILY HISTORY

There are many reasons to collect FHHx. Family history may clarify the cause of a disease through recognition of a hereditary cancer syndrome. FHHx can influence eligibility for genetic testing or inform screening and management decisions for both affected patients and their unaffected extended family members. Often, the purpose of the FHHx is to assess the need for a genetic referral. Therefore, an initial FHHx is usually cursory and targeted to the condition of interest to address that limited decision. However, a FHHx is important as a factor in many common, chronic diseases to inform the following:

- A differential diagnosis in a patient with signs and symptoms
  - An example is the evaluation of chest pain in a 45-year-old man who reports myocardial infarction in his father at the age of 45 years. This evaluation will move angina higher up on the list.
  - In another example, decisions about subtotal colectomy for polyposis are typically informed by the polyp burden and whether there is a history of polyposis or colorectal cancer in family.
- Surveillance and prevention options
  - When evaluating a patient to determine if antiestrogens (tamoxifen, raloxifene) are appropriate for chemoprevention of breast cancer, the Gail model assesses the 5-year and lifetime risk for breast cancer based on FHHx and other factors such as age, reproductive history, and breast biopsy history.
  - In another instance, first degree relatives of individuals with early onset colon cancers may be advised to initiate colon cancer screening earlier than the population recommendation of age 50.

THE PROCESS OF COLLECTING AND DOCUMENTING CANCER FAMILY HISTORY

Like much of medicine, there is both a science and an art to collecting an FHHx. When the unaffected female patient presented at the beginning of this article requests prophylactic mastectomy because of her strong family history, genetic testing, regardless of the number of genes analyzed, may not provide a sufficient answer to guide that decision. If she has a deleterious mutation in a gene that predisposes to breast cancer, such as *BRCA1, BRCA2,* or *TP53*, making the decision to undergo prophylactic surgery may be easier. Alternatively, if a familial breast cancer gene mutation could be excluded, there would be no indication for prophylactic mastectomy, in the absence of an assessment of personal risk factors. However, testing her and finding no mutation does not exclude her familial risk. Thus, a family history is different from knowing of a familial mutation that predisposes to breast cancer. Knowing what constitutes her strong family history will help direct decisions for supportive counseling to emotionally deal with the cancers in her family or a possible referral for genetic evaluation.

How to Start

Family histories begin with the patient: the consultand.[12] If the plan is to draw a graphic representation while collecting the FHHx, the patient is often designated with an arrow or a C ("today, you are the Center of this universe"). The patient's personal history of cancer, if any, may already be known. If not, any cancer history should be documented because this could help to inform the likelihood of an inherited cancer syndrome.

Next, the person in the family who has cancer and his or her relationship to the patient needs to be identified. Asking questions about the aggregate family (does anyone in the family have X type of cancer?) is quickest, although asking questions about each individual in the family (does your mother have any type of cancer?) will likely allow the patient to reflect and provide a more comprehensive response. Then knowing the age of the person at the time of the diagnosis and current age or age at death will help with the risk assessment.

Information about the first-degree relatives (parents, siblings, children) and second-degree relatives (grandparents, aunts/uncles) allows for recognition of the pattern of cancers that are most relevant and is usually sufficient to assess the need for a more comprehensive genetic evaluation. Most hereditary cancer syndromes are inherited in an autosomal dominant manner.

More comprehensive cancer histories often include cousins, as well as great aunts and uncles and lead to expansion of histories around affected individuals. For instance, a cousin with breast cancer may have a relevant family history on the side of the family not related to the patient, but would be important to a risk assessment, because an apparent inherited predisposition may be clearly demonstrated in the lineage not related to the patient.

Since genes—and environmental behaviors—come from both sides of the family, it is important to collect FHHx information from both the maternal and paternal sides. Especially with gender-specific cancers (ovarian, prostate), the second- and third-degree relatives are more important if the genetic predisposition seems to be inherited from the side of the family in which the gender-specific cancer would not be manifest in the parent.

An example of a chart note documenting family history for a 45-year-old woman with a recent diagnosis of breast cancer might read as follows:

A three-generation pedigree was obtained. All diagnoses are by patient report; no records confirming diagnoses were obtained.

- *Children: 1 son aged 23 years; 3 daughters, (25, 21, 19 years old), all healthy. No grandchildren.*
- *Siblings: 5 male siblings: 3 brothers alive (52, 48, and 43 years old), 1 had colon cancer at the age of 51 years, 1 brother died as infant, and another died at the age of 24 years, because of a motor vehicle accident. Another brother had colonoscopy with 6 benign polyps removed at the age of 48 years. One sister, aged 54 years, had breast cancer, with age at onset of 50 years.*
- *Maternal: Mother, 78 years old, good health. Normal mammograms until age 75 years, no colon screenings. Four siblings, 1 died of breast cancer, with age at onset of 67 years. Grandparents died in their late 70s/early 80s of heart complications.*
- *Paternal: Father, 78 years old, prostate cancer at the age of 70 years. Nine siblings, lived into their 80s, some with heart problems; no known history of cancer. Grandfather died of lung cancer, worked in coal mines. Grandmother died of heart problems.*

Ancestry: Northern European, no Ashkenazi Jewish ancestry.

Knowing how many individuals are unaffected with any type of cancer allows for the assessment of penetrance in the family. Lack of understanding of penetrance is one of the many reasons people overestimate their risk of developing cancer. Although a patient may present with a perception of a strong family history, it may be that her mother and 2 favorite aunts (1 from mother's side and 1 from father's side) developed breast cancer and that she does not take into consideration the other 12 females who lived to their 70s cancer free (**Fig. 1**).

There are many examples of how to collect FHHx in the public domain to encourage the general public (and surgeons!) to better understand the importance of collecting this information. Short videos demonstrate the importance and process from organizations such as Kaiser Permanente (https://www.youtube.com/watch?v=xSuMkrhzXGA) and National Coalition for Health Professional Education in Genetics (https://www.youtube.com/watch?v=TS45BJ7YnC0) and can also be used by clinicians to quickly refresh the process of quickly collecting this information.

CIRCUMSTANCES THAT MAKE FAMILY HISTORY COLLECTION A CHALLENGE

- Incongruous information: Families share health stories, and patients may not understand if they are providing misleading information. Polyps are not the same as

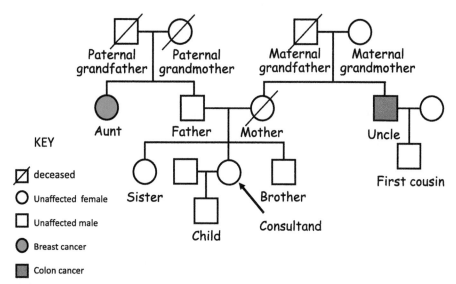

Fig. 1. Graphical representation of first-, second-, and third-degree family members in a pedigree, with a legend identifying several cancers.

cancer. "Female" cancer is not a diagnosis, and a gynecologic cancer diagnosed in a 24-year-old woman that was resolved by surgery was more likely cervical than ovarian. Although genetic professionals might request medical records to confirm these incongruities, a few additional questions regarding the management of that diagnosis may clarify the type of cancer being reported.

- Adoption: One of the most common reasons adoptees search for birth parents is to learn about their ancestry and medical histories. In the past few decades, some adoption agencies collected cursory health history, but health history is typically limited.[13] From a counseling perspective, it can help patients to remember that only about 10% to 20% of cancers occur as a result of a genetic predisposition to a highly penetrant cancer syndrome, so over 80% of cancers will not have an identifiable inherited component.
- Small family size: Sometimes an individual is an only child; this may be by parental choice, infertility, or other reasons. Collecting information about miscarriages and stillbirths can be important in the genetic evaluation of some conditions. It is not as relevant in the evaluations of most cancer syndromes, but small family size could result in limited information from which to conduct a risk assessment.[14]
- Death in a family: Sometimes the death of an individual at an early age (the exact reason the history is needed) creates an environment where one side of the family history becomes totally unavailable. On further questioning, there is often an aunt or a cousin who stayed in touch and might be of help in fleshing out sufficient information to conduct a risk assessment. Individuals with Jewish heritage may not know family members who died in the Holocaust, and more recently, political refugees from war-torn countries may not know or have access to information about their kin.
- Disenfranchised families: It happens. Families separate or disown members. Long-standing anger puts patients in a position of being unwilling or unable to obtain family health information; this can especially be true if the patient is under

the erroneous belief that genetic testing will provide a comprehensive answer and that obtaining an accurate FHHx is unnecessary.[15]

In the face of a truncated history, it is important to clarify the patient expectations. Many unaffected individuals overestimate their risks of developing cancer.[16,17] Understanding why the patient is asking questions about risk assessment and what the eventual goal is can lead to conversations about a realistic outcome. It can also help start the conversation about genetic testing and who the most appropriate candidate can be.

For those individuals, referral for a genetic consultation can help them put their risk into perspective and include a discussion about the nongenetic causes of cancer. Genetic testing in the absence of an FHHx or clinical indication may result in a challenging interpretation in an era in which knowledge of genetic mutations is rapidly changing.

UPDATING A FAMILY HEALTH HISTORY

Family health histories are dynamic. Between clinical visits for any one patient, extended family members may have died or been newly diagnosed with cancer. Sometimes the questions asked at an initial visit prompt a patient to ask more specific questions about relatives. As additional FHHx becomes available, risk assessment can easily change. Therefore, if the original FHHx information is available during subsequent visits, it can be used to review the initial report and update as new information is collected by the patient.

Once the brief family history is collected, at-risk individuals could then be referred for cancer genetic consultations. One barrier to this step is a lack of understanding of the referral criteria. Organizations such as the National Comprehensive Cancer Network have developed guidelines, as have many other national and professional organizations. These guidelines can be accessed for free by registering at www.nccn.org, and the Web site provides a wealth of information. Their guidelines change with new genetic discoveries.

A task force that included members of both the American College of Medical Genetics and the National Society of Genetic counselors recently published a comprehensive review that details referral indications.[1] These practice guidelines are organized by the cancer of interest and include rare tumors in addition to common cancers. This useful resource includes brief summaries of the syndromes and reviews the rationale for the referral criteria.

The US Preventive Services Task Force has also published recommendations regarding genetic risk assessment for unaffected women with a focus on BRCA-related cancers. This group identifies several familial risk scoring tools to assess the need for referral and specifically does not routinely recommend genetic counseling or testing women with an unremarkable family history.[18]

REQUESTING A GENETIC CONSULT BASED ON THE FAMILY HEALTH HISTORY

Genetics is about families, as is a cancer diagnosis, albeit in different ways. When an individual is diagnosed with cancer, the family is often involved in the journey to wellness. In some families, when an individual is diagnosed with cancer, family members wonder about their own risk of developing that cancer, and it is often overestimated.[16,19] In general, with most common cancers, about 10% to 20% of individuals with that cancer have a strong family history of cancer, meaning 80% to 90% do not have a strong family history. However, for families with a known hereditary cancer syndrome, the mode of inheritance identifies at-risk family members. For an autosomal dominant hereditary cancer syndrome, siblings and children are appropriate testing candidates for the known familial mutation. Once it is established that the mutation is from the maternal or paternal lineage, then aunts, uncles, and cousins can also be referred for counseling and testing. However, a few hereditary cancer syndromes are inherited as an autosomal recessive condition, such as polyposis due to mutations in the *MUTYH* gene. In these families, full siblings would be at greatest risk for having a similar genotype.

AVERAGE/POPULATION RISK

After obtaining an FHHx, it may be assessed that a patient has an average risk of developing cancer based on the family history provided. Average risk applies to individuals who may have only a few affected family members, usually at least second- or third-degree relatives with cancers diagnosed at older (or typical) ages. Remembering that 1 in 2 to 1 in 3 individuals develop cancer, it might not be unusual in a family of 30 to 40 individuals to find a maternal grandmother with breast cancer in her 60s, an uncle with prostate cancer at the age of 71 years, and a paternal uncle with colon cancer at the age of 57 years. Average-risk family history can be characterized by the following:

- Few individuals with cancer in a family (number of cancers appropriate for number of people in family)
- More common cancers
- Typical age at which that cancer is diagnosed

These individuals are more likely to be at average risk if the affected person is a second-degree or more distant degree relative (uncle, grandparent), especially in the absence of cancer in the parents. This type of family history may increase the patient's concern about a personal cancer risk, especially if there are emotional ties with an affected family member. In those cases, counseling by the primary or specialty care provider may help the patient understand that he or she has a risk similar to others in the general population. A genetic referral is not necessary, and usually genetic testing does not provide additional risk information.

INCREASED RISK

This group can be subdivided into 2 groups: those whose cancers may be due to multifactorial inheritance of genes of small effect interacting with each other and nongenetic risk factors (eg, lifestyle habits, exposures, hormonal milieu) and those with a known hereditary cancer syndrome due to a highly penetrant single gene. Referral to a genetic professional to differentiate between these 2 groups can be useful to determine whether patients in the increased risk category would benefit from enhanced cancer surveillance, prophylactic surgery, chemoprevention, and/or genetic testing.

An individual with increased familial cancer risk is typically characterized as having at least 1 first-degree relative with a cancer at a later age, 2 first- or second-degree relatives with the same cancer, or 1 first-degree relative with a less-common cancer, such as medullary thyroid cancer or a pheochromocytoma, all at ages typical for that particular cancer. These individuals may have a 2- to 3-fold increased risk for developing the cancer seen in other family members. These individuals may not need a formal genetic referral, but a clinician-to-clinician communication (e-consult) to confirm if enhanced intervention is warranted.

In situations in which genetic consultation or testing may not be indicated for the patient (or the relatives), there may still be a benefit from enhanced cancer screening and education about risk-reducing lifestyle modifications. Typically, counseling and education to help the patient understand the many environmental or lifestyle factors related to the development of cancer might empower the patient toward those health changes. Risk models that include minimal history, but other lifestyle factors (such as the one found at www.cancer.gov/bcrisktool/), can identify patients who would benefit from chemoprevention. In some circumstances, earlier or more frequent cancer screening might also be appropriate.

Individuals who are more likely to have a hereditary cancer syndrome are members of families in which there are multiple affected family members, usually in multiple generations, and have at least 1 family member with a cancer at a young age.

Sometimes a family may unexpectedly be at a higher risk for a hereditary cancer syndrome than is evident from the family history. In the absence of an extensive family history of cancer, having a single family member with cancer could indicate a hereditary cancer syndrome if the relative were diagnosed with cancer at a younger-than-average age or had features of a hereditary cancer syndrome. In these cases, genetic evaluation can be helpful to elucidate a possible hereditary cancer syndrome, particularly if the family member affected with cancer is available for evaluation.

- For example, a woman may have a sister with ovarian cancer, but no other relatives with breast or ovarian cancer. However, her father was an only child. If a paternal *BRCA1* or *BRCA2* mutation existed in this family, it would make sense that no other cancers have presented in the family.
- A few cancer syndromes present de novo, where the affected patient presenting does not have a family history, such as Li-Fraumeni syndrome, Cowden syndrome, and familial adenomatous polyposis.
- In addition, individuals of certain ancestries (such as Ashkenazi Jewish) can be at a higher risk than the general population for certain cancer predispositions, even in the face of a moderate-risk family history.

Individuals who are members of a family with a known hereditary cancer syndrome are appropriate for a genetic consultation referral. There are well over 50 known inherited syndromes associated with an increased risk for developing cancer. Affected individuals in high-risk families are the ideal genetic testing candidates because their results can allow for improved interpretation when testing unaffected family members. For unaffected family members who are concerned about their risk, the genetic consultation often includes a conversation about the value of initially testing an affected family member.

Several organizations, including the US Preventive Services Task Force and the Commission on Cancer, recommend that genetic testing be performed in the context of pretest and posttest genetic counseling by qualified clinicians, especially for families with a hereditary cancer syndrome.[18] The National Cancer Institute offers an online genetic services directory at http://www.cancer.gov/cancertopics/genetics/directory. The National Society of Genetic Counselors has a link to find a genetic counselor at http://nsgc.org, as does the American College of Medical Genetics and Genomics at https://www.amcg.net. Several companies and laboratories have hired genetic counselors, although many serve in a sales or marketing role, so they may target their conversations on a focused number of testing products; their perspective should be considered when partnering to arrange for genetic testing. Some facilities and insurance companies have aligned with telephone counseling services. Preliminary studies report that genetic counseling in selected situations can be effectively and efficiently delivered by phone.[20–24]

WHO CAN BENEFIT FROM A REFERRAL FOR GENETIC CONSULTATION?

Both affected and unaffected family members can potentially benefit from a genetic evaluation. Many people with cancer wonder why a cancer developed. While that is sometimes a spiritual or metaphysical question, it can also be a biological question. Understanding if there is a genetic etiology to a diagnosis can be important with respect to understanding the cause, knowing if there are other management options to consider, and informing extended family members about risk. Unaffected, extended family members often ask their providers what a cancer diagnosis might mean to their personal risk, and they often overestimate that risk.[16,17] Often, unaffected individuals are hesitant to bother someone who is currently involved with cancer treatment. However, a genetic referral can help the unaffected patient understand the challenges of interpreting genetic testing in the absence of knowledge about the mutation status of the affected individual. And although most cancers occur in adults, some cancer syndromes are associated with childhood ages of onset, so obtaining the family history in the pediatric setting can benefit the family as well.

A NOTE ABOUT CONFIDENTIALITY

Patients hold information private until they share it with a clinician. At that point, there is an expectation that the clinician will hold that information confidential. FHHx carries a few special concerns because patients sometimes provide sensitive information, with the expectation that it will remain confidential, about another family member who might have held that same information fully private and would never have revealed it to a clinician.

There is no question that publication of pedigrees warrants a level of caution.[25,26] Clinically, an EHR may actually provide an additional level of security if sections of the record can be accessed only with permission. Some sensitive information, such as mental health or substance abuse issues, can be locked to only those with need-to-know permissions. While it is unlikely that this level of restriction is useful for FHHx, attention to the amount of identifiable information collected on extended family members is important. Although ages of cancer onset are important, documenting full names of family members may not be necessary. Collecting first names is helpful because it allows the conversation to flow more naturally—rather than asking, "now, about your third brother, the one with pancreatic cancer," one can ask about Steven.

FORMATS AND PLACEMENT OF A DOCUMENTED FAMILY HISTORY

Traditionally, a statement regarding FHHx was often included in the history section of a progress note. "No family history" may be true if the patient is adopted, but even then a patient may have knowledge about some of the biological family members.[13] A "noncontributory" family history reveals that the clinician asked questions about a particular condition (ie, breast and ovarian cancer history in a woman with a breast mass) to learn that no one in the immediate family has related conditions. However, it is more informative to document pertinent negatives—knowing the woman with the breast mass has 3 older sisters and 6 maternal aunts with no cancer is more informative than if she were in a sibship of 2 with parents who were both an only child. Once the history is obtained, a written list of family members and their cancer history is typically documented, usually with abbreviations (eg, mgm = maternal grandmother), or a list of cancer types followed by family members with those cancers is documented. Often, specialist (cardiologist, surgical oncologist) target the FHHx collection to their specialty area, whereas primary care providers are typically more general in their approach. Members of the genetics community complete a pedigree/graphic representation and may use a different colored pen or marker to update the pedigree. The transition to electronic records poses a challenge because now that diagram is scanned, making it static and difficult to search or update.[27]

FHHx is often collected with an initial history and physical examination or in a progress note and is embedded in that clinic note. Several EHRs are developing a family history or genetic tab where the FHHx can be located, sometimes along with genetic test results. Alternately, if the data are collected in a format with structured elements, they could be captured from any note and inform CDS.

An ideal format would capture structured data elements (age, date of birth, relationship to the patient, gender, etc.), all tied to Systematized Nomenclature of Medicine (SNOMED) terms. SNOMED is an international effort of which the National Library of Medicine is the US Member and which designates nomenclature standards for the electronic exchange (and interoperability) of clinical health information. This format could also be used to inform CDS tools. Clinical reminders, such as one that alerts to the need for colon cancer screening if there is documentation of a first-degree relative with colon cancer, is but one example of the usefulness of this format.

Teams that are developing programs to incorporate family histories into electronic records are exploring many of the steps from the data input to the decision support, which includes clinical reminders for screening or referrals.[3,28–33] With the growth of genealogy as one of the top 5 hobbies in the United States, many individuals are becoming more comfortable with identifying family relationships and using Web-based services to document family information. With appropriate patient confidentiality information in place, several might grow to include FHHx. At present, EHR software packages such as EPIC are field testing family history modules. Several resources, such as the Surgeon General's Family History tool (familyhistory.hhs.gov), are patient friendly and can allow the information to be captured before a clinic visit.[33–35] **Box 1** lists several tools that have been developed to capture information in an electronic manner; some have associated decision support guidance. Most tools

---

Box 1
Examples of validated computerized FHHx tools

- Breast Care Center, UCSF: GRACE[30]
- Brigham and Women's Hospital[28]
- Cambridge: GRAIDS[40]
- CDC: My Family Health Portrait[11,34,35]
- Cleveland Clinic: MyFamily, GREAT[27,41,42]
- Duke Cancer Institute: MeTree[29,43]
- Georgia Breast Cancer Genomic Health Consortium: B-RST[44]
- Greater Los Angeles VA Medical Center[33]
- University of Virginia Health System: Health Heritage[32]

Abbreviations: B-RST, breast cancer genetics referral screening tool; CDC, Centers for Disease Control and Prevention; GRACE, Genetic Risk Assessment in the Clinical Environment; GRAIDS, Genetic Risk Assessment on the Internet and Decision Support; GREAT, Genetic Risk Easy Assessment Tool; UCSF, University of California, San Francisco; VA, Veterans Affairs.

are still being evaluated and are proprietary or specific to the organization that developed it.

Genetically guided personalized health care is one of NIH's major current focuses. The goal is to deliver individually tailored medical care that leverages information about each person's unique genetic characteristics, identified in both family history and genetic testing. A significant reason to implement CDS tied to the family history is that it can translate evidence into practice relatively quickly and help bridge the promise of personalized medicine.[36,37] The CDS field is relatively new, but some of the first outcome evaluations were linked to FHHx. Ideally, systems could be developed to allow for patient-entered FHHx. The next step, once those data were entered, would allow for a CDS integrated into an EHR that would support genetic referrals, genetic testing, and screening reminders based on either family history or mutation status.

While many of the currently available FHHx collection programs have demonstrated effectiveness, the only one widely available (free and available online) is the Surgeon General's Web tool.[38] One of the most significant challenges to date is that almost every system is designed to work within specific institutions. This fact limits scalability and interoperability. A resolution will only come if designers (and their clinical customers) can agree on a standardized representation of the relevant patient data and use standard approaches to leverage the variety of programs currently being developed.[36] The Health Level Seven (HL7) International standards are currently accepted as the data standard for transmitting FHHx information.[39] Several groups, such as the Surgeon General's Web tool, use HL7 standards, but they are not yet universal. Use of standards would enhance the utility and potential universal application of this vital component of genetic care.

SUMMARY

Taking a relatively short time during an initial consultation can reveal key factors to benefit not only the patients but also their family members. This information can be used to determine the need for a more extensive evaluation, or it can have the potential to impact surgical, screening, and psychological care. Assuring that patients understand the value of their FHHx and encourage that they share it with health care providers, including pediatric providers, can make a difference for the extended family. For affected individuals, the FHHx may make a difference regarding treatment options; for the unaffected family members, this information might lead to early detection of cancer or prevention. Although a family history is often static in a medical record, more active patient involvement and interest will facilitate periodic updates. As tools are developed to capture and help interpret FHHx data in the EHR, clinicians will have improved ability to conduct risk assessment for cancer and make decisions regarding management options or the need for genetic referrals for more extended evaluation and discussion about germline genetic testing.

REFERENCES

1. Hampel H, Bennett RL, Buchanan A, et al. A practice guideline from the American College of Medical Genetics and Genomics and the National Society of Genetic Counselors: referral indications for cancer predisposition assessment. Genet Med 2015;17(1):70–87.
2. Scheuner MT, Wang SJ, Raffel LJ, et al. Family history: a comprehensive genetic risk assessment method for the chronic conditions of adulthood. Am J Med Genet 1997;71(3):315–24.

3. Acheson LS, Wiesner GL, Zyzanski SJ, et al. Family history-taking in community family practice: implications for genetic screening. Genet Med 2000;2(3):180–5.
4. Blumenthal D, Causino N, Chang YC, et al. The duration of ambulatory visits to physicians. J Fam Pract 1999;48(4):264–71.
5. Wattendorf DJ, Hadley DW. Family history: the three-generation pedigree. Am Fam Physician 2005;72(3):441–8.
6. Qureshi N, Wilson B, Santaguida P, et al. Collection and use of cancer family history in primary care. Evid Rep Technol Assess (Full Rep) 2007;(159):1–84.
7. Foo W, Young JM, Solomon MJ, et al. Family history? The forgotten question in high-risk colorectal cancer patients. Colorectal Dis 2009;11(5):450–5.
8. Murff HJ, Byrne D, Syngal S. Cancer risk assessment: quality and impact of the family history interview. Am J Prev Med 2004;27(3):239–45.
9. Murff HJ, Greevy RA, Syngal S. The comprehensiveness of family cancer history assessments in primary care. Community Genet 2007;10(3):174–80.
10. Grover S, Stoffel EM, Bussone L, et al. Physician assessment of family cancer history and referral for genetic evaluation in colorectal cancer patients. Clin Gastroenterol Hepatol 2004;2(9):813–9.
11. Giovanni MA, Murray MF. The application of computer-based tools in obtaining the genetic family history. Curr Protoc Hum Genet 2010. Chapter 9:Unit 9.21.
12. Bennett RL, French KS, Resta RG, et al. Standardized human pedigree nomenclature: update and assessment of the recommendations of the National Society of Genetic Counselors. J Genet Couns 2008;17(5):424–33.
13. Venne VL, Botkin JR, Buys SS. Professional opportunities and responsibilities in the provision of genetic information to children relinquished for adoption. Am J Med Genet A 2003;119A(1):41–6.
14. Weitzel JN, Lagos VI, Cullinane CA, et al. Limited family structure and BRCA gene mutation status in single cases of breast cancer. JAMA 2007;297(23):2587–95.
15. Julian-Reynier C, Eisinger F, Chabal F, et al. Disclosure to the family of breast/ovarian cancer genetic test results: patient's willingness and associated factors. Am J Med Genet 2000;94(1):13–8.
16. Katapodi MC, Lee KA, Facione NC, et al. Predictors of perceived breast cancer risk and the relation between perceived risk and breast cancer screening: a meta-analytic review. Prev Med 2004;38(4):388–402.
17. Woloshin S, Schwartz LM, Black WC, et al. Women's perceptions of breast cancer risk: how you ask matters. Med Decis Making 1999;19(3):221–9.
18. Moyer VA, U.S. Preventive Services Task Force. Risk assessment, genetic counseling, and genetic testing for BRCA-related cancer in women: U.S. Preventive Services Task Force recommendation statement. Ann Intern Med 2014;160(4):271–81.
19. Valente J, Stybio T, Hyde S, et al. Factors affecting informed decision-making in women with increased breast cancer risk or DCIS pursuing contralateral prophylactic mastectomy. Cancer Epidemiol Biomarkers Prev 2015;24(4):761.
20. Butrick M, Kelly S, Peshkin BN, et al. Disparities in uptake of BRCA1/2 genetic testing in a randomized trial of telephone counseling. Genet Med 2015;17(6):467–75.
21. Baumanis L, Evans JP, Callanan N, et al. Telephoned BRCA1/2 genetic test results: prevalence, practice, and patient satisfaction. J Genet Couns 2009;18(5):447–63.
22. Bradbury AR, Patrick-Miller L, Fetzer D, et al. Genetic counselor opinions of, and experiences with telephone communication of BRCA1/2 test results. Clin Genet 2011;79(2):125–31.

23. Kinney AY, Butler KM, Schwartz MD, et al. Expanding access to BRCA1/2 genetic counseling with telephone delivery: a cluster randomized trial. J Natl Cancer Inst 2014;106(12) [pii:dju328].
24. Schwartz MD, Valdimarsdottir HB, Peshkin BN, et al. Randomized noninferiority trial of telephone versus in-person genetic counseling for hereditary breast and ovarian cancer. J Clin Oncol 2014;32(7):618–26.
25. Botkin J. Protecting the privacy of family members in survey and pedigree research. JAMA 2001;285(2):207–11.
26. Byers PH, Ashkenas J. Pedigrees-publish? or perish the thought? Am J Hum Genet 1998;63(3):678–81.
27. Doerr M, Edelman E, Gabitzsch E, et al. Formative evaluation of clinician experience with integrating family history-based clinical decision support into clinical practice. J Pers Med 2014;4(2):115–36.
28. Baer HJ, Schneider LI, Colditz GA, et al. Use of a web-based risk appraisal tool for assessing family history and lifestyle factors in primary care. J Gen Intern Med 2013;28(6):817–24.
29. Buchanan AH, Christianson CA, Himmel T, et al. Use of a patient-entered family health history tool with decision support in primary care: impact of identification of increased risk patients on genetic counseling attendance. J Genet Couns 2015; 24(1):179–88.
30. Braithwaite D, Sutton S, Mackay J, et al. Development of a risk assessment tool for women with a family history of breast cancer. Cancer Detect Prev 2005;29(5): 433–9.
31. Braithwaite D, Sutton S, Smithson WH, et al. Internet-based risk assessment and decision support for the management of familial cancer in primary care: a survey of GPs' attitudes and intentions. Fam Pract 2002;19(6):587–90.
32. Cohn WF, Ropka ME, Pelletier SL, et al. Health Heritage(c) a web-based tool for the collection and assessment of family health history: initial user experience and analytic validity. Public Health Genomics 2010;13(7–8):477–91.
33. Scheuner MT, Hamilton AB, Peredo J, et al. A cancer genetics toolkit improves access to genetic services through documentation and use of the family history by primary-care clinicians. Genet Med 2014;16(1):60–9.
34. Facio FM, Feero WG, Linn A, et al. Validation of My Family Health Portrait for six common heritable conditions. Genet Med 2010;12(6):370–5.
35. Feero WG, Facio FM, Glogowski EA, et al. Preliminary validation of a consumer-oriented colorectal cancer risk assessment tool compatible with the US Surgeon General's My Family Health Portrait. Genet Med 2014. [Epub ahead of print].
36. Kawamoto K, Del Fiol G, Orton C, et al. System-agnostic clinical decision support services: benefits and challenges for scalable decision support. Open Med Inform J 2010;4:245–54.
37. Bates DW, Kuperman GJ, Wang S, et al. Ten commandments for effective clinical decision support: making the practice of evidence-based medicine a reality. J Am Med Inform Assoc 2003;10(6):523–30.
38. de Hoog CL, Portegijs PJ, Stoffers HE. Family history tools for primary care are not ready yet to be implemented. A systematic review. Eur J Gen Pract 2014; 20(2):125–33.
39. Feero WG, Bigley MB, Brinner KM, Family Health History Multi-Stakeholder Workgroup of the American Health Information Community. New standards and enhanced utility for family health history information in the electronic health record: an update from the American Health Information Community's Family Health History Multi-Stakeholder Workgroup. J Am Med Inform Assoc 2008;15(6):723–8.

40. Emery J. The GRAIDS Trial: the development and evaluation of computer decision support for cancer genetic risk assessment in primary care. Ann Hum Biol 2005;32(2):218–27.
41. Acheson LS, Wang C, Zyzanski SJ, et al. Family history and perceptions about risk and prevention for chronic diseases in primary care: a report from the family healthware impact trial. Genet Med 2010;12(4):212–8.
42. Acheson LS, Zyzanski SJ, Stange KC, et al. Validation of a self-administered, computerized tool for collecting and displaying the family history of cancer. J Clin Oncol 2006;24(34):5395–402.
43. Beadles CA, Ryanne Wu R, Himmel T, et al. Providing patient education: impact on quantity and quality of family health history collection. Fam Cancer 2014;13(2): 325–32.
44. Brannon Traxler L, Martin ML, Kerber AS, et al. Implementing a screening tool for identifying patients at risk for hereditary breast and ovarian cancer: a statewide initiative. Ann Surg Oncol 2014;21(10):3342–7.

Certified Genetic Counselors

A Crucial Clinical Resource in the Management of Patients with Suspected Hereditary Cancer Syndromes

Zohra Ali-Khan Catts, MS, LGC[a],*, Heather Hampel, MS, LGC[b]

KEYWORDS

- Cancer genetic counseling • Genetic counselor • Cancer genetics • Genetic testing

KEY POINTS

- The cancer genetic counselor is critical in the management of patients with cancer who may have an inherited susceptibility to cancer.
- Patients with cancer with an early age at diagnosis, multiple primary tumors, rare tumors, or a family history of multiple cases of the same or related cancers should be referred for cancer genetic counseling.
- The identification of patients with hereditary cancer susceptibility syndromes can aid in surgical decision-making.

WHAT IS GENETIC COUNSELING?

The National Society of Genetic Counseling defines genetic counseling as "The process of helping people understand and adapt to the medical, psychological, and familial implications of genetic contributions to disease." This process integrates interpretation of family and medical histories to assess the chance of disease occurrence or recurrence; education about inheritance, testing, management, prevention, resources, and research; and counseling to promote informed choices and adaptation to the risk or condition.[1]

The authors have nothing to disclose.
[a] Christiana Care Health System, Helen F. Graham Cancer Center and Research Institute, 4701 Ogletown Stanton Road, Suite 2231, Newark, DE 19713-2079, USA; [b] The Ohio State University Comprehensive Cancer Center, 2001 Polaris Parkway, Columbus, OH 43240, USA
* Corresponding author.
E-mail address: ZAli-KhanCatts@Christianacare.org

Surg Oncol Clin N Am 24 (2015) 653–666
http://dx.doi.org/10.1016/j.soc.2015.06.005

WHAT IS A CERTIFIED GENETIC COUNSELOR?

A certified genetic counselor is a master's level trained health care professional with a specialized degree in genetic counseling from an accredited genetic counseling training program that has passed the National Board Examination for Certification administered currently by the American Board of Genetic Counseling (ABGC) and previously by the American Board of Medical Genetics. At the time of this publication there are 31 accredited training programs for genetic counseling in the United Sates and three in Canada. A complete and up-to-date list is found at http://gceducation. org/Pages/Accredited-Programs.aspx. Genetic counselors are experienced in areas of medical genetics and counseling. By combining their knowledge of basic science, medical genetics, epidemiologic principles, and counseling theory with their skills in genetic risk assessment, education, interpersonal communication, and counseling, they provide services to clients and their families for a diverse set of genetic or genomic indications. Certification of genetic counselors provides assurance that the individual has met the minimum standards and competencies to practice.

Why Is Certification Important

Certification is important because it ensures a genetic counselor has graduated from an accredited genetic counseling program,[2] which means they have met the established standards for professional practice through documentation of specialized training as required for graduation from an accredited training program, and received a passing score on the ABGC Certification Examination. Once this has been done, the Certified Genetic Counselor credential is granted by the ABGC. Genetic counselors certified before 1996 by ABGC or the American Board of Medical Genetics do not have a time-limited certification; however, voluntary recertification is strongly encouraged and demonstrates an ongoing commitment to lifelong learning in a rapidly growing and dynamic field. Recertification is required for genetic counselors that were certified in 1996 or later and is important to ensure that skills and knowledge are maintained. In addition, certification and recertification is becoming more significant for licensing, insurance reimbursement, credentialing, hospital credentialing, and professional advancement and employment opportunities.[3]

ARE GENETIC COUNSELORS LICENSED?

Genetic counselors are required to hold a license to practice in 15 states at the time of this publication. Four additional states have passed licensure and are in the process of drafting the rules and regulations. The current up-to-date list of states that license genetic counselors is found at http://nsgc.org/p/cm/ld/fid=19. There is an increasing need to obtain licensure in the remaining 31 states. Licensure of genetic counselors is paramount because it aids in protecting the public from potential harms that may result from this occupation remaining unregulated. Harm caused by untrained individuals attempting to provide genetic counseling includes the following:

- Misinformation regarding genetic risk or lack of risk
- Misunderstanding of the implications of genetic information, such as family history or test results, which can lead to
  - Unnecessary medical treatment and/or surgery
  - Lack of prevention or disease-monitoring strategies
  - Irreversible management decisions
  - Avoidable fear, anxiety, and guilt

- Potential discrimination from insurance companies with no federally mandated protection including but not limited to life insurance, long-term care, short-term care, and disability insurance
- Inappropriately undertaking costly genetic testing[4,5]

Ensuring providers are up-to-date on the new technologies and testing options for cancer syndromes with the advent of gene panels, exome sequencing, and whole genome sequencing is critical for ordering the appropriate test and interpreting the results that are received.

WHO SHOULD BE REFERRED FOR CANCER GENETIC COUNSELING?

There are several hallmarks of the hereditary cancer susceptibility syndromes that can serve as "red flags" for when to refer patients for cancer genetic counseling. The red flags are (see **Box 1**) early onset cancer diagnosis (younger than age 50), multiple primary cancers in the same patient, multiple cases of the same or related cancers on the same side of the family, and rare tumor types (ie, male breast cancer, paraganglioma, medullary thyroid cancer, pheochromocytoma).

For specific syndrome-related referral criteria, the American College of Medical Genetics and Genomics and the National Society of Genetic Counselors have just published a joint practice guideline that includes referral criteria by cancer type.[6] This includes an easy-to-use table where one can look up the cancers in a patient's family history and then determine whether or not they meet any criteria that would warrant referral. In addition, there are many on-line tools available to help determine which patients could benefit from a referral to cancer genetics. My Family Health Portrait (familyhistory.hhs.gov) is a tool from the Surgeon General that allows patients to enter a family health history, to learn about their risk for conditions that can run in families, to print their family history to share with family or health care providers, and to save it so it can be updated over time.

HOW DOES USE OF GENETIC COUNSELING SERVICES IMPROVE THE QUALITY OF CARE PROVIDED BY THE PRACTICING SURGICAL ONCOLOGIST?

Individuals with hereditary cancer susceptibility syndromes have a very high risk for second primary cancers. As a result, they may elect to pursue a more aggressive surgery for a current cancer to prevent a second malignancy. For example, an individual with colorectal cancer who is diagnosed with Lynch syndrome may elect to pursue subtotal colectomy versus segmental resection or hemicolectomy. (See The Genetics of Colorectal Cancer).[7] Most cancer genetics clinics hold surgical decision-making appointments open each week so they can quickly accommodate any patient who needs testing before surgery. Furthermore, the diagnosis of a hereditary cancer syndrome may affect decisions about chemotherapy. For example, PARP inhibitors are approved by the Food and Drug Administration for the third-line treatment of women with ovarian cancer and a *BRCA1/2* mutation. In addition, once these patients have completed treatment of their current cancer, they may be at risk for multiple different new primary cancers. At a minimum, this requires intensive cancer surveillance. Some individuals may also elect to pursue risk-reducing surgeries to lower or eliminate their risk for some of these second primary cancers, such as bilateral salpingo-oophorectomy in a patient with breast cancer with a *BRCA1/2* mutation. Furthermore, this enables the unaffected at-risk relatives of patients with cancer to benefit from predictive testing. Those who test positive also need intensive cancer surveillance and possibly risk-reducing surgeries.

WHAT HAPPENS IN PRETEST CANCER GENETIC COUNSELING?

Pretest genetic counseling and consultation typically consists of an appointment in which genetic counselors have a one-on-one interaction (face to face, teleconference, and/or telemedicine) with the patient. There are five main components of a pretest genetic counseling session. The first component and most critical of the pretest genetic counseling session is eliciting and documenting the individual's medical and family history. Genetic counselors adhere to the gold standard of obtaining a family history that consists of three generations or greater and they elicit the ages of diagnosis of cancer and other medical conditions in the family. Most centers use a family history questionnaire that can be sent out before their appointment. Some examples are found at the National Society of Genetic Counselors Web site (http://nsgc.org/p/cm/ld/fid=239). This is a tool that aids the individual in collecting the medical history of relatives and allows the individual to contact family members and confirm cancer history and ages of diagnosis before their appointment allowing for a more accurate cancer risk assessment. Multiple studies have shown that in nongenetic practices less than 70% of patients with breast and colon cancer have the minimum standard family history documented,[8–10] and only 41.7% had the age of cancer diagnosis documented in these histories.[8] The minimum adequate cancer family history recommended by the American Society of Clinical Oncology is all first- and second-degree relatives on the maternal and paternal side of the family including ethnicity and for each cancer case in the family the establishment of age at diagnosis, type of primary tumor, and results of any cancer predisposition testing in any relative.[8] Because family histories are dynamic they should be updated periodically.

The second component of the pretest counseling is to provide education on genetic concepts related to diagnosis or family history. Genetic counselors provide education on the basic genetic concepts including chromosomes, genes, and DNA. They provide education on cancer genetics discussing sporadic versus familial or hereditary cancer and use the family history to demonstrate to the individual how their family history is more consistent with sporadic, familial, or hereditary cancer. The features of hereditary cancer syndromes (**Box 1**) and inheritance patterns for the syndromes are discussed in detail with the patient. Most hereditary cancer syndromes are inherited in an autosomal-dominant fashion with a 50% chance or one in two probability of passing it on to offspring. The main hereditary cancer syndrome that is inherited in an autosomal-recessive fashion is MutYH-associated polyposis and constitutional balletic mismatch repair mutations; however, with the use of multigene panel testing

---

Box 1
Features of hereditary cancer syndromes

Early age onset cancers; cancer that occurs at a younger age than the population mean (eg, breast or colon cancer before the age of 50)

Multiple primary cancers

Bilateral or multifocal cancers

Cancer in the less commonly affected sex (eg, male breast cancer)

Clustering of rare cancers

Multiple affected family members with the same cancer or cancers related to a specific genetic syndrome (eg, breast and ovarian cancer or colon and uterine cancers)

Ethnicities with a higher carrier incidence (eg, Ashkenazi Jewish ancestry)

other gene mutations that can lead to an autosomal-recessive condition include genes in the Fanconi anemia pathway, ataxia telangiectasia, and other chromosome breakage syndromes. Autosomal-recessive syndromes occur in 25% of offspring provided both parents carry one copy of the disease-associated allele.

The third component for discussion is genetic testing options and detailed discussion of risks, limitations, and benefits to testing. There are currently more than 50 hereditary cancer syndromes[11] that genetic counselors assess when taking a family history. This assessment drives the testing options that are presented to the patient. If the family history is suggestive of more than one syndrome then the testing strategy may vary from single gene/syndrome testing to a small panel of genes versus a large panel of genes for complex family histories that encompass many cancer types. The most common hereditary cancer syndromes are listed in **Table 1**. The methodology of testing varies from Sanger sequencing for single gene/syndrome testing; next-generation sequencing for small and large panels; and, in the future, exome sequencing and whole genome sequencing for families with hereditary cancer where a gene alteration has not been identified.

The fourth component of the pretest counseling is risk assessment to determine probability of carrying a mutation and/or lifetime risk of developing cancer. There are several models that are used to determine the probability of carrying a pathogenic variant in BRCA1, BRCA2, MLH1, MSH2, MSH6, PTEN, TP53, CDKN2A, and/or lifetime risk of developing cancer (**Table 2**); however, each model has benefits and limitations and there is no one perfect model. Cancer genetic counselors are trained to select the best model for each particular patient to most accurately assess risk.

The fifth component of pretest counseling is obtaining informed consent. Genetic counselors are trained to adhere to the 14 components of informed consent recommended by the American Society of Clinical Oncology, as reviewed in detail next[26]:

1. Discuss the purpose of the testing. This includes discussion of the genetic test being offered based on personal and/or family history and incorporates the risk assessment models when appropriate in the explanation of why a genetic test is being offered or not being offered.
2. Provide education and information on the specific gene/genetic mutations or genomic variants being tested, including whether the range of risk associated with the variant impacts medical care. Discussion of the cancer risk associated with specific genes has become somewhat more complicated with the advent of multigene panels. When offering a multigene panel test discussion of high-, moderate-, and low-penetrant genes components of the panel and their associated risks of developing cancer should be discussed.
3. Discussion of the implications of a pathogenic (mutation confirmed to be deleterious), negative (no identified change in the genetic sequence), or uncertain (genetic variant of unknown clinical significance) result.
4. Education and clear discussion on the possibility the test will not be informative. Cancer genetic testing is limited to the genes available using current technology. Testing of a family that clearly displays autosomal-dominant inheritance of a cancer phenotype may yield no identifiable alteration. The clinical implications of this possible scenario need to be discussed before testing
5. Discussion and plan regarding risk to children and/or other family members who may have inherited the genetic condition.
6. Technical accuracy of the test including where required by law, licensure of the testing laboratory, and sensitivity and specificity of the particular test.

Table 1
A list of the top 10 cancer syndromes

Cancer Syndrome	Genes	Associated Cancers (Not All-Inclusive)	Other Associated Features (Not All-Inclusive)
Familial adenomatous polyposis	APC	Colon, liver, small bowel, stomach, pancreas, thyroid, central nervous system	Multiple colonic polyps, desmoid tumor, osteomas, congenital hypertrophy of the retinal pigment epithelium
Hereditary breast and ovarian cancer	BRCA1, BRCA2	Breast, ovarian, prostate, pancreatic, melanoma	—
Hereditary nonpolyposis colorectal cancer	MLH1, MSH2, MSH6, PMS2, EPCAM	Colon, uterine, stomach, ovarian, hepatobiliary tract, urinary tract, small bowel, brain/central nervous system	Sebaceous adenomas
Juvenile polyposis syndrome	BMPR1A, SMAD4	Colon, upper gastrointestinal tract, stomach, pancreas	Hamartomatous polyps in the gastrointestinal tract
Hereditary diffuse gastric cancer	CDH1	Gastric, breast (lobular), Colorectal	—
Familial atypical multiple mole and melanoma	CDK4, CDKN2A	Melanoma, pancreas, breast	Moles
MutYH-associated polyposis	MutYH	Colorectal, endometrial, gastric, liver	Colorectal adenomas
Cowden/PTEN hamartoma tumor syndrome	PTEN	Breast, endometrial, thyroid, colon, and renal	Macrocephaly, trichilemmomas, papillomatous papules, lipomas, colon polyps, endometrial fibroids, thyroid goiter
Peutz-Jeghers syndrome	STK11	Gastrointestinal, breast, ovarian, cervical, pancreatic	Mucocutaneous pigmentation, gastrointestinal polyposis, gonadal tumors
Li-Fraumeni syndrome	TP53	Sarcomas, osteosarcoma, adrenocortical carcinomas, breast, brain	—

7. All fees including possible "copays" involved in testing and counseling. For direct-to-consumer testing, the financial relationship of the counselor to the testing company must be disclosed.
8. Discussion of psychological implications of test results exploring how they would handle a positive, negative, or variant result; emotional status; life stressors; coping strategies and resources; and support structure or network I.[27]

Table 2
Commonly used Risk Assessment Models

Model	Factors That Are Incorporated Into Model
Hereditary Breast and Ovarian Cancer Syndrome Models	
These models calculate probability of carrying a BRCA1/2 alteration and in women who are unaffected calculates lifetime risk of developing breast cancer	
BRCApro model[12]: http://bcb.dfci.harvard. edu/bayesmendel/ brcapro.php	Computer-based Bayesian probability model that uses first- and second-degree family history of breast and/or ovarian cancer and number of unaffected, and takes into account Ashkenazi Jewish ancestry.
Tyrer-Cuzick model[13]	A computer-based model for unaffected individuals that takes into account first-, second-, and some third-degree female relatives with breast and/or ovarian cancer and epidemiologic factors.
Boadicea model[14]: http://ccge.medschl. cam.ac.uk/boadicea/web-application/	A computer-based model that takes into account up to fourth-degree relatives with breast, ovarian, pancreatic, and prostate cancers and number of unaffected relatives.
These models calculate only probability of carrying a BRCA1/2 alteration	
Myriad Prevalence tables[15]: https://www. myriadpro.com/hereditary-cancer-testing/hereditary-breast-and-ovarian-cancer-hboc-syndrome/prevalence-tables/	A set of tables derived from data submitted to Myriad on test requisition form (age of diagnosis, cancer history, and Ashkenazi Jewish ancestry).
Couch model[16]	BRCA1 alteration probability is calculated by mean age at breast cancer onset in a family, presence or absence of ovarian cancer, and Ashkenazi Jewish Ancestry.
Penn II model[17]: http://www.afcri.upenn. edu/itacc/penn2	A World Wide Web–based model that takes into account, first-, second-, and third-degree male and female relatives with breast, ovarian, prostate, and/or pancreatic cancer.
These models calculate only the lifetime risk of developing breast cancer in unaffected women	
Gail model[18]: http://www.cancer.gov/ bcrisktool/	This model takes into account current age, number of first-degree female relatives with breast cancer, age at first menstrual cycle, age at first live birth, number of breast biopsies and results.
Claus model[19,20]	This model takes into account two relatives that are either first- or second-degree who have had breast cancer or first-degree relatives with ovarian cancer.

(*continued on next page*)

9. Risks and protections against genetic discrimination by employers or insurers. Currently there is federal and some state legislation to aid in protecting against genetic discrimination. Two of the main federal legislations are the Health Insurance Portability and Accountability Act and Genetic Information Nondiscrimination Act.[27] (See Confidentiality & the Risk of Genetic Discrimination: What Surgeons Need to Know)[28]

Table 2 (*continued*)	
Model	**Factors That Are Incorporated Into Model**
Lynch syndrome models	
These models calculate probability of carrying a MLH1, MSH2, or MSH6 alteration and in unaffected individuals calculates lifetime risk of developing colon cancer and in addition for unaffected women calculates lifetime risk of endometrial and ovarian cancer	
MMRpro model[21] (MLH1, MSH2, MSH6): http://bcb.dfci.harvard.edu/ bayesmendel/mmrproqa.html	Computer-based Bayesian probability model that uses first- and second-degree family history of colon and/or uterine cancer and the number of unaffected individuals.
These models only calculate probability of carrying a MLH1, MSH2, or MSH6 alteration	
PREMM1,2, 6 model[22] (MLH1, MSH2, MSH6): http://premm.dfci.harvard.edu	Computer-based model that takes into account colon and/or uterine cancer in the proband, and colon, uterine, and other Lynch-related cancers in first- and second-degree relatives.
Myriad Prevalence tables (MLH1 and MSH2)[23]: https://www.myriadpro.com/ hereditary-cancer-testing/hereditary-colon-and-gynecologic-cancers/ lynch-syndrome-hnpcc/mlh1-and-msh2-prevalence-table/	A set of tables categorized by age at onset (<50 or ≥50 years old) of colon, uterine, and other Lynch-(HNPCC) associated cancers in the patients and/or first- or second-degree relatives, based on test data from Myriad Genetics Laboratories Inc.
Wijnen model (MLH1 and MSH2)[24]: http://bcb.dfci.harvard.edu/bayesmendel/ mmrproqa.html	A World Wide Web–based model that takes into account first- and second-degree male and female relatives with colon, uterine, and HNPCC-associated cancers.
Cowden syndrome model	
This model calculates the probability of a carrying a PTEN alteration	
PTEN risk model[25]: http://www.lerner.ccf.org/gmi/ccscore/	Calculates probability of carrying a PTEN alteration. A computer-based model that takes into account personal history (sex, age, head circumference, cancer history, and other medical conditions).

Abbreviation: HNPCC, hereditary nonpolyposis colorectal cancer.

10. Discuss confidentiality issues, including direct-to-consumer testing companies, policies related to privacy, and data security.
11. Discuss possible use of DNA samples for future research and coordination of testing. Most laboratory consent forms have an opt-in or opt-out of future research on samples that need to be documented during the signing of the consent form.
12. Discussion of options and limitations of medical surveillance and strategies for prevention after genetic or genomic testing. Discuss appropriate evidence-based screening, management, and risk-reducing strategies based on genetic test results and/or family history (this is typically done in the posttest genetic counseling and consultation session). Screening and management guidelines have not been established for all genes.

13. Discussion and documentation of importance of sharing genetic and genomic test results with at-risk relatives so that they may benefit from this information because they may be at increased risk for cancer and single-site genetic testing is recommended.

14. Discuss plans for disclosing the test result and providing follow-up including how results will be disclosed (whether they will be in person or by telephone). Discuss how follow-up plan will be communicated based on results and family history.

WHAT HAPPENS IN POSTTEST CANCER GENETIC COUNSELING?

Posttest genetic counseling generally occurs at the results disclosure session. Some centers prefer to do this in person, whereas most now provide this service via telephone.[29] At this time, the genetic test results are shared with a patient who has already undergone pretest genetic counseling (generally pretest counseling is performed in person) and had testing ordered. Perhaps more importantly, the genetic test results are interpreted in the context of that individual's personal medical and family history. For example, someone who has a very strong family history consistent with a hereditary cancer syndrome may still have a significantly increased risk for cancer even if they receive normal genetic test results.

With the increased use of multigene panels for cancer genetic testing, it is also possible that the patient is diagnosed with a hereditary cancer syndrome that was not fully discussed during the pretest genetic counseling session because of time constraints given the large number of genes and syndromes included on these panels.[30] In these cases, the posttest genetic counseling becomes even more important because all of the details about the particular diagnosis are explained to the patient including cancer risks and management recommendations. Any necessary referrals for cancer surveillance or risk-reducing surgeries can be discussed during posttest genetic counseling. In addition, patients can be referred to any on-line or in-person support groups for individuals with that particular cancer syndrome.

In some cases, information regarding the exact cancer risks associated with certain genes and syndromes or consensus guidelines about the appropriate management for the condition may be limited. Patients should be counseled regarding these ambiguities given the limited information currently known about their particular diagnosis and encouraged to stay in touch with the genetic counselor in the future to learn about any updates with regard to their cancer risks and management options.

Variants of uncertain significance (VUS) are found in 20% to 40% of individuals undergoing multigene cancer panel test.[31,32] These results are challenging because they may or may not lead to an increased risk for cancer. Management for patients and families with VUS results includes cancer surveillance based on their family history of cancer and not on the VUS. In addition, although other affected family members and parents may sometimes be offered free segregation testing to determine whether or not the VUS is segregating with the disease in the family (that is to say, all those affected by a related cancer have the VUS and those without cancer do not have the VUS), unaffected at-risk relatives should not be offered predictive testing for a VUS. It is important to prepare people for VUS results during pretest counseling so the result is not too disconcerting. VUS are common, should be expected, and most are eventually reclassified as benign.[33]

For families found to have a pathogenic mutation in a cancer susceptibility gene, posttest counseling is the ideal time to discuss so-called "cascade testing" for other at-risk family members. Testing is offered to all at-risk first-degree family members (including children and siblings) who are older than age 18. In some cases, the side of the family from which the mutation was inherited is obvious based on family history. In these cases, testing can be offered to that parent if they are still living and to any living aunts and uncles. When it is not obvious, both parents can be tested one at a time to determine from which side of the family the mutation was inherited. "Cascade testing" refers to genetic testing that should start as high up in the family as possible and proceed to the children of that individual only if they test positive.[34] For example, if someone who inherited a cancer gene mutation from their mother has a maternal aunt with seven children it is much more cost-effective to test the aunt first if possible. If she does not have the mutation, her seven children do not need to undergo testing. If she does have the mutation, then her seven children need to undergo testing.

HOW CAN A CANCER GENETICS DATABASE OR REGISTRY HELP?

Secure registries or databases of cancer genetics patients and genetic testing results are useful to patients and providers.[35] For the clinic, it is important to track patient numbers over time to gauge the growth of the clinic and the need for additional cancer genetic counseling staff. In addition, it is a way to track referral patterns so that those physicians who are not referring or those who are referring lower-risk individuals are targeted for additional education about the program and appropriate referrals. This can also be useful for quality assurance to ensure that test results have been received on all tested patients and that letters have been mailed to the referring physician and patient. With regard to mutation status, it is helpful to keep track of all mutations that are identified in the patient population for the clinic and the patients. Because some laboratories classify the same VUS differently, a database or registry can allow one to quickly identify all the patients in the clinic who have the same mutation so that they can all be informed when the VUS is reclassified as benign or pathogenic. Similarly, a database can help to link a patient to another more distant branch of the family that may already have a known mutation in a cancer susceptibility gene. In these cases, with the appropriate signed release from the original family member, the mutation result can be shared with the new patient and they can benefit from much less expensive single mutation testing rather than full genetic testing possibly including a large panel of genes. A database or registry can also be used to identify all patients with the same syndrome for mailings about additional testing or research studies, changes to management recommendations, newsletters, or patient education conferences. This is much easier than going through hundreds of charts after the fact to identify mutation-positive individuals.

Numerous international mutation databases have been developed. Examples include PROMPT (Prospective Registry of Multiplex Testing, a commercial enterprise with strong participation from leading academic institutions; www.promptsudy.org) and the Leiden Open Variation Database (www.lovd.nl). In addition cancer family registries for colorectal cancer are listed on the Collaborative Group of the Americas on Inherited Colorectal Cancer Web site (www.cgaicc.com). Beyond obvious clinical utility the role of expertly curated international collaborative mutation databases in facilitating research into basic questions regarding the biologic processes that control genotype phenotype interactions, penetrance, and many other fundamental genetic issues cannot be overstated.

HOW TO FIND OR HIRE A CANCER GENETIC COUNSELOR?

If access to a certified genetic counselor is not available multiple options exist to facilitate provision of comprehensive care with genetic counseling. Options include (1) referring to a local cancer genetics program, (2) partnering with a local cancer genetics program to provide on-site services, (3) using a national telephone genetic counseling service to provide cancer genetics services, or (4) hiring a cancer genetic counselor. Each of these options is explored next.

It is important to have cancer genetics services available because this is now a required standard for accreditation by the American College of Surgeons' Commission on Cancer (Standard 2.3, Risk Assessment and Genetic Counseling, of the 2012 Cancer Program Standards; http://www.facs.org/cancer/coc/cocprogramstandard2012.pdf). This standard requires that accredited hospitals provide cancer risk assessment, genetic counseling, and testing services to patients by a qualified genetics professional, either on-site or by referral.

It has also been shown that patient demand for cancer genetics services is increasing and cancer genetic counseling reduces inappropriate testing and erroneous interpretations of genetic test results.[36,37] Also importantly, genetic counseling services are increasingly sought and used by newly diagnosed patients with breast cancer for surgical decision-making among, for example, those found to have hereditary breast-ovarian cancer syndrome and considering bilateral mastectomy instead of breast-conservation therapy for their management.[38]

Multiple professional organizations (Evaluation of Genomic Applications in Practice and Prevention [EGAPP], the US Multi-Society Task Force on Colorectal Cancer, the American College of Gastroenterology, the National Comprehensive Cancer Network, and the Society of Gynecologic Oncology) have recommended that all newly diagnosed patients with colorectal cancer (and the latter has recommended that all endometrial) undergo tumor screening for Lynch syndrome at the time of diagnosis.[39–42] To follow these guidelines, it is best to make sure that there is a relationship with a cancer genetics provider who can coordinate the genetic counseling and follow-up genetic testing for those with abnormal tumor screen results that indicate they are more likely to have Lynch syndrome.

Referral to a Local Cancer Genetics Program

Generally there are cancer genetic counselors in every large city in the United States. Depending on the state, most patients should not have to drive more than 2 hours to receive services. To find a nearby cancer genetic counselor, visit the National Society of Genetic Counselors Find a Counselor page on their Web site (www.nsgc.org). Genetic counselors can be searched for by state, by city and state, or by zip code. Select "cancer" from the Types of Specialization list, then hit search.

A local cancer genetic counselor can also be found through the National Cancer Institute Cancer Genetics Services Directory at http://www.cancer.gov/cancertopics/genetics/directory. At that site, cancer genetics providers are found by cancer type, syndrome name, city, state, or country. All of the providers listed specialize in cancer genetics.

Partnering with a Local Cancer Genetics Program to Provide On-Site Services

Clinics can also choose to set up a formal relationship with local cancer genetics centers. For example, many academic medical centers cancer genetics programs have successfully partnered with community hospitals to provide cancer genetic counseling services on-site via telemedicine and video medicine. This allows for collaboration with experts in cancer genetics while patients stay close to their communities. The setup required to counsel patients via video conference is inexpensive, and accomplished relatively quickly. For example, The Ohio State cancer genetics service offers a 1- to 2-hour genetic counseling appointment with risk assessment, a results disclosure and posttest appointment or telephone call if the patient pursues genetic testing, review of all cases at a multidisciplinary case conference, and a thorough consultation summary report for the referring provider and patient.

Using a National Telephone Genetic Counseling Service for Patients

There are at least two companies (Informed DNA at www. informeddna.com and DNA Direct at www.dnadirect.com) that provide telephone genetic counseling for patients who would not otherwise have access. They can either develop partnerships with hospitals to provide their genetic counseling services or they can work directly with patients, billing their insurance for the service. Hospital systems that would like to speak to a representative about adding genetic counseling to their hospital system should contact representatives from these companies directly.

Hiring a Cancer Genetic Counselor

Although hiring a full-time cancer genetic counselor may seem too costly, a cancer genetics program can grow very quickly with a knowledgeable staff member identifying high-risk patients and providing them with services. The average salary for a cancer genetic counselor is between $50,000 and $60,000 per year. Once patient volume is high enough, this option may become the most cost-effective way of providing services and allows an institution to bill for these services. The best way to find a cancer genetic counselor is to post the position with the National Society of Genetic Counselors Job Connection service (http://nsgc.org/p/cm/ld/fid=92).

REFERENCES

1. About Genetic Counselors: What is genetic counseling? Available at: http://nsgc. org/p/cm/ld/fid=175. Accessed February 2, 2015.
2. ACGC (Accreditation Council for Genetic Counseling) Standards of Accreditation for Graduate Programs in Genetic Counseling. 2013. Available at: http:// gceducation.org/Documents/Standards%20Final%20approved%20Feb%202013. pdf. Accessed February 1, 2015.
3. American Board of Genetic Counseling. Certification. Copyright 2013. Available at: http://www.abgc.net/Certification/certification.asp. Accessed February 1, 2015.
4. Testimony of Angela Trepanier, GCG, Assistant Professor, Director Genetic Counseling Graduate Program, Wayne State University, Past President National Society of Genetic Counselors before the State of Michigan House of Representatives Health Policy Committee. 2014. Available at: http://www.senate.michigan.gov/ committees/files/2014-SCT-HP__-05-28-1-08.PDF. Accessed February 5, 2015.
5. The Virginia Board of Health Professions, The Virginia Department of Health Professions. Study into the need to regulate genetic counselors in the commonwealth of Virginia. 2011. Available at: http://www.dhp.virginia.gov/dhp_studies/ GeneticCounselorsFINAL_June2011.pdf. Accessed February 3, 2015.
6. Hampel H, Bennett RL, Buchanan A, et al. A practice guideline from the American College of Medical Genetics and Genomics and the National Society of Genetic Counselors: referral indications for cancer predisposition assessment. Genet Med 2015;17(1):70–87.
7. Jasperson K, Burt RW. The Genetics of Colorectal Cancer. Surg Oncol Clin N Am, in press.
8. Wood ME, Kadlubek P, Pham TH, et al. Quality of cancer family history and referral for genetic counseling and testing among oncology practices: a pilot test of quality measures as part of the American Society of Clinical Oncology Quality Oncology Practice Initiative. J Clin Oncol 2014;32(8):824–9.

9. Tyler CV Jr, Snyder CW. Cancer risk assessment: examining the family physician's role. J Am Board Fam Med 2006;19(5):468–77.
10. Sweet KM, Bradley TL, Westman JA. Identification and referral of families at high risk for cancer susceptibility. J Clin Oncol 2002;20(2):528–37.
11. Lindor NM, McMaster ML, Lindor CJ, et al, National Cancer Institute, Division of Cancer Prevention, Community Oncology and Prevention Trials Research Group. Concise handbook of familial cancer susceptibility syndromes - second edition. J Natl Cancer Inst Monogr 2008;38:1–93.
12. Berry DA, Iversen ES Jr, Gudbjartsson DF, et al. BRCApro validation, sensitivity of genetic testing of BRCA1/BRCA2 and prevalence of other breast cancer suscep-tibility genes. J Clin Oncol 2002;20:2701–12.
13. Tyrer J, Duffy SW, Cuzick J. A breast cancer prediction model incorporating famil-ial and personal risk factors. Stat Med 2004;23(7):1111–30.
14. Antoniou AC, Pharoah PP, Smith P, et al. The BOADICEA model of genetic sus-ceptibility to breast and ovarian cancer. Br J Cancer 2004;91(8):1580–90.
15. Frank TS, Deffenbaugh AM, Reid JE, et al. Clinical Characteristics of individuals with germline mutations in BCA1 and BRCA2: analysis of 10,000 individuals. J Clin Oncol 2002;20:1480–90.
16. Couch FJ, DeShano ML, Blackwood MA, et al. BRCA1 mutations in women attending clinics that evaluate the risk of breast cancer. N Engl J Med 1997; 336:1409–15.
17. The Penn II BRCA1 and BRCA2 Mutation Risk Evaluation Model. Philadelphia: University of Pennsylvania Abramson Cancer Center. Available at: http://www. afcri.upenn.edu/itacc/penn2. Accessed February 2, 2015.
18. Gail MH, Brinton LA, Byar DP, et al. Projecting individualized probabilities of developing breast cancer for white females who are being examined annually. J Natl Cancer Inst 1989;81(24):1879–86.
19. Claus EB, Risch N, Thompson WD. Autosomal dominant inheritance of early-onset breast cancer. Implications for risk prediction. Cancer 1994;73(3):643–51.
20. Claus EB, Risch N, Thompson WD. The calculation of breast cancer risk for women with a first degree family history of ovarian cancer. Breast Cancer Res Treat 1993;28(2):115–20.
21. Chen S, Wang W, Lee S, et al, Colon Cancer Family Registry. Prediction of germ-line mutations and cancer risk in the Lynch syndrome. JAMA 2006;296:1479–87.
22. Kastrinos F, Steyerberg EW, Mercado R, et al. The PREMM(1,2,6) model predicts risk of MLH1, MSH2, and MSH6 germline mutations based on cancer history. Gastroenterology 2011;140(1):73–81.
23. Myriad Prevalence Table. 2007. Available at: https://www.myriadpro.com/hereditary-cancer-testing/hereditary-colon-and-gynecologic-cancers/lynch-syndrome-hnpcc/mlh1-and-msh2-prevalence-table/. Accessed February 5, 2015.
24. Wijnen JT, Vasen HF, Khan PM, et al. Clinical findings with implications for genetic testing in families with clustering of colorectal cancer. N Engl J Med 1998;339(8): 511–8.
25. Tan MH, Mester J, Peterson C, et al. A clinical scoring system for selection of pa-tients for PTEN mutation testing is proposed on the basis of a prospective study of 3,042 probands. Am J Hum Genet 2011;88:42–56.
26. Robson M, Storm C, Weitzel J, et al. American Society of Clinical Oncology policy statement update: genetic and genomic testing for cancer susceptibility. J Clin Oncol 2010;28(5):893–901.
27. Schneider K. Counseling about cancer strategies for genetic counseling. 3rd edi-tion. Hoboken (NJ): Wiley-Blackwell; 2012.

28. Gammon A, Neklason DW. Confidentiality & the Risk of Genetic Discrimination What Surgeons Need to Know. Surg Oncol Clin N Am, in press.

29. Trepanier AM, Allain DC. Models of service delivery for cancer genetic risk assessment and counseling. J Genet Couns 2014;23(2):239–53.

30. HIraki S, Rinella ES, Schnabel F, et al. Cancer risk assessment using genetic panel testing: considerations for clinical application. J Genet Couns 2014;23: 604–17.

31. Tung N, Battelli C, Allen B, et al. Frequency of mutations in individuals with breast cancer referred for BRCA1 and BRCA2 testing using next-generation sequencing with a 25-gene panel. Cancer 2015;121(1):25–33.

32. LaDuca H, Stuenkel AJ, Dolinsky JS, et al. Utilization of multigene panels in hereditary cancer predisposition testing: analysis of more than 2,000 patients. Genet Med 2014;16(11):830–7.

33. Eggington JM, Burbidge LA, Roa B, et al. Current variant of uncertain significance rates in BRCA1/2 and Lynch syndrome testing (MLH1, MSH2, MSH6, PMS2, EPCAM). Presented at the American College of Medical Genetics and Genomics annual education conference. Charlotte, March 27–31, 2012.

34. George R, Kovak K, Cox SL. Aligning policy to promote cascade genetic screening for prevention and early diagnosis of heritable diseases. J Genet Couns 2015;24(3):388–99.

35. Birch P, Friedman JM. Utility and limitations of genetic disease databases in clinical genetics research: a neurofibromatosis 1 database example. Am J Med Genet C Semin Med Genet 2004;125C(1):42–9.

36. Lewis KM. Identifying hereditary cancer: genetic counseling and cancer risk assessment. Curr Probl Cancer 2014;38(6):216–25.

37. Miller CE, Krautscheid P, Baldwin EE, et al. Genetic counselor review of genetic test orders in a reference laboratory reduces unnecessary testing. Am J Med Gen A 2014;164A(5):1094–101.

38. Palit TK, Miltenburg DM, Brunicardi FC. Cost analysis of breast conservation surgery compared with modified radical mastectomy with and without reconstruction. Am J Surg 2000;179(6):441–5.

39. Evaluation of Genomic Applications in Practice and Prevention (EGAPP) Working Group. Recommendations from the EGAPP Working Group: genetic testing strategies in newly diagnosed individuals with colorectal cancer aimed at reducing morbidity and mortality from Lynch syndrome in relatives. Genet Med 2009; 11(1):35–41.

40. Lancaster JM, Powell CB, Chen LM, et al, SGO Clinical Practice Committee. Society of Gynecologic Oncology statement on risk assessment for inherited gynecologic cancer predispositions. Gynecol Oncol 2015;136(1):3–7.

41. Giardiello FM, Allen JI, Axilbund JE, et al. Guidelines on genetic evaluation and management of Lynch syndrome: a consensus statement by the US Multisociety Task Force on colorectal cancer. Am J Gastroenterol 2014;109(8): 1159–79.

42. Syngal S, Brand RE, Church JM, et al, American College of Gastroenterology. ACG clinical guideline: Genetic testing and management of hereditary gastrointestinal cancer syndromes. Am J Gastroenterol 2015;110(2):223–62.

Confidentiality & the Risk of Genetic Discrimination
What Surgeons Need to Know

Amanda Gammon, MS, Deborah W. Neklason, PhD*

KEYWORDS

- Genetic discrimination • Privacy • Genetic Information Nondiscrimination Act
- Health Insurance Portability and Accountability Act • Genetic testing • Legal
- Hereditary cancer

KEY POINTS

- Federal and state laws are now in place to prohibit many forms of genetic discrimination including health insurance eligibility, coverage, and rates, and employment.
- Patient health information including genetic testing and family history are protected under the Health Insurance Portability and Accountability Act and the Genetic Information Nondiscrimination Act.
- Some groups are not covered by current regulations.
- Physicians have a duty to warn patients that they and their relatives are at risk from a genetically transferable condition, but they must rely on the patient to communicate with family members.

INTRODUCTION

Fears about genetic discrimination plague patients and providers alike. These concerns can arise throughout the genetic testing process: before testing, after results are received, and when patients are deciding what type of cancer screening or risk reduction measures they should take based on their results. Some of the major concerns expressed by patients and providers around genetic discrimination include

- "Could I lose my health insurance if my genetic test comes back positive?"
- "If I have genetic testing, will my insurance premiums increase?"
- "What if my employer finds out I'm at high risk for cancer; could I be fired or demoted?"

The authors have nothing to disclose.
Department of Internal Medicine, High Risk Cancer Research, Huntsman Cancer Institute at University of Utah, 2000 Circle of Hope, Salt Lake City, UT 84112, USA
* Corresponding author.
E-mail address: deb.neklason@hci.utah.edu

Surg Oncol Clin N Am 24 (2015) 667–681
http://dx.doi.org/10.1016/j.soc.2015.06.004
1055-3207/15/$ – see front matter

surgonc.theclinics.com

- "Should I recommend genetic testing for my patient if it could cause him/her problems obtaining health insurance?"

When genetic testing for hereditary cancer risk first became clinically available in the mid-1990s, comprehensive legal protections prohibiting genetic discrimination did not exist. Both patients and clinicians were wary of the potential for genetic discrimination.

The current state of affairs in the United States is quite different. Both federal and state laws are now in place to prohibit many forms of genetic discrimination. Despite this, many patients and clinicians are unaware of these protections. A 2010 study conducted by Parkman and colleagues[1] used questions added to the Behavioral Risk Factor Surveillance System (BRFSS) survey in 4 states to assess public knowledge regarding legal protections from genetic discrimination. Only 13.3% to 19.1% of respondents indicated that they were aware of laws (such as the Genetic Information Nondiscrimination Act, GINA) that "prevent genetic test results from being used to determine health insurance coverage and costs."[1] In 2009, Laedtke and colleagues[2] sent surveys to 1500 members of the American Academy of Family Physicians assessing their knowledge of GINA and their concerns regarding genetic discrimination. Of the 401 physicians who responded, over half (54.5%) were not aware of GINA, and 44% were "highly concerned" about their patients' potential risk for genetic discrimination in health insurance.[2]

This article reviews the current legal protections against genetic discrimination, how they can affect both patients and their families, and perspectives on how current protections will be applied to an ever-changing genetic testing landscape. It will focus on how this information can be used by surgeons to help reassure their patients regarding the protections that exist and also educate them about loopholes where safeguards are not currently in place.

CURRENT LEGAL FRAMEWORK IN THE UNITED STATES REGARDING GENETIC DISCRIMINATION AND GENETIC INFORMATION PRIVACY
The Americans with Disabilities Act

The Americans with Disabilities Act (ADA) was passed in 1990.[3] The primary purpose of the ADA is to prevent discrimination against individuals with disabilities in the workplace and to set enforceable standards for accessibility in public and commercial buildings, transportation, and communication services (specifically telecommunications device for the deaf/telephone relay services).[3,4] It provides some limited protections regarding genetic discrimination with regard to hereditary cancer predispositions to individuals employed by an employer with 15 or more employees.[3] Some state laws also ban employers from discriminating against individuals on the basis of disability. If an individual has a genetic disease that causes symptoms that significantly impair a person's ability to perform one or more functions, then their disease qualifies as a disability under the ADA.[3,5–7] This would then afford an individual protection from employment discrimination under the ADA, as long as they are able to perform the duties of their job with reasonable accommodations. Some hereditary cancer syndromes can be associated with cognitive impairment (such as *PTEN* hamartoma tumor syndrome), which may classify as a disability for some individuals.[8,9] Others may have experienced debilitating effects following their cancer treatment that could potentially rise to the level of a disability.[10,11] However, most individuals with hereditary predispositions to cancer do not have disease effects that rise to the level of disability.

Confidentiality and the Health Insurance Portability and Accountability Act

The Health Insurance Portability and Accountability Act (HIPAA) was passed in 1996. The primary goal of the law is to make it easier for people to keep health insurance

(Title 1, Portability), protect the confidentiality and security of health care information and help the health care industry control administrative costs (Title II, Administrative Simplification).[12] In 2013, the HIPAA privacy rule was modified to prohibit most health plans from using or disclosing genetic information (individual or family) for underwriting purposes.[12] This includes determining eligibility, benefits under the plan, coverage, and premiums.

The portability section
The portability section of HIPAA provides rules for continuity in health insurance coverage for individuals and their families if they change jobs. It limits restrictions that a group health plan can place on benefits for preexisting conditions. Health plans cannot consider pre-existing conditions if there is no more than a 63-day lapse in coverage.

The Health Insurance Portability and Accountability Act privacy rule
The HIPAA privacy rule provides federal protection for individually identifiable health information. This includes information in patient health record, conversations with care providers, billing information, and information that the patient is seen at the clinic. It has 3 major components: how data are protected, when data can be disclosed, and the patient's rights to this information.

Data protection
The HIPAA security rule establishes national security standards for protecting health information that is held or transferred in electronic form. In general, these laws apply to covered entities, which include health plans, most health care providers, business associates and subcontractors of covered entities, and health care clearinghouses.

Disclosure
Disclosure of health information is permitted for treatment, care, and payment. It can also be disclosed to others the patient identifies as involved with health care, termed personal representatives. It can be disclosed to protect the public's health (eg, contagious conditions) and in police reports (eg, gunshot wounds).

Patient rights
Patients have the right to see and obtain a copy of health records, have corrections added, receive notice of how their information may be used and shared, receive a report on when and why health information was shared, and file a complaint with the health provider, insurer or US government.

Organizations exempt from following privacy and security rules
Examples of other organizations exempt from following privacy and security rules include: life insurers, schools, workers compensation carriers, law enforcement, and many state agencies like child protective services. An employer can also ask for a doctor's note or other information if an employer needs information to administer sick leave, worker's compensation, wellness programs, or health insurance. However, the health care provider can not release this without authorization from the patient.

State laws prohibiting genetic discrimination
Prior to the enactment of GINA in 2008, many states had laws prohibiting genetic discrimination.[6,7] One difficulty with these laws is that they differed from state to state. Some laws only extended protection to people with individual health care policies and not group policies, or vice versa.[13] Other laws were very narrow (eg, only focusing on requiring patient consent before genetic information could be shared with his or her

health insurance company).[13] Because hereditary cancer predispositions are by nature a family affair, under such laws the proband initially seeking genetic testing could live in a state with strong legislative protections while his or her potentially at-risk relatives could reside in states with no protections.[6] This presented quandaries for patients whose families were spread throughout the United States before GINA provided a baseline level of protection across the nation.

As of 2014, 48 states plus Washington D.C. have laws in place that prohibit forms of genetic discrimination in health insurance.[14] Regarding employment protections, 35 states plus Washington D.C. have laws prohibiting some types of genetic discrimination.[14] Of note, some state laws provide stronger protections than GINA, or prohibit genetic discrimination in other areas not covered by GINA (such as life insurance or long-term disability insurance). GINA is explicitly written so that the most comprehensive law in effect for an individual person (whether that be GINA or a stronger local law) takes precedence.[15] For a complete list of the state protections regarding genetic discrimination in health insurance enacted prior to GINA, please see the list compiled by the National Conference of State Legislatures.[13]

Genetic Information Nondiscrimination Act

GINA was the culmination of 13 years of debate at the federal level regarding the best way to provide genetic discrimination protections to the American public.[7,15–17] The first such bill was introduced to Congress in 1995, but it was not until May 21, 2008, that the final bill, GINA, was enacted; GINA's protections fully came into effect over the course of the next 3 years. Lauded as the "first major civil rights bill of the century" by Senator Edward Kennedy (D, Massachusetts), GINA provides the majority of the American public a baseline level of protection against genetic discrimination in the workplace and health insurance realms.[16]

As its name suggests, GINA involves regulations regarding the collection and use of genetic information as well as prohibitions on genetic discrimination.[15,17] GINA specifically applies to health insurance plans and employers (with a few exceptions noted later). It is important to note that GINA does not provide legal protections against genetic discrimination in other types of insurance underwriting or enrollment, including life insurance and short-/long-term disability insurance.[6,15,17]

GINA defines genetic information broadly, including not only genetic test results, but also genetic services (such as documentation of a patient meeting with a genetic counselor, and family health history) (**Box 1** and **2**).[17] With few exceptions (**Box 3**), it prohibits health insurance plans and employers from requesting, requiring, or collecting genetic information on an individual or his or her family members (out to fourth-degree relatives).[15,17] One exception is that a health insurance plan may request the results of an individual's genetic test (or family history) to determine coverage of a procedure. Also, if no genetic testing has been performed and an individual is requesting a specific procedure because of his or her family's history of cancer, a health insurance plan may request that genetic testing be completed. This could apply to a woman with a *BRCA1* mutation requesting that her insurance cover an annual breast MRI or prophylactic mastectomy due to her high lifetime risks for breast cancer. Her insurance company may request to see a copy of her *BRCA1* genetic test results in order to confirm that she is truly at high risk for breast cancer and that the requested screening/surgery is warranted. Under GINA, employers are also allowed to collect genetic information in certain limited circumstances (eg, collecting family health history as part of a workplace wellness program).[17]

Box 1

Genetic Information Nondiscrimination Act protections regarding genetic information privacy

Individual and group health insurance plans cannot

- Require an individual to undergo genetic testing for underwriting or enrollment purposes (ie, determining premiums or starting/terminating coverage)
- Request genetic information (genetic test results, information on genetic assessment services pursued by the patient, or family history information) for underwriting or enrollment purposes

Most employers cannot

- Request an individual to undergo genetic testing for hiring, termination, promotion, or placement decisions
- Request information (genetic test results, information on genetic assessment services pursued by the patient, or family history information) on an individual for hiring, termination, promotion, or placement decisions

---

Regarding health insurance protections, GINA prohibits most health insurance policies from using an individual's genetic information for underwriting purposes.[6,17] Under GINA, a person's current health insurance policy cannot be terminated because of genetic information, nor can their premiums be raised.[15,17] When an individual is applying for health insurance coverage or changing policies, genetic information cannot be used to decide whether or not that individual will be covered. GINA applies to most group and individual health insurance policies; some notable exceptions include health insurance provided through the military, Veteran's Administration (VA), Indian Health Services, or to federal employees.[17] Many of these organizations have other protections in place that are similar to GINA, but may have some restrictions or gaps in protection. If an individual has served in the military for at least 6 months and is later found to have a genetic condition, he or she typically is still eligible for health insurance benefits.[18] The VA follows a similar policy; veterans generally cannot be denied benefits through the VA on the basis of a genetic disease that was diagnosed after the individual started military service.

GINA also provides protections against genetic discrimination in the workplace. Most employers with 15 or more employees fall under GINA's provisions. Under

---

Box 2

Genetic Information Nondiscrimination Act protections from genetic discrimination

Health insurance

Most individual and group health insurance plans cannot

- Use an individual's genetic information for underwriting or enrollment purposes (ie, determining premiums or starting/terminating coverage)

Most individual and group health insurance plans can:

- Request genetic information (ie, genetic test results or family history) for the purpose of determining coverage of a specific procedure/claim (ie, a cancer screening or prophylactic surgery)

Employers

Most employers with more than 15 employees cannot use an employee's genetic information for hiring, termination, promotion, or placement decisions

---

Box 3
Insurance providers and employers who do not need to comply with the Genetic Information Nondiscrimination Act

Health insurance providers: federal government employees, military, VA, Indian Health Services

Employers: military, federal government, employers with fewer than 15 employees

Other forms of insurance: life insurance, short-/long-term disability insurance

---

GINA, employers are not allowed to use genetic information in hiring, firing, or promotion decisions. The military does not fall under GINA's employment provisions, but as mentioned previously has some similar protections in place. The military reserves the right to potentially use an individual's genetic information to assist with duty assignments.[18] Some genetic testing can be required by the military, such as mandatory testing for sickle cell anemia.[18] Individuals employed by the federal government are not covered under GINA either. However, they have protections under Executive Order 13145 (To Prohibit Discrimination in Federal Employment Based on Genetic Information), issued by President Bill Clinton in 2000.[19] Although employers with fewer than 15 employees are exempt from GINA's provisions, prospective employees are not required to disclose genetic information in most situations.

One important nuance of GINA is that it was written specifically to provide protections against genetic discrimination based on the use of a person's genetic information and not symptoms of his or her disease.[17] For example, a 40-year-old man who was recently diagnosed with Lynch syndrome, but has never developed cancer, would be protected from genetic discrimination with regard to health insurance and employment in most cases. However, if he later developed colon cancer, he could become at risk for adverse changes to his health insurance or employment on the basis of his cancer diagnosis. His employer and health insurance policy could not cite Lynch syndrome as the cause for such actions, as this is still protected genetic information under GINA, but his colon cancer diagnosis could be used. There are many other laws that can protect patients from this discrimination on the basis of health status. As explained in detail in the next section, the Affordable Care Act now prevents most individuals from experiencing discrimination in health insurance underwriting on the basis of pre-existing conditions, such as a cancer diagnosis.[20] The ADA prohibits most employers from using an individual's health status against him or her unless it is compromising his or her work duties in a way that cannot be resolved through reasonable accommodations.[3] Other programs available to workers to help when they are unable to perform their job due to medical problems include Family and Medical Leave Act (FMLA) and short- or long-term disability coverage.

Interaction of the Genetic Information Nondiscrimination Act with the Affordable Care Act

With the passing of the Affordable Care Act in 2010, GINA's protections were strengthened in an important way: by stating that individuals could not face health insurance discrimination on the basis of a pre-existing health condition, individuals whose hereditary cancer syndrome had manifested could now be protected.[5,20] This manifestation could include a malignancy (such as breast cancer in a woman with a *BRCA1/2* mutation) or a premalignant lesion (such as a colon polyp in an individual with familial adenomatous polyposis) or a benign feature (macrocephaly in a man with Cowden syndrome). Although GINA prohibited health insurance discrimination on the basis of genetic test results, once an individual manifested symptoms of the cancer predisposition, GINA alone could no longer protect the individual from facing potential health insurance discrimination, since the symptoms could be considered a pre-existing condition.[5,17] Now that the ACA outlaws the use of a person's pre-existing conditions to determine health insurance coverage or premium determination, both pre-symptomatic and symptomatic individuals are protected.[20] Through ACA, health insurance no longer needs to be tied to the employer. This relieves some concerns of losing health insurance because of genetic information when employed by a company of 15 or less employees. However, the enactment of the ACA does not make GINA irrelevant – GINA still provides important protections against genetic discrimination in employment. Given the mixed political sentiment regarding the ACA, some patients may be wary of relying on its protections regarding genetic discrimination. Given the low level of public awareness of GINA in comparison to the ACA, some patients can conflate the two when clinicians are discussing their protections. It is often beneficial to highlight to patients that GINA is an entirely separate piece of legislation, with wide support in Congress and among the public.

WADING THROUGH THE MISCONCEPTIONS TO DELIVER OPTIMAL MEDICAL CARE

Now that we have discussed the current legal protections against genetic discrimination, as well as the existing gaps in coverage, how can this information be applied to patients' surgical needs? Asking a few basic questions of your patients regarding their health insurance and employment can assist you in determining whether or not GINA's protections will apply. The following vignettes serve to highlight ways in which surgeons can help their patients navigate questions regarding genetic discrimination:

1. Before genetic testing occurs. A 30-year-old woman presents to the clinic due to her family history of cancer. Her paternal aunt and paternal grandmother were both diagnosed with breast cancer in their mid-30s/early 40s and passed away from metastatic disease. Her father has recently developed pancreatic cancer at age 60. The patient is very worried about developing cancer and is interested in prophylactic mastectomy to reduce her breast cancer risk. She has considered genetic testing previously, but had heard she would lose her health insurance if she pursued it.
2. After genetic testing. A 40-year-old woman recently tested positive for a *BRCA1* mutation after her sister was diagnosed with breast cancer at 38. She is interested in pursuing a prophylactic salpingo-oophorectomy and bilateral mastectomy as soon as possible. However, she fears that if her employer finds out that she is at high risk for cancer, she will be let go, and is thus worried about taking time off to have the surgeries.
3. When symptoms are present. A 20-year-old man is referred for colectomy; he was recently found to have hundreds of adenomatous colon polyps. He is currently covered by his parents' health insurance plan. His new diagnosis makes him worry about his ability to obtain his own health insurance policy later in life.

   Table 1 helps to summarize the key points related to genetic discrimination protections and gaps that apply to each of the previously described patients, as well as some additional points regarding management. Most patients can be reassured that the combined protections of the laws described earlier in this article will protect them from genetic discrimination in the areas of health insurance and employment. In a busy surgical practice, an in-depth, lengthy discussion of every legal protection and loophole is not feasible, nor should it be necessary, for all patients. A brief explanation will suffice in most instances. When a patient has a question that requires more

	Patient #1	Patient #2	Patient #3
Table 1			
Patient vignettes—current protections and additional considerations			
Benefit to using genetic information as part of surgical decisions	Genetic testing could help clarify patient's cancer risks	Prophylactic salpingo-oophorectomy and bilateral mastectomy are reasonable risk-reducing surgeries for a woman with a *BRCA1* mutation	Colectomy is warranted in this patient based on his colonic polyp phenotype
	Insurance may be more likely to cover prophylactic surgery if she is found to have a specific hereditary cancer predisposition	—	—
Legal protections from discrimination	Patient is most likely protected by GINA, HIPAA, ACA, and applicable state laws	GINA makes it illegal for most employers to use her *BRCA1* mutation status to terminate her employment	The ACA makes it illegal for most health insurance companies to use his clinical diagnosis of polyposis as a pre-existing condition to deny him health insurance coverage in the future
	Her health insurance policy would be prohibited from using her genetic test results to alter or terminate her coverage	In most situations, her employer cannot require her to reveal information regarding her *BRCA1*-positive status	—
Exceptions to legal protection	If patient receives her health insurance through one of the entities not covered by GINA (see **Box 3**), there may be other protections in place that would apply (on the state level or through her insurance provider)	If patient is in the military, or works for an employer with fewer than 15 employees, she could be at risk for genetic discrimination by her employer	The ACA should allow him to receive coverage by a health insurance plan in the future (either through an employer or via an individual policy)

(continued on next page)

	Patient #1	Patient #2	Patient #3
Table 1 **(*continued*)**			
Medical management options	Patient's father would be the ideal person in the family to first pursue genetic testing.	Salpingo-oophorectomy is recommended, as there is no current effective screening for ovarian cancer	Genetic testing could potentially clarify his type of polyposis (likely familial adenomatous polyposis or *MUTYH* associated polyposis)
	—	Breast cancer screening with mammogram and MRI is a reasonable alternative	Medical insurance more likely to cover additional screening for associated cancers (eg, upper gastrointestinal tract) when genetic diagnosis can be made
Other considerations	If her father tests positive for a hereditary cancer predisposition, genetic testing for the patient will be more targeted, less costly, and more likely covered by her insurance	Filing for FMLA for her surgery recovery period would further help to secure her employment	—

research or he or she possibly falls into a gap in genetic discrimination protection, local genetics specialists are an excellent source of current knowledge and information. For example, some states have laws restricting use of genetic information to determine life, disability, and long-term care insurance. Individuals who are concerned about obtaining life insurance should consider obtaining a policy prior to genetic testing, but understand that life insurance can use family history to determine eligibility. **Box 4** includes the listing for the National Society of Genetic Counselors' Web site,

Box 4 **Resources for providers and patients**
National Conference of State Legislatures: list of state laws regarding genetic discrimination: http://www.ncsl.org/research/health/genetic-nondiscrimination-in-health-insurance-laws.aspx
GINAhelp.org: patient-friendly information on GINA, its protections, and gaps: http://www.ginahelp.org/
HIPAA policies: summary of HIPAA and its protections: http://www.hhs.gov/ocr/privacy/hipaa/understanding/index.html
National Society of Genetics Counselors: resource for identifying genetic counselors in one's local area: http://www.nsgc.org

where local genetic counselors specializing in cancer genetics can be found. This box also lists other resources that may assist patients with additional information.

FAMILY IMPLICATIONS

Management of a patient with a positive genetic test extends to the family members as well. In most cases, the genetic cause of the patient's condition is inherited from the mother or father. As most hereditary cancer predispositions are inherited in an autosomal-dominant manner, siblings and biologic children typically have a 50% chance of carrying the mutation, with more extended family members having a risk as well. A few hereditary cancer predispositions have other patterns of inheritance, including MAP (MUTYH-associated polyposis), which is autosomal recessive, and SDHD mutations causing hereditary parganglioma/pheochromocytoma syndrome, which demonstrate a maternal imprinting effect. Another exception is when a patient has a de novo mutation, a mutation that arose in that individual shortly after conception but was not inherited from a parent. Other articles in this issue have addressed these inheritance patterns. Risk perception can also influence whom patients inform about their genetic test results. Multiple studies have shown that individuals with a BRCA1/2 mutation are more likely to inform their female relatives about the mutation than their male relatives, due to higher lifetime cancer risks seen in women who have a BRCA1/2 mutation.[21,22] This is in spite of the fact that men have increased cancer risks associated with BRCA1/2 mutations and are just as likely to pass the mutation on to their children. It is important for clinicians to help educate their patients about the inheritance pattern of the syndrome within their family to assist in correctly identifying at-risk relatives.

The clinical provider has an obligation to maintain the confidentiality of his or her patient's genetic test result under HIPAA guidelines. In an ideal situation, the patient is willing to share the genetic results and has the tools to properly communicate this to family members who may be at risk for carrying the genetic mutation. This becomes an ethical challenge when the individual tested does not share the information with family members.

Key points to empower family communication include

- Physician has a duty to warn the patient that his or her relatives are at risk from a genetically transferable condition.[23]
- Patients should tell family members about their genetic test results, because it is not just their individual result; it affects the health of their biologic relatives.[24,25]
- Patients should be provided with a copy of the test report so that it can be easily shared with family members without having to sign medical record release forms.
- When an individual presents for genetic testing for a known syndrome within his or her family, an official copy of one of their relative's positive genetic test results is needed to ensure the individual's test are ordered correctly and in the most cost-effective manner.
- Identify a plan for communicating genetic information upon the patient's death.
- Ultimately it is the patient's choice of what information he or she will share and what procedures he or she will undergo.

Benefits and Challenges to Family Members

The benefits of germline genetic testing are that if the mutation is known, conclusive genetic testing can be offered to family members at a fraction of the cost, and medical management will be specific to their genetic status. When the specific mutation is known, the appropriate technology can be applied so that a false-negative result can be avoided. Mutation carriers will be educated on appropriate cancer screening and risk reduction, and noncarriers can avoid unnecessary worry and procedures.

Most patients elect to communicate their test results to relatives. A 2013 study showed that *BRCA1/2* mutation carriers shared their test results with 73% of their at-risk first- and second-degree relatives.[22] Family dynamics, however, can present challenges that can get in the way of sharing results. Some patients may be estranged or have lost contact from some or all of their relatives, inhibiting disclosure of test results. Some patients may have cultural factors that influence their willingness to share genetic test results or undergo genetic testing.

Conversely, a patient may be eager to share his or her genetic test results, but may run into resistance from family members. Some individuals do not want to know if they have a hereditary cancer risk, or they may wish to block other relatives, like children, from learning the information.[26] A recent review by Sharaf and colleagues[27] in 2013 summarized 8 published studies looking at uptake of genetic testing for Lynch syndrome among relatives of individuals who had tested positive. Importantly, each of the studies covered in this review paper recruited patients during the mid-1990s to mid-2000s.[27] Genetic testing uptake reported among first-degree relatives in these reviewed studies ranged from 34% to 52%.[27] Some studies that did not delineate between uptake in first-degree or extended relatives showed higher uptake rates, up to 75%.[27] These numbers may improve with the more recent improved legal protections regarding genetic discrimination.

A genetic diagnosis also has the potential to change family relationships in positive and negative ways.[28] Some individuals experience guilt and worry about whether or not they could have passed the condition on to their children.[28,29] Patients sometimes experience conflict with family members over their decision to pursue genetic testing or certain management decisions (ie, prophylactic surgery).[28,29] Relatives who are found not to carry the mutation can also experience guilt, wondering why they were spared from having increased cancer risks. Genetic counselors and other clinicians are trained to help patients prepare for a range of potential reactions from their family members.

Maintain Confidentiality in Light of Sharing Information with Family Members

Does a physician have a duty to warn patients' relatives of their risk for a hereditary condition?[30,31] Two legal cases Pate v. Threlkel (1995) and Safer v. Estate of Pack (1996) found that the physician has a duty to inform the patient that his or her genetic condition was transferable to offspring, and Safer v. Estate of Pack extended the duty to warn to members of the patient's immediate family.[23] Under the HIPAA privacy rule, which followed these legal decisions, divulging the genetic result to third parties without patient's permission is not allowed, so the physician is left with relying on the patient to facilitate this communication.

Disclosure of Result if the Patient Dies

One may consider genetic information belonging to the family, especially after the death of a patient; however, the laws surrounding privacy change over time and are by no means consistent across different jurisdictions.[32] There is a fine balance between respecting the privacy and wishes of the deceased versus the health interests and needs of the family. The obstacle has been that the HIPAA privacy rule applies to both alive and deceased, and the interpretation continues to evolve. In 2013, HIPAA was modified to extend privacy protection of health information for 50 years after death, but considered the needs of family and care takers. Disclosure is now permitted to family members or others involved in an individual's care before death, even when this person is not the designated personal representative.[33] The exceptions are if the deceased has expressed otherwise or if the practitioner is uncomfortable doing so. In order to disclose genetic results upon patient death, providers must make reasonable assurances that the requester is a relative or involved in the care through documents, past interactions, or reasonable discretion, and check for patient's preferences about disclosure.

Interestingly, a survey of research biobank participants showed that 52% would want their results returned to their nearest biologic relative after death; 30% would designate someone other than a biological relative, and 9% would not want results disclosed after death.[34]

EMERGING ISSUES
Genome Sequencing

With the increasing access to affordable whole-genome sequencing, the genomes of patients and their tumors are being sequenced as standard clinical care.[35]

Sequencing of the tumor will become increasingly common and important to precisely target chemotherapy. Sequencing of the tumor can reveal germline genetic predispositions as well. This may include mutations in cancer syndrome genes that explain the origins of the cancer as well as completely unrelated but medically actionable findings such as mutations leading to cardiac failure.

Sequencing of individual genomes is being requested clinically when there is concern of an underlying condition in patients or their children.[36,37] It can also be requested by individuals for preventative measures or even curiosity through physicians. A time may be coming when everyone will be sequenced at birth and use this information to manage their care throughout their lifetime.[38] Although this would create a broader opportunity for misuse, the HIPAA, GINA, and ADA laws in place should still offer protection.

Now, with newer HIPAA rules, the patient has rights to access his or her medical records, including complete access to the DNA sequence report and interpretation. Additionally, the ordering physician has a duty to warn the patient of the findings. One challenge is management and reporting of medically actionable incidental findings, that is, findings that are unrelated to the original reason for performing sequencing, are unexpected, and have immediate implications for clinical management. Up to 5% of the time, incidental findings result from sequencing, and clinical providers should be prepared to help the patient manage these through education and referral.[36] Ideally the risk of these findings should be discussed prior to sequencing. Engaging a genetic counselor early in the process of genome sequencing (tumor or germline) is of enormous benefit in that the counselor can address these unanticipated risks, educate, and facilitate communication.

Social Media/Scenarios

Under GINA, federal protections are in place that disallow intentional acquisition of genetic information, and this includes social media and Web sites.[39] The key to this is intentional, which opens the door to different levels of interpretation. It is not uncommon for employers and prospective employers to review the Internet and social media sites when considering someone for a position. This could lead to unintentional acquisition of genetic information, on which, legally, they could not act. However, the burden of proof that an employer intentionally viewed this information and/or used it for an employment decision is on the individual who suspects such a violation.

Patients concerned about confidentiality of their genetic information should practice caution when sharing on the Internet.

SUMMARY

Overall, significant protections are currently in place for individuals residing in the United States related to genetic discrimination in employment and health insurance. Other countries have also pursued legislation prohibiting genetic discrimination. Although reviewing all countries' protections/gaps is beyond the scope of this article, it is encouraging that the worldwide community is considering this important issue. As genetic testing becomes a greater part of all individuals' health care management, current laws are likely to change to address the evolving understanding of genetics. The authors encourage all clinicians to reach out to local genetics specialists to keep abreast of the evolving legal landscape surrounding genetic discrimination.

REFERENCES

1. Parkman AA, Foland J, Anderson B, et al. Public awareness of genetic nondiscrimination laws in four states and perceived importance of life insurance protections. J Genet Couns 2015;24(3):512–21.
2. Laedtke AL, O'Neill SM, Rubinstein WS, et al. Family physicians' awareness and knowledge of the Genetic Information Non-Discrimination Act (GINA). J Genet Couns 2012;21(2):345–52.
3. Division USDoJCR. Americans with Disabilities Act of 1990, as amended. 2009.
4. Division USDoJCR. Information and technical assistance on the Americans with disabilities act. 2015. Available at: http://www.ada.gov/2010_regs.htm. Accessed March 17, 2015.
5. Prince AE, Berkman BE. When does an illness begin: genetic discrimination and disease manifestation. J Law Med Ethics 2012;40(3):655–64.
6. Prince AE, Roche MI. Genetic information, non-discrimination, and privacy protections in genetic counseling practice. J Genet Couns 2014;23(6): 891–902.
7. Slaughter LM. The Genetic Information Nondiscrimination Act: why your personal genetics are still vulnerable to discrimination. Surg Clin North Am 2008;88(4): 723–38, vi.
8. McBride KL, Varga EA, Pastore MT, et al. Confirmation study of PTEN mutations among individuals with autism or developmental delays/mental retardation and macrocephaly. Autism Res 2010;3(3):137–41.
9. Busch RM, Chapin JS, Mester J, et al. Cognitive characteristics of PTEN hamartoma tumor syndromes. Genet Med 2013;15(7):548–53.
10. Commission USEEO. Questions & Answers about Cancer in the Workplace and the Americans with Disabilities Act (ADA). 2013.
11. Nachreiner NM, Ghebre RG, Virnig BA, et al. Early work patterns for gynaecological cancer survivors in the USA. Occup Med 2012;62(1):23–8.
12. Health Insurance Portability and Accountability Act of 1996 (HIPAA). Code of Federal Regulations (CFR) 45 C.F.R. Part 160, Part 162, and Part 1641996.
13. Legislatures NCoS. Genetics and health insurance state anti-discrimination laws. 2008. http://www.ncsl.org/research/health/genetic-nondiscrimination-in-health-insurance-laws.aspx. Accessed March 17, 2015.
14. Institute NHGR. Genetic discrimination. 2014. Available at: http://www.genome.gov/10002077. Accessed July 31, 2014.

15. Payne PW Jr, Goldstein MM, Jarawan H, et al. Health insurance and the Genetic Information Nondiscrimination Act of 2008: implications for public health policy and practice. Public Health Rep 2009;124(2):328–31.
16. Hudson KL, Holohan MK, Collins FS. Keeping pace with the times–the genetic information nondiscrimination act of 2008. N Engl J Med 2008;358(25):2661–3.
17. Congress t. Genetic Information Nondiscrimination Act of 2008. 2008.
18. Baruch S, Hudson K. Civilian and military genetics: nondiscrimination policy in a post-GINA world. Am J Hum Genet 2008;83(4):435–44.
19. Clinton P. Executive order 13145, to prohibit discrimination in federal employment based on genetic information. 2000. Available at: http://www.eeoc.gov/eeoc/history/35th/thelaw/13145.html. Accessed March 19, 2015.
20. Counsel OotL. Compilation of Patient Protection and Affordable Care Act. 2010:1–974.
21. Montgomery SV, Barsevick AM, Egleston BL, et al. Preparing individuals to communicate genetic test results to their relatives: report of a randomized control trial. Fam Cancer 2013;12(3):537–46.
22. Fehniger J, Lin F, Beattie MS, et al. Family communication of BRCA1/2 results and family uptake of BRCA1/2 testing in a diverse population of BRCA1/2 carriers. J Genet Couns 2013;22(5):603–12.
23. Schleiter KE. A physician's duty to warn third parties of hereditary risk. Virtual Mentor 2009;11(9):697–700.
24. Vadaparampil ST, McIntyre J, Quinn GP. Awareness, perceptions, and provider recommendation related to genetic testing for hereditary breast cancer risk among at-risk Hispanic women: similarities and variations by sub-ethnicity. J Genet Couns 2010;19(6):618–29.
25. Sussner KM, Thompson HS, Jandorf L, et al. The influence of acculturation and breast cancer-specific distress on perceived barriers to genetic testing for breast cancer among women of African descent. Psychooncology 2009; 18(9):945–55.
26. Ackermann S, Lux MP, Fasching PA, et al. Acceptance for preventive genetic testing and prophylactic surgery in women with a family history of breast and gynaecological cancers. Eur J Cancer Prev 2006;15(6):474–9.
27. Sharaf RN, Myer P, Stave CD, et al. Uptake of genetic testing by relatives of Lynch syndrome probands: a systematic review. Clin Gastroenterol Hepatol 2013;11(9): 1093–100.
28. van Oostrom I, Meijers-Heijboer H, Duivenvoorden HJ, et al. A prospective study of the impact of genetic susceptibility testing for BRCA1/2 or HNPCC on family relationships. Psychooncology 2007;16(4):320–8.
29. MacDonald DJ, Sarna L, Weitzel JN, et al. Women's perceptions of the personal and family impact of genetic cancer risk assessment: focus group findings. J Genet Couns 2010;19(2):148–60.
30. Laberge AM, Burke W. Duty to warn at-risk family members of genetic disease. Virtual Mentor 2009;11(9):656–60.
31. Milner LC, Liu EY, Garrison NA. Relationships matter: ethical considerations for returning results to family members of deceased subjects. Am J Bioeth 2013; 13(10):66–7.
32. Tasse AM. The return of results of deceased research participants. J Law Med Ethics 2011;39(4):621–30.
33. Kels CG, Kels LH. Medical privacy after death: implications of new modifications to the health insurance portability and accountability act privacy rule. Mayo Clinic Proc 2013;88(10):1051–5.

34. Allen NL, Karlson EW, Malspeis S, et al. Biobank participants' preferences for disclosure of genetic research results: perspectives from the OurGenes, Our-Health, Our Community project. Mayo Clinic Proc 2014;89(6):738–46.
35. Biesecker LG, Green RC. Diagnostic clinical genome and exome sequencing. N Engl J Med 2014;371(12):1170.
36. Yang Y, Muzny DM, Xia F, et al. Molecular findings among patients referred for clinical whole-exome sequencing. JAMA 2014;312(18):1870–9.
37. Lee H, Deignan JL, Dorrani N, et al. Clinical exome sequencing for genetic identification of rare Mendelian disorders. JAMA 2014;312(18):1880–7.
38. Topol EJ. Individualized medicine from prewomb to tomb. Cell 2014;157(1): 241–53.
39. Soo-Jin Lee S, Borgelt E. Protecting posted genes: social networking and the limits of GINA. Am J Bioeth 2014;14(11):32–44.

The Genetics of Colorectal Cancer

Kory Jasperson, MS[a],*, Randall W. Burt, MD[b]

KEYWORDS

- Hereditary colon cancer • Lynch syndrome • Familial adenomatous polyposis
- MUTYH-associated polyposis • Peutz-Jeghers syndrome • Juvenile polyposis

KEY POINTS

- Multigene tests using next-generation sequencing technologies are becoming more widely used in clinical practice.
- Multigene tests do not replace the need for genetic counseling or a thorough evaluation of the personal and family history.
- Universal tumor testing of all colorectal and endometrial cancers is cost-effective and therefore recommended by many societal guidelines.
- Involvement of genetics in the development, implementation, and tracking of these programs is important for the success of these programs.
- The colonic polyposis conditions are a heterogeneous group; a detailed reporting of all endoscopy findings, including the histopathology of polyps, skin findings, and cancer history, is critical in making a correct diagnosis.

INTRODUCTION

The hereditary colorectal cancer (CRC) syndromes comprise a heterogeneous group of conditions with varying cancer risks, gastrointestinal (GI) polyp types, nonmalignant findings, and inheritance patterns. Although each one is unique in its own right, these syndromes often have overlapping features, making diagnoses difficult in select cases. Obtaining accurate polyp history (histologic type, number, location, and age of onset), cancer history (location, type, and age of onset), and other nonmalignant features is imperative in determining the likely disease diagnosis and thereby the appropriate genetic tests for precise diagnosis in a timely fashion. This process often necessitates collaboration among surgical oncology team members and genetic counselors.

The authors have nothing to disclose.
[a] Department of Internal Medicine, Huntsman Cancer Institute, The University of Utah, 2000 Circle of Hope Drive, Room 1166, Salt Lake City, UT 84112, USA; [b] Department of Internal Medicine, Huntsman Cancer Institute, The University of Utah, 2000 Circle of Hope Drive, Salt Lake City, UT 84112, USA
* Corresponding author.
E-mail address: kory.jasperson@hci.utah.edu

Surg Oncol Clin N Am 24 (2015) 683–703
http://dx.doi.org/10.1016/j.soc.2015.06.006
1055-3207/15/$ – see front matter © 2015 Elsevier Inc. All rights reserved.
surgonc.theclinics.com

Advances in genetic testing technologies have improved the detection of various hereditary CRC syndromes. Here, some of these improvements, including the current state of genetic testing for hereditary CRC syndromes, are highlighted. Lynch syndrome (LS), familial adenomatous polyposis (FAP), MUTYH-associated polyposis (MAP), juvenile polyposis, and Peutz-Jeghers syndrome (PJS) are reviewed in detail. The genetic causes, inheritance patterns, cancer risks, and additional characteristic features are covered. **Table 1** includes a summary of the characteristic features of these syndromes, in addition to other causes of hereditary CRC, which will not be addressed in this review in detail. Last, also highlighted are the management issues revolving around various syndromes (**Table 2**), genetic testing guidelines are reviewed, and the implications of newer genetic testing technologies on clinical practice, especially as it relates to surgical oncology, are highlighted.

LYNCH SYNDROME

The understanding of LS has greatly increased since 1885, when pathologist Aldred Warthin first made the astute observation that his seamstress had a striking family history of cancer, particularly colon, uterine, and small bowel.[1] This particular kindred, which was called family G, was later confirmed to have LS.[1] Various names have been used for LS; the most notable was hereditary nonpolyposis colorectal cancer (HNPCC), which helped differentiate it from FAP.[2] LS is now deemed a more fitting name, given it is well-known that CRC is only one of many associated cancers.

LS is the most common cause of hereditary colon and endometrial cancer, accounting for 2% to 6% of all cases.[3–5] LS is also one of, if not the most, common cancer-related syndromes known,[1] even more prevalent than hereditary breast and ovarian cancer caused by *BRCA1* or *BRCA2* mutations. Like most other hereditary CRC predispositions, LS is inherited in an autosomal-dominant manner. It is caused by mutations in one of the mismatch repair (MMR) genes (*MLH1*, *MSH2*, *MSH6*, *PMS2*). LS may also occur from mutations in the *EPCAM* gene, as 3′ deletions in *EPCAM* result in *MSH2* hypermethylation, thereby acting like an *MSH2* mutation. CRC is the characteristic tumor, although the risk of endometrial cancer (EC) in some LS families is higher than the risk of CRC.[6] The incidence of LS is estimated at 1 in 370 individuals or even higher.[7] Other cancers are also increased in LS, including gastric, ovarian, urinary tract, hepatobiliary, brain, pancreas, and sebaceous skin (see **Table 1**). It is still questionable whether breast and prostate are LS cancers. A systematic review of the literature in 2013 was inconclusive as to whether breast cancer is associated with LS, although microsatellite instability (MSI) was found in some of the tumors, highlighting the possible link between the two.[8] In a similar review, it was revealed that prostate cancer risk was moderately elevated in LS,[9] although selection biases may have influenced those data.

Features

Although LS is defined as a single condition, the clinical phenotypes can vary quite significantly depending on the gene involved. As outlined in **Table 1**, not only do many different types of cancers occur in LS, but also the cancer risks are variable depending on the underlying genetics. In *MLH1* and *MSH2* mutation carriers, early estimates of CRC risk approached 80%, while the risk of EC was 40% to 60%.[10] These early studies were weighted toward high-risk families, which likely resulted in overestimations of cancer risk. Recent estimates are assuredly more precise. In a large study of more than 17,500 members of *MLH1* and *MSH2* families, the CRC risk to age 70 was estimated to be 34% to 47%, while the EC risks were 18% to

30%.[11] Compare these risks to *PMS2* mutation carriers, which have an estimated 19% CRC risk for men and an 11% and 12% risk for CRC and EC, respectively, for women.[12] Even though the risks are substantially lower for *PMS2* mutation carriers, the age of CRC and EC can be very young in some cases.[12,13] Recent evidence also suggests that for *MLH1* or *MSH2* mutations there may be certain individuals at very high cancer risk, while others are at much lower risk, even with the same gene mutation.[14] The reasons for these differing risk cohorts are largely unknown. Modifying factors, such as diet, smoking, exercise, or other environmental factors, in addition to other genetic modifiers, could be influencing risk. More work is clearly needed in this area.

Other features of LS include cancers occurring at younger ages than the general population, higher chance of metachronous and synchronous cancers,[15–17] and tumors that characteristically have MSI.[1] MSI is the result of expansions or contractions of repetitive DNA sequences called microsatellite repeats. MSI in colorectal or endometrial cancers indicates a deficiency in the MMR system, although these defects can be somatic or germline (Lynch syndrome).[18] The most common somatic cause of MMR deficiency in tumors is hypermethylation of *MLH1*, which is present in 10% to 15% of all colon and endometrial cancers.[18] Greater than 90% of CRCs and ECs in LS patients are MSI-high or have absent MMR protein staining via immunohistochemistry (IHC) analysis.[19]

Testing

Guidelines
Testing strategies for LS have evolved over the years. The Amsterdam criteria (AC I) were originally developed to identify high-risk families for recruitment into research, but later used to identify families appropriate for genetic testing.[20] Given that more than half of individuals with LS fail to meet AC I, the Bethesda guidelines were developed.[21] The Bethesda guidelines were originally used to identify CRC patients appropriate for tumor testing via MSI analysis.[21] The AC were subsequently amended to include certain extracolonic cancers and called AC II.[22] Unfortunately, the AC still misses up to 78% of LS cases.[23] The most recent version of the Bethesda guidelines, called the revised Bethesda guidelines, are the most sensitive of the group, although they still miss at least 1 in 4 LS cases.[5] The revised Bethesda guidelines are primarily used to identify CRC patients appropriate for tumor tissue testing with MSI and IHC analysis. IHC and MSI analyses are not only used to screen CRCs, but also they are widely used to screen ECs for MMR deficiency. MSI and IHC analyses can be used in other LS tumors, such as sebaceous adenomas/carcinomas, adenomatous colon polyps, ovarian cancer, urothelial malignancies, and other GI cancers beyond colon.[24–31] However, the results of MSI and IHC analyses on tumors beyond CRC and EC should be interpreted with caution.

Additional testing criteria and probability models
Other guidelines, such as those updated annually by the National Comprehensive Cancer Network (NCCN), take into account additional indications for testing, such as endometrial cancer diagnosed at young ages, or those with at least a 5% probability of having an LS gene mutation on one of the MMR probability models.[32] Models such as PREMM(1,2,6), MMRpro, and MMRpredict estimate probability of finding an MMR gene mutation depending on various personal and family history features.[33–36] Validation of these models has been promising. However, the utilization of these models to identify LS testing candidates is likely very low in clinical practice possibly in part due to the logistics in filling out the required information for some of

Table 1
Hereditary colorectal cancer syndromes: characteristic features and associated cancer phenotypes

Syndrome: Inheritance	Gene(s)	Associated Cancers (Lifetime Risk, %)	Nonmalignant Features	References
LS: Autosomal dominant	MLH1, MSH2, EPCAM	Colorectal (22%–74%), Endometrial (14%–54%), Stomach (0.2%–13%), ovary (4%–20%), urinary tract (0.2%–25%), hepatobiliary tract (0.02%–4%), small bowel (0.4%–12%), brain (1%–4%), sebaceous tumors (0.4%–4%)	Some colon adenomas; sebaceous gland adenomas and epitheliomas	12,23,51,52
	MSH6	Colorectal (10%–22%), Endometrial (17%–71%), Other malignancies possibly increased		
	PMS2	Colorectal (9%–20%), Endometrial (10%–15%), Other malignancies possibly increased		
FAP: Autosomal dominant	APC	Colorectal (~100%), Duodenal/periampullary (4%–12%), thyroid (1%–2%) gastric (0.5%–1%), hepatoblastoma (<1%), medulloblastoma (1%–2%), other cancers: pancreatic, biliary, distal small bowel	Colonic adenomatous polyposis, gastric polyposis (fundic gland), Duodenal polyps (adenomas), Desmoid tumors, epidermoid cysts, fibromas, osteomas, congenital retinal pigment epithelial hypertrophy, adrenal adenomas, dental abnormalities, pilomatrixomas, nasal angiofibromas	32,51,52
AFAP: Autosomal dominant		Colorectal (69%), Duodenal/periampullary (4%–12%), thyroid (1%–2%)	Colonic adenomatous polyposis, gastric polyposis (fundic gland), duodenal polyps/polyposis (adenomas)	32,51,52
MAP: Autosomal recessive	MUTYH	Colorectal (80%), Duodenal (4%), Other malignancies possibly increased	Colonic polyposis (adenomas, hyperplastic, and sessile serrated polyps), sebaceous gland adenomas, and epitheliomas	32,51,52,116
PJS: Autosomal dominant	STK11	Breast (32%–54%), pancreatic (11%–36%), gastric (29%), small bowel (13%), ovarian (21%), uterine (9%), lung (7%–17%), testes (9%), cervix (10%)	Petuz-Jeghers-type polyps throughout GI tract, mucocutaneous melanin pigment spots	32,51,52

Syndrome: Inheritance	Gene	Cancer risk	Features	Ref
JPS: Autosomal dominant	SMAD4, BMPR1A	Stomach and duodenum combined up to 21% (mainly in SMAD4 carriers) Other malignancies possibly increased	Juvenile-type polyps predominantly in the colon, gastric polyposis; congenital abnormalities, arteriovenous malformations, telangiectasia, and epistaxis	32,51,52
PTEN hamartoma tumor syndrome: Autosomal dominant	PTEN	Breast (25%–50%) Thyroid (3%–10%) Endometrial (7%–17%) Colon (9%–16%) Other malignancies possibly increased	Juvenile, ganglioneuromas, adenomatous, inflammatory, leiomyomatous, lipomatous, and lymphoid polyps Macrocephaly, Lhermitte-Duclos disease, trichelemmomas, oral papillomas, cutaneous lipomas, macular pigmentation of the glans penis, autism spectrum disorder, esophageal glycogenic acanthosis, multinodular goiter	132
Li-Fraumeni Syndrome: Autosomal dominant	TP53	By age 50, 80% have cancer and the risk goes up with age. Core cancers are sarcomas, breast, brain, and adrenocortical cancers. Colon cancer and various other cancers increased	—	133
Polymerase proofreading-associated polyposis: Autosomal dominant	POLE, POLD1	Colorectal (increased but specific risk unknown), possibly endometrial cancer in POLD1 carriers	Multiple colon polyps (adenomas)	134
Hereditary mixed polyposis syndrome: Autosomal dominant	GREM1	Colorectal (specific risk unknown)	Multiple colon adenomas, hamartomas, and serrated polyps (polyps with more than one histologic type) Ashkenazi Jewish ancestry	135,136
Constitutional mismatch repair deficiency syndrome: Autosomal recessive	MLH1, MSH2, MSH6, PMS2, EPCAM	Very high risks, typically hematological and brain, in addition to other LS tumors, exact risks not known	Café-au-lait macules, axillary/inguinal freckling, Lisch nodules, neurofibromas; colonic adenomatous polyposis; hepatic adenomas, pilomatricomas, congenital malformations	137

Table 2
Management considerations for hereditary colorectal cancer syndrome

Syndrome	Management Recommendations	References
LS: *MLH1*, *MSH2*, and *EPCAM*	Colonoscopy every 1–2 y at age 20–25 y Consider prophylactic hysterectomy and bilateral salpingo-oophorectomy if childbearing complete Consider esophagogastroduodenoscopy every 3–5 y at age 25–30 y Annual physical/neurologic examination at age 25–30 y	23,32,51,52,67,68
LS: *MSH6 and PMS2*	Colonoscopy every 1–2 y at age 25–30 y Consider prophylactic hysterectomy and bilateral salpingo-oophorectomy if childbearing complete	
FAP	Annual colonoscopy/sigmoidoscopy by 10–12 y until colectomy (total colectomy with IPAA often preferred) Upper endoscopy with side-viewing instrument every 1–4 y by 25–30 y Annual physical examination, with particular attention to the thyroid	32,51,52
AFAP	Colonoscopy every 2–3 y by late teens Total colectomy with ileal rectal anastomosis often preferred with advanced polyp/polyposis Upper endoscopy with side-viewing instrument every 1–4 y by 25–30 y Annual physical examination, with particular attention to the thyroid	
MUTYH-associated polyposis	Colonoscopy every 2–3 y by 25–30 y Upper endoscopy with side-viewing instrument every 1–4 y by 30–35 y	32,51,52
PJS	Colonoscopy every 2–3 y starting in late teens Breast MRI annually at 25 y, mammogram and breast MRI annually starting at age 30 y Magnetic resonance cholangiopancreatography and/or endoscopic ultrasound every 1–2 y at 30–35 y Upper endoscopy starting in late teens; consider small-bowel visualization (computed tomography or MRI enterography) by 8–10 y Annual pelvic examination and Pap smear, consider transvaginal ultrasound at 18–20 y Annual testicular examination	32,52
JPS	Colonoscopy by age 15 y repeating annually if polyps are present and every 2–3 y if no polyps Upper endoscopy by age 15 y repeating annually if polyps are present (particularly in *SMAD4* carriers) and every 2–3 y if no polyps Screen for vascular lesions associated with HHT at 6 mo in *SMAD4* carriers	32,52

these models. Using both probability models and clinical criteria, such as those outlined by NCCN, may prove successful in certain settings.

Universal tumor testing

Recently, King and colleagues[37] recommended that all women over the age of 30 undergo genetic testing of the BRCA1 and BRCA2 genes, regardless of personal or family history of breast or ovarian cancer. This broad-reaching population-based testing has not gained very much support in the medical community. However, it has resulted in more discussions about population-based testing for hereditary cancer syndromes. Although not general population-based testing, testing all CRC and EC tumor tissues for evidence of LS is gaining support across the United States.[38–41] This screening strategy, which often uses IHC, and sometimes MSI analysis, is referred to as universal tumor testing. In addition to CRCs, universal testing is also being performed on all ECs at various hospitals across the United States.[41] The pivotal studies on universal tumor testing revealed that 1 in 35 CRCs are due to LS.[5,42] Universal tumor testing of ECs revealed promising results as well.[43,44] Multiple studies have subsequently shown that universal tumor testing of all CRCs is cost-effective.[45–48] As a result, the Evaluation of Genomic Applications in Practice and Prevention (EGAPP) Working Group found enough evidence to recommend that all newly diagnosed CRCs be evaluated for LS.[19,49] Although EGAPP did not find sufficient evidence to recommend IHC over MSI or vice versa, IHC is the preferred method because it can direct germline genetic testing to the appropriate gene, when necessary, thereby reducing genetic testing costs. MSI testing is not useful in determining which of the 5 LS genes may be responsible for an MMR-deficient tumor. Importantly, MSI analysis is not known to be affected by neoadjuvant chemoradiation, whereas IHC analysis can be.[50] This finding is, of course, particularly important for many patients with rectal cancer that receive neoadjuvant therapy before resection. If only MSH6 deficiency is found on IHC analysis of the rectal cancer following neoadjuvant therapy, MSI analysis may be useful in determining whether the abnormal IHC result is due to a true MSH6 mutation or was the result of treatment. Given the uncertainties just described, biopsy of rectal cancer *before* neoadjuvant therapy should be considered preferable. Also, importantly, colonoscopic biopsies of CRC to facilitate MSI/IHC analyses or germline genetic testing should be sought before surgery in individuals suspected of having LS given that a proven diagnosis of genetic LS before a CRC resection may change the extent of surgery. As genetic panel testing advances, this may provide a less logistically challenging option, allowing providers to pursue a genetic diagnosis when LS is suspected.

Since the EGAPP recommendations were first made, multiple other societal guideline recommendations have supported universal tumor testing of CRCs.[23,32,51–53] Although most guidelines focus on CRCs, the data also suggest that universal tumor testing in ECs should also be performed.[54–57] Therefore, as hospitals are considering universal tumor testing of CRCs, ECs should not be overlooked. Many hospitals have already started this transition to testing all CRC and ECs.[41] Even with growing support for universal tumor testing, implementing a program at a hospital is not always an easy task.[23] It is very important to include a multidisciplinary team when setting up a universal tumor testing program. Some of the stakeholders that are often involved include surgeons, oncologists, pathologists, genetic counselors, nurses, hospital administrators, and other allied health care staff. Some of the resources that have been used by other hospitals in their program include LS factsheets that can be handed to patients before testing, example letters that can be sent to patients with normal or abnormal results, protocols that outline the various tumor tests that can be used and the order in which they occur, in addition to the protocol for following up on results. The Lynch Syndrome Screening Network has compiled various resources on their Web site (http://www.lynchscreening.net/) to help assist with this process.[41] Cragun and colleagues[58] have put together an excellent review that highlights many of the potential outcomes of universal tumor testing, in addition to ethical considerations that must be taken into account with developing a universal program. They also highlight and compare these public health initiatives to newborn screening.[40,58]

Multigene testing

LS testing ideally should start with an individual who has a personal history of CRC, EC, or other LS cancer. Of course, this may not always be possible for a variety of reasons. Some of the barriers for testing include deceased relatives, lack of contact with affected family members, archived tumor tissue destroyed, inadequate cancer tissue remaining, out-of-pocket expenses for patients, limited access to care for family members, or even just a family member who is disinclined to undergo testing for whatever reason. In these scenarios, LS testing in an unaffected individual may be necessary.[32] Historically, genetic testing of multiple genes, 5 in the case of LS, has been cost prohibitive. With the advent of next-generation sequencing technologies, testing for multiple genes simultaneously (called panel or multigene testing) is now comparable in price to testing 1 or 2 genes using older technologies.[59] Various multigene testing options are available clinically. Although current CRC NCCN guidelines[32] do not state when multigene testing should be performed, this has been partially addressed in the NCCN Genetic/Familial High-Risk Assessment: Breast and Ovarian guidelines (www.nccn.org). Examples of when to consider multigene testing are provided, such as a 49-year-old patient with both colorectal and ovarian cancer. This patient would meet guidelines for both LS and BRCA1/2 genetic testing. Multigene testing in this example seems cost-effective compared with tumor testing or germline genetic testing for LS, in addition to targeted genetic testing of *BRCA1* and *BRCA2*. Multiple other situations may warrant multigene testing, and these considerations will assuredly change in the next few years as multigene testing becomes more commonplace. Early-onset CRC with few to no polyps is one of the situations in which multigene testing may be used more often in the near future; this is in part due to attenuated familial adenomatous polyposis (AFAP) and MAP presenting with this phenotype.[60,61] In addition, there are multiple examples of individuals having more than one hereditary CRC syndrome.[62–66]

It is important that clinicians understand that multigene testing is not a replacement for a thorough genetic risk assessment. Pretest and posttest counseling by a professional with genetic expertise is even more important in the setting of multigene testing given the higher chance of getting results with uncertainty. There are many moderate or intermediate penetrant genes on various multigene tests. The actionability of these lower penetrant genes is often unclear. In addition, the rate of detecting variants of unknown significance (VUS) increases with each gene added to a test. One of the first clinically based studies using multigene tests for hereditary CRC found a 20% VUS rate.[59] It is also possible to get more than one VUS in different genes in a single individual when using multigene tests. Finding VUS or mutations in indeterminate risk genes may cause uncertainty for the patient and provider, which may lead to overscreening patients even though current guidelines do not support it.

Management

Screening recommendations

Various guidelines have addressed screening- and risk-reducing recommendations for individuals and families with LS. Some of the guidelines that have been updated or published within the last 2 years include the Mallorca group,[67] the NCCN,[32] the American College of Gastroenterology,[52] the American College of Obstetricians and Gynecologists,[68] the American Society of Clinical Oncology,[51] and the US Multi-Society Task Force.[23] There are differing opinions on management among the groups. A summary of different screening and management considerations for LS is included in **Table 2**.

The mainstay for cancer surveillance and prevention in LS is undoubtedly annual or biennial colonoscopies initiating at young ages. The hallmark study on colonoscopy surveillance in LS revealed that colonoscopic surveillance at 3-year intervals halved the risk of CRC and prevented CRC-related deaths.[69] Because not all of the CRCs were prevented using colonoscopies every 3 years, screening guidelines now include more frequent intervals, every 1 to 2 years. However, newer evidence suggests that the risk-benefit ratio of screening is very dependent on age.[14]

Given the cancer risks are substantially lower for *PMS2* compared with other LS genes, the effectiveness of screening *PMS2* mutation carriers in their 20s is certainly even less effective than what is seen for *MLH1* and *MSH2*. *PMS2* mutation carriers can develop cancer at very young ages.[12,13] Still, not everyone agrees that screening recommendations should differ among genes.[70] Given there are multiple types of cancers increased in LS, it is important to keep in mind the burden of frequent screenings. The balance between missed versus detected or prevented cancers must be weighed, but the final decision of when to offer or start screening is not straightforward. Given hereditary CRC syndromes are relatively rare, evidence-based data on screenings for cancer may be limited or nonexistent. Guidelines for screening may be based on expert opinion only, which has limitations and controversies. Ultimately, with the growing interest regarding personalize medicine, it seems prudent to not only make recommendations based on the specific gene involved but also adjust recommendations based on the patient's age and sex-adjusted risk level.[12,14] It is hoped that with time, more data will be available to make recommendations based on these factors.

Surgical decision-making following colorectal cancer diagnosis in Lynch syndrome

It is well-known that individuals with LS have an increased risk for synchronous and metachronous cancers. In one study, 22% of patients with LS who underwent segmental resections for colon cancer were diagnosed with metachronous CRC compared with none of the patients with extensive colectomies.[71] Interestingly, the risk of metachronous CRC was reduced by 31% for every 10 cm of bowel removed.[71] In another large study of individuals with LS who underwent proctectomy for rectal cancer, the risk of metachronous colon cancer was 19% at 10 years and up to 69% at 30 years.[17] These data highlight that more extensive surgeries, such as total colectomy with ileorectal anastomosis (IRA) or proctocolectomy, should be considered in patients with colon or rectal cancer with LS. Colectomy with IRA in LS is also endorsed by several national guidelines/societies for individuals with colon cancer or colonic neoplasia that cannot be endoscopically removed.[23,32,52] Some of the factors that should be considered when determining the extent of surgery include the very high rate of metachronous CRC, patient age, patient choice, patient ability to undergo frequent surveillance after surgery, and other factors that may influence functional outcome.

Chemoprevention

The Colorectal Adenoma/carcinoma Prevention Programme 2 (CAPP2) was the first large-scale randomized, double-blind, placebo-controlled chemoprevention trial in individuals with likely LS. The primary outcome of interest was the effect of aspirin on the incidence of CRC.[72] Initially, findings did not find that the use of aspirin, resistant starch, or both for up to 4 years had an effect on the incidence of CRC or even adenomas in LS.[73] Additional analysis did reveal a delayed effect of aspirin on reducing CRC incidence in LS. At this time, there is not sufficient evidence to support universal use of aspirin as a chemopreventative agent in LS, although the CAPP2 study results are promising. In addition, the CAPP3 study is currently underway, which will be a non-inferiority, dose-finding trial in LS[74] that may provide the additional evidence necessary to implement aspirin use as chemoprevention on a larger scale in LS.

FAMILIAL ADENOMATOUS POLYPOSIS AND ATTENUATED FAMILIAL ADENOMATOUS POLYPOSIS
Background

FAP and AFAP are hereditary polyposis conditions due to germline mutations in the *APC* gene. FAP is characterized by hundreds to thousands of colonic polyps, whereas AFAP is less severe and has on average 25 polyps, but also can vary greatly (0–470 polyps).[60,75,76] The prevalence of FAP varies from 1 in 6850 to 1 in 31,250 individuals.[77–83] AFAP is often more difficult to diagnose given the lower polyp load, and as a result, the prevalence of AFAP is currently unknown. Approximately 0.5% of all CRCs historically were due to FAP; however, current numbers are likely lower given current cancer prevention interventions in FAP.[78,79] The clinical diagnosis of FAP is designated by finding at least 100 colorectal adenomas. Currently, a clinical diagnosis of AFAP has not been agreed on, and therefore, a diagnosis relies on the identification of an *APC* mutation, in addition to the personal and family history of polyps or lack thereof.[32]

Features

Given the sheer number of adenomatous colon polyps in FAP, CRC is unavoidable without colon removal. In AFAP, the risk of CRC approaches 70% and can be drastically reduced with early and frequent colonoscopy, polypectomies, and risk-reducing surgeries.[84] The average age of CRC onset is 39 for FAP and in the 50s for AFAP.[60] Both FAP and AFAP have increased risk for extracolonic polyps and tumors (see **Table 1**). The upper GI phenotype, such as gastric and duodenal polyposis and cancer, seems similar between FAP and AFAP. Gastric fundic gland polyposis is present in 23% to upward of 100% of patients.[85–88] Adenomas and cancers may also occur in the stomach, but the risk of gastric cancer seems to be only slightly increased above the general population in most families. Duodenal polyps are all adenomas and occur in 50% to possibly greater than 90% of patients.[85,87,89] The risk for duodenal and peri-ampullary cancer ranges from 4% to 12%.[77,85,87,90,91]

Desmoid tumors, which are exceptionally infrequent in the general population, are seen in 3.6% to 25% of patients with FAP.[92–98] Desmoid tumors were one of the main extracolonic features used for Gardner syndrome, which is now more of a historical term because it is known that it is also caused by *APC* mutations. Other features of Gardner syndrome included osteomas, epidermoid cysts, and fibromas.[99] Desmoids do not metastasize; however, they can be locally invasive, aggressive, and challenging to diagnose and manage. Because of these features, desmoids frequently result in significant morbidity and remain the second leading cause of mortality in FAP.[100] Various other malignant and nonmalignant findings can be seen in FAP and AFAP (see **Table 1**).

Testing

Genetic testing of *APC* is considered for individuals with greater than 10 colonic adenomas.[32] Given the rate of finding *APC* mutations is still low in this group, waiting for testing until a cumulative 20 adenomas occurs is the preferred starting point for testing in many cases. Age of onset of polyps and family history of polyps and CRC may influence the decision to offer testing. Up to 10% of individuals with hepatoblastoma have FAP.[101–103] This situation is similar for desmoid tumors.[104] Genetic testing in individuals with hepatoblastoma or desmoid tumors should also be considered.[32] Although individuals with early-onset CRC and few to no polyps may have AFAP,[84] genetic testing for APC in these cases has not been widely adopted. Given that 10% to 30% of FAP cases are the result of de novo (new mutation) APC mutations, a family history may be lacking.[105,106] Even in individuals with a clinical diagnosis of FAP, genetic testing is helpful to confirm the diagnosis because individuals with MAP may have an overlapping polyp presentation. In addition, other syndromes may be misdiagnosed as FAP. AFAP may be misdiagnosed as many conditions as well, the most notable are MAP and LS. Genetic testing in probands can also help clarify risk for family members through cascade genetic testing (testing for known mutations in at-risk family members).

Management
Screening and risk-reducing strategies
Except for the ages at which to start, screening recommendations for FAP and AFAP are very similar (see **Table 2**). Given the preponderance of proximal colonic polyps in AFAP, colonoscopy is necessary, whereas sigmoidoscopies can be used in FAP until polyps start to develop. For FAP, annual sigmoidoscopies/colonoscopies begin around age 10 and continue until the polyp load becomes endoscopically unmanageable, or advanced polyps are found.[32] Colonoscopies can be delayed until the late teens in AFAP and annual examinations can decrease the need for colectomy in many patients. Total colectomy with IRA is often preferred for AFAP given there is often rectal sparing, whereas total proctocolectomy with ileal pouch-anal anastomosis (IPAA) is preferred in FAP. Upper GI endoscopies with side viewing instruments to examine the duodenal papilla are preferred. The age to begin is not known, but screening by 25 to 30 years of age is commonly performed. Although gastric polyps are prominent in FAP and AFAP, complete polyp removal is not advised given the low rate of malignancy. Large gastric polyps, or polyps with other features concerning for malignancy, should be biopsied. Duodenal polyps should be removed when feasible. The Spigelman criteria (stages 0 to IV) are used to determine the frequency at which upper GI screening is needed based on duodenal polyp findings. As an example, individuals with stage III or IV have up to a 36% risk of duodenal cancer and require more aggressive therapy,[87,107] whereas those with lower stages (0–2) have much lower risks and can be followed less frequently. Thyroid cancer screening should also be considered. Screening for other tumors and malignancies in FAP and AFAP can be considered on a case-by-case basis, but is not routinely recommended.

MUTYH-ASSOCIATED POLYPOSIS
Background

MAP was first discovered when 3 siblings with multiple adenomas or CRC were reported in 2002.[108] Of the conditions described thus far, this is the only one inherited in an autosomal-recessive manner. MAP is caused by biallelic (homozygous or compound heterozygous) mutations in the MUTYH gene. MAP is even less common than FAP and AFAP. It accounts for less than 1% of all CRCs.[109] In one study of more than one thousand population-based CRC cases, 0.4% had MAP.[110] Monoallelic MUTYH mutations are found in 1% to 2% of the general population.[111] Although a slight increased risk for CRC has been suggested in monoallelic *MUTYH* carriers in some studies, this is not been verified in other studies.[111]

Features

Similar to FAP and AFAP, multiple colonic adenomas are the characteristic feature. The most common colon presentation for MAP is between 20 and 100 polyps.[111,112] Rarely do they have more than 500 polyps, which is a common feature of FAP. Hyperplastic or sessile serrated polyps were found in about half (47%) of MAP patients, and ~18% in one study met criteria for serrated polyposis (previously referred to as hyperplastic polyposis).[113] Similar to LS, individuals with MAP may also have MSI-high CRCs, although this is not common.[111] Dissimilar to sporadic cases, MAP CRC tissues have a near-diploid karyotype,[111] and a specific and characteristic *K-ras* mutation is frequently observed in adenomas and cancers in MAP. The risk of CRC in MAP is approximately 28-fold, with CRC occurring in 19% by age 50, 43% by 60, and 80% by 70 years.[114,115] As previously mentioned, individuals with MAP may present with early-onset CRC and few to no polyps.[33] The risk of duodenal cancer in MAP is 4%, which is similar to that of FAP.[116] It is still unclear whether individuals with MAP are at increased risk of other cancers.

Genetic Testing

As is the case for AFAP/FAP, genetic testing for MAP is also considered in individuals with greater than 10 adenomas. In the absence of germline *APC* mutations, biallelic *MUTYH* mutations were found in 1.7% of individuals 50 years of age or younger with CRC; 14% of individuals with 20 to 49 adenomas; 20% of those with 50 to 99 adenomas; 20% if there were 100 to 499 adenomas, but in no individuals with greater than 500 adenomas.[61] Given the high rate of biallelic mutations in the 20 or more polyp group, this is often the preferred criterion used for when to consider testing. Although many different testing algorithms have been suggested, individuals with at least 20 adenomas are often tested simultaneously for *APC* and *MUTYH* mutations. Two common *MUTYH* mutations are seen in most individuals of European ancestry; however, many other mutations occur.[111] Therefore, comprehensive testing of *MUTYH* is preferred. Unlike FAP and AFAP, which often have multigenerational affected individuals, individuals with MAP frequently have no affected family members, or affected siblings only (autosomal-recessive inheritance). Diligent documentation and informed thoughtful review of family history information can be helpful in identifying MAP. A pedigree with multiple affected siblings in one generation and no prior or subsequent generations affected may be a valuable clue suggesting consideration of MAP.

Management

Screening and risk-reducing recommendations for GI malignancies (see **Table 2**) in MAP are similar to FAP/AFAP.

PEUTZ-JEGHERS SYNDROME AND JUVENILE POLYPOSIS SYNDROME
Background

PJS and juvenile polyposis syndrome (JPS) are 2 of the most well-known of the hamartomatous polyposis syndromes. They are both autosomal-dominant conditions and exceptionally rare. PJS occurs in about 1 in 50,000 to 200,000 births,[117] whereas JPS is estimated to occur in 1 in 100,000 to 160,000.[118] PJS is caused by mutations in the *STK11* gene, whereas *SMAD4* or *BMPR1A* mutations result in JPS.

Features

As suggested by their names, the characteristic GI polyps in PJS are Peutz-Jeghers polyps, whereas juvenile-type hamartomas are seen in JPS. The GI polyps in PJS occur in 88% to 100% of cases and are distributed through the stomach (24%), small bowel (96%), colon (27%), and rectum (24%).[119,120] In JPS, the polyps are distributed through the colorectum (98%), stomach (14%), jejunum and ileum (7%), and duodenum (7%).[118,120–122] Both JPS and PJS have an increased risk for CRC (see **Table 1**), and PJS also has exceptionally high risk for other cancers as well, most notably, pancreatic and breast cancer.[123,124] PJS is most recognizable because of the mucocutaneous melanin pigmentation that occurs in more than 95% of cases of PJS. Arteriovenous malformations and other features of hereditary hemorrhagic telangiectasia (HHT) occur in some JPS individuals with mutations in *SMAD4*, but not *BMPR1A*.[125] Individuals with JPS who have gastric polyposis have an increased risk of gastric cancer, although this is typically only seen in *SMAD4* mutation carriers.[125]

Genetic Testing and Diagnosis

Clinical diagnostic criteria have been developed for both PJS and JPS (**Box 1**). Genetic testing for the associated gene(s) is indicated for anyone meeting criteria. *SMAD4* and *BMPR1A* mutations are still only found in up to 60% of individuals meeting clinically defined JPS criteria.[126] The detection rate of *STK11* mutations in individuals meeting PJS criteria is as high as 94%.[127,128] In most cases, a diagnosis of PJS and JPS relies on the polyp history. Because the polyps that are found in PJS and JPS are often misdiagnosed as other polyp types, polyps may need to be reviewed by a GI pathologist when a polyposis condition is considered.[129]

Laugier-Hunziker syndrome is an acquired condition that has perioral pigmentation similar to that seen in PJS.[130] Unlike PJS, Laugier-Hunziker syndrome typically

---

Box 1
Diagnostic criteria for Peutz-Jeghers syndrome and juvenile polyposis syndrome

Peutz-Jeghers syndrome

A clinical diagnosis of PJS is considered when any of the following are met:

1. Greater than 3 histologically confirmed Peutz-Jeghers polyps

2. Any number of Peutz-Jeghers polyps and a family history of PJS

3. Characteristic, prominent, mucocutaneous pigmentation and a family history of PJS

4. Greater than 1 Peutz-Jeghers polyp and characteristic, prominent, mucocutaneous pigmentation

Juvenile polyposis syndrome

A clinical diagnosis of JPS is considered when any of the following are met:

1. Three to 5 juvenile polyps of the colorectum

2. Juvenile polyps throughout the GI tract

3. Greater than 1 juvenile polyp in an individual with a family history of JPS

Modified from Burt RW, Cannon JA, David DS, et al. Colorectal cancer screening. J Natl Compr Canc Netw 2013;11(12):1538–75; and Syngal S, Brand RE, Church JM, et al. ACG clinical guideline: genetic testing and management of hereditary gastrointestinal cancer syndromes. Am J Gastroenterol 2015;110(2):223–62.

presents in adulthood and is not known to be at increased risk for polyps or cancer.[131] Both PJS and JPS may also be misdiagnosed as many other hereditary polyposis syndromes, in addition to acquired conditions.

Management

Screening recommendations for children and young adults with PJS and JPS are mainly targeting nonmalignant findings and complications, such as GI bleeding and small bowel intussusception. Cancer screening in JPS is mainly focused on CRC, or in the case of *SMAD4* (because *BMPR1A* mutation carriers are not known to be at increased risk of gastric cancer), mutation carriers, gastric cancer risk, and findings of HHT.

SUMMARY

Hereditary CRC syndromes vary quite substantially in their presentations. A detailed personal and family history is the first key step in identification. The clinical diagnosis of hereditary CRC syndromes also may in part depend on the total number of cumulative polyps, the histologic type, and the age of onset of the polyps. Total proctocolectomy with IPAA is standard of care in FAP; however, total colectomy with IRA is preferred for AFAP given there is often rectal sparing. Given the high metachronous CRC risk in LS, total colectomy with IRA is recommended in those with LS and colon cancer, although consideration must be given to segmental resection based on patient age, choice, and ability to undergo frequent surveillance after surgery.

Given that a substantial proportion of LS cases will not meet current testing criteria, testing of all CRC and endometrial cancers should be considered regardless of age of onset or family history. As multigene testing becomes more commonplace, it is increasingly important for health care providers with experience in genetics to be involved in the evaluation, testing, and clinical management of affected and at risk individuals.

REFERENCES

1. Lynch HT, Snyder CL, Shaw TG, et al. Milestones of Lynch syndrome: 1895-2015. Nat Rev Cancer 2015;15(3):181–94.
2. Kravochuck SE, Kalady MF, Burke CA, et al. Defining HNPCC and Lynch syndrome: what's in a name? Gut 2014;63(9):1525–6.
3. Ferguson SE, Aronson M, Pollett A, et al. Performance characteristics of screening strategies for Lynch syndrome in unselected women with newly diagnosed endometrial cancer who have undergone universal germline mutation testing. Cancer 2014;120(24):3932–9.
4. Hampel H. Point: justification for Lynch syndrome screening among all patients with newly diagnosed colorectal cancer. J Natl Compr Canc Netw 2010;8(5): 597–601.
5. Hampel H, Frankel WL, Martin E, et al. Feasibility of screening for Lynch syndrome among patients with colorectal cancer. J Clin Oncol 2008;26(35): 5783–8.
6. Lu KH, Broaddus RR. Gynecologic cancers in Lynch syndrome/HNPCC. Fam Cancer 2005;4(3):249–54.
7. Hampel H, de la Chapelle A. How do we approach the goal of identifying everybody with Lynch syndrome? Fam Cancer 2013;12(2):313–7.
8. Win AK, Lindor NM, Jenkins MA. Risk of breast cancer in Lynch syndrome: a systematic review. Breast Cancer Res 2013;15(2):R27.

9. Ryan S, Jenkins MA, Win AK. Risk of prostate cancer in Lynch syndrome: a systematic review and meta-analysis. Cancer Epidemiol Biomarkers Prev 2014; 23(3):437–49.

10. Vasen HF, Wijnen JT, Menko FH, et al. Cancer risk in families with hereditary non-polyposis colorectal cancer diagnosed by mutation analysis. Gastroenterology 1996;110:1020–7.

11. Dowty JG, Win AK, Buchanan DD, et al. Cancer risks for MLH1 and MSH2 mutation carriers. Hum Mutat 2013;34(3):490–7.

12. Ten Broeke SW, Brohet RM, Tops CM, et al. Lynch syndrome caused by germline PMS2 mutations: delineating the cancer risk. J Clin Oncol 2015;33(4): 319–25.

13. Senter L, Clendenning M, Sotamaa K, et al. The clinical phenotype of Lynch syndrome due to germ-line PMS2 mutations. Gastroenterology 2008;135(2): 419–28.

14. Jenkins MA, Dowty JG, Ait Ouakrim D, et al. Short-term risk of colorectal cancer in individuals with Lynch syndrome: a meta-analysis. J Clin Oncol 2015;33(4): 326–31.

15. Win AK, Lindor NM, Winship I, et al. Risks of colorectal and other cancers after endometrial cancer for women with Lynch syndrome. J Natl Cancer Inst 2013; 105(4):274–9.

16. Win AK, Lindor NM, Young JP, et al. Risks of primary extracolonic cancers following colorectal cancer in Lynch syndrome. J Natl Cancer Inst 2012; 104(18):1363–72.

17. Win AK, Parry S, Parry B, et al. Risk of metachronous colon cancer following surgery for rectal cancer in mismatch repair gene mutation carriers. Ann Surg Oncol 2013;20(6):1829–36.

18. Yamamoto H, Imai K. Microsatellite instability: an update. Arch Toxicol 2015; 89(6):899–921.

19. Palomaki GE, McClain MR, Melillo S, et al. EGAPP supplementary evidence review: DNA testing strategies aimed at reducing morbidity and mortality from Lynch syndrome. Genet Med 2009;11(1):42–65.

20. Vasen HF, Mecklin J, Merra Khan P, et al. The International Collaborative Group on Hereditary Non-Polyposis Colorectal Cancer (ICG-HNPCC). Dis Colon Rectum 1991;34:424–5.

21. Rodriguez-Bigas MA, Boland CR, Hamilton SR, et al. A National Cancer Institute workshop on hereditary nonpolyposis colorectal cancer syndrome: meeting highlights and Bethesda guidelines. J Natl Cancer Inst 1997;89:1758–62.

22. Vasen HF, Watson P, Mecklin J-P, et al. New clinical criteria for hereditary non-polyposis colorectal cancer (HNPCC, Lynch syndrome) proposed by the International Collaborative Group on HNPCC. Gastroenterology 1999;116: 1453–6.

23. Giardiello FM, Allen JI, Axilbund JE, et al. Guidelines on genetic evaluation and management of Lynch syndrome: a consensus statement by the US Multi-Society Task Force on Colorectal Cancer. Am J Gastroenterol 2014;109(8): 1159–79.

24. Chui MH, Gilks CB, Cooper K, et al. Identifying Lynch syndrome in patients with ovarian carcinoma: the significance of tumor subtype. Adv Anat Pathol 2013; 20(6):378–86.

25. Chui MH, Ryan P, Radigan J, et al. The histomorphology of Lynch syndrome-associated ovarian carcinomas: toward a subtype-specific screening strategy. Am J Surg Pathol 2014;38(9):1173–81.

26. Eckert A, Kloor M, Giersch A, et al. Microsatellite instability in pediatric and adult high-grade gliomas. Brain Pathol 2007;17(2):146–50.

27. Ericson KM, Isinger AP, Isfoss BL, et al. Low frequency of defective mismatch repair in a population-based series of upper urothelial carcinoma. BMC Cancer 2005;5:23.

28. Gylling A, Abdel-Rahman WM, Juhola M, et al. Is gastric cancer part of the tumour spectrum of hereditary non-polyposis colorectal cancer? A molecular genetic study. Gut 2007;56(7):926–33.

29. Kastrinos F, Mukherjee B, Tayob N, et al. Risk of pancreatic cancer in families with Lynch syndrome. JAMA 2009;302(16):1790–5.

30. Roberts ME, Riegert-Johnson DL, Thomas BC, et al. Screening for Muir-Torre syndrome using mismatch repair protein immunohistochemistry of sebaceous neoplasms. J Genet Couns 2013;22(3):393–405.

31. Yurgelun MB, Goel A, Hornick JL, et al. Microsatellite instability and DNA mismatch repair protein deficiency in Lynch syndrome colorectal polyps. Cancer Prev Res (Phila) 2012;5(4):574–82.

32. Burt RW, Cannon JA, David DS, et al. Colorectal cancer screening. J Natl Compr Canc Netw 2013;11(12):1538–75.

33. Backes FJ, Hampel H, Backes KA, et al. Are prediction models for Lynch syndrome valid for probands with endometrial cancer? Fam Cancer 2009;8(4):483–7.

34. Chen S, Wang W, Lee S, et al. Prediction of germline mutations and cancer risk in the Lynch syndrome. JAMA 2006;296(12):1479–87.

35. Dinh TA, Rosner BI, Atwood JC, et al. Health benefits and cost-effectiveness of primary genetic screening for Lynch syndrome in the general population. Cancer Prev Res (Phila) 2011;4(1):9–22.

36. Kastrinos F, Steyerberg EW, Mercado R, et al. The PREMM1,2,6 model predicts risk of MLH1, MSH2, and MSH6 germline mutations based on cancer history. Gastroenterology 2011;140(1):73–81.e75.

37. King MC, Levy-Lahad E, Lahad A. Population-based screening for BRCA1 and BRCA2: 2014 Lasker Award. JAMA 2014;312(11):1091–2.

38. Beamer LC, Grant ML, Espenschied CR, et al. Reflex immunohistochemistry and microsatellite instability testing of colorectal tumors for Lynch syndrome among US cancer programs and follow-up of abnormal results. J Clin Oncol 2012;30(10):1058–63.

39. Cohen SA. Current Lynch syndrome tumor screening practices: a survey of genetic counselors. J Genet Couns 2014;23(1):38–47.

40. Cragun D, DeBate RD, Vadaparampil ST, et al. Comparing universal Lynch syndrome tumor-screening programs to evaluate associations between implementation strategies and patient follow-through. Genet Med 2014;16(10):773–82.

41. Mange S, Bellcross C, Cragun D, et al. Creation of a network to promote universal screening for Lynch syndrome: the Lynch syndrome screening network. J Genet Couns 2014;24(3):421–7.

42. Hampel H, Frankel WL, Martin E, et al. Screening for the Lynch syndrome (hereditary nonpolyposis colorectal cancer). N Engl J Med 2005;352(18):1851–60.

43. Hampel H, Frankel W, Panescu J, et al. Screening for Lynch syndrome (hereditary nonpolyposis colorectal cancer) among endometrial cancer patients. Cancer Res 2006;66(15):7810–7.

44. Hampel H, Panescu J, Lockman J, et al. Comment on: screening for Lynch syndrome (hereditary nonpolyposis colorectal cancer) among endometrial cancer patients. Cancer Res 2007;67(19):9603.

45. Gausachs M, Mur P, Corral J, et al. MLH1 promoter hypermethylation in the analytical algorithm of Lynch syndrome: a cost-effectiveness study. Eur J Hum Genet 2012;20(7):762–8.
46. Gudgeon J, Williams JL, Burt RW, et al. Lynch syndrome screening implementation: business analysis by a healthcare system. Am J Manag Care 2011;17(8): e288–300.
47. Ladabaum U, Wang G, Terdiman J, et al. Strategies to identify the Lynch syndrome among patients with colorectal cancer: a cost-effectiveness analysis. Ann Intern Med 2011;155(2):69–79.
48. Mvundura M, Grosse SD, Hampel H, et al. The cost-effectiveness of genetic testing strategies for Lynch syndrome among newly diagnosed patients with colorectal cancer. Genet Med 2010;12(2):93–104.
49. Evaluation of Genomic Applications in Practice and Prevention (EGAPP) Working Group. Recommendations from the EGAPP Working Group: genetic testing strategies in newly diagnosed individuals with colorectal cancer aimed at reducing morbidity and mortality from Lynch syndrome in relatives. Genet Med 2009; 11(1):35–41.
50. Ondrejka SL, Schaeffer DF, Jakubowski MA, et al. Does neoadjuvant therapy alter KRAS and/or MSI results in rectal adenocarcinoma testing? Am J Surg Pathol 2011;35(9):1327–30.
51. Stoffel EM, Mangu PB, Gruber SB, et al. Hereditary colorectal cancer syndromes: American Society of Clinical Oncology Clinical Practice Guideline endorsement of the familial risk-colorectal cancer: European Society for Medical Oncology Clinical Practice Guidelines. J Clin Oncol 2015;33(2):209–17.
52. Syngal S, Brand RE, Church JM, et al. ACG clinical guideline: genetic testing and management of hereditary gastrointestinal cancer syndromes. Am J Gastroenterol 2015;110(2):223–62.
53. Weissman SM, Burt R, Church J, et al. Identification of individuals at risk for Lynch syndrome using targeted evaluations and genetic testing: National Society of Genetic Counselors and the Collaborative Group of the Americas on Inherited Colorectal Cancer Joint Practice Guideline. J Genet Couns 2011;21: 484–93.
54. Kwon JS, Scott JL, Gilks CB, et al. Testing women with endometrial cancer to detect Lynch syndrome. J Clin Oncol 2011;29(16):2247–52.
55. Ma J, Ledbetter N, Glenn L. Testing women with endometrial cancer for Lynch syndrome: should we test all? J Adv Pract Oncol 2013;4(5):322–30.
56. Mills AM, Liou S, Ford JM, et al. Lynch syndrome screening should be considered for all patients with newly diagnosed endometrial cancer. Am J Surg Pathol 2014;38(11):1501–9.
57. Snowsill T, Huxley N, Hoyle M, et al. A systematic review and economic evaluation of diagnostic strategies for Lynch syndrome. Health Technol Assess 2014;18(58): 1–406.
58. Cragun D, DeBate RD, Pal T. Applying public health screening criteria: how does universal newborn screening compare to universal tumor screening for Lynch syndrome in adults with colorectal cancer? J Genet Couns 2015;24(3):409–20.
59. Cragun D, Radford C, Dolinsky JS, et al. Panel-based testing for inherited colorectal cancer: a descriptive study of clinical testing performed by a US laboratory. Clin Genet 2014;86(6):510–20.
60. Burt RW, Leppert MF, Slattery ML, et al. Genetic testing and phenotype in a large kindred with attenuated familial adenomatous polyposis. Gastroenterology 2004;127(2):444–51.

61. Wang L, Baudhuin LM, Boardman LA, et al. MYH mutations in patients with attenuated and classic polyposis and with young-onset colorectal cancer without polyps. Gastroenterology 2004;127(1):9–16.

62. Lindor NM, Smyrk TC, Buehler S, et al. Multiple jejunal cancers resulting from combination of germline APC and MLH1 mutations. Fam Cancer 2012;11(4):667–9.

63. Okkels H, Sunde L, Lindorff-Larsen K, et al. Polyposis and early cancer in a patient with low penetrant mutations in MSH6 and APC: hereditary colorectal cancer as a polygenic trait. Int J Colorectal Dis 2006;21(8):847–50.

64. Scheenstra R, Rijcken FE, Koornstra JJ, et al. Rapidly progressive adenomatous polyposis in a patient with germline mutations in both the APC and MLH1 genes: the worst of two worlds. Gut 2003;52(6):898–9.

65. Soravia C, DeLozier CD, Dobbie Z, et al. Double frameshift mutations in APC and MSH2 in the same individual. Int J Colorectal Dis 2005;20(5):466–70.

66. van Puijenbroek M, Nielsen M, Reinards TH, et al. The natural history of a combined defect in MSH6 and MUTYH in a HNPCC family. Fam Cancer 2007;6(1): 43–51.

67. Vasen HF, Blanco I, Aktan-Collan K, et al. Revised guidelines for the clinical management of Lynch syndrome (HNPCC): recommendations by a group of European experts. Gut 2013;62(6):812–23.

68. Committee on Practice Bulletins-Gynecology, Society of Gynecologic Oncology. ACOG Practice Bulletin No. 147: Lynch syndrome. Obstet Gynecol 2014;124(5): 1042–54.

69. Järvinen HJ, Aarnio M, Mustonen H, et al. Controlled 15-year trial on screening for colorectal cancer in families with hereditary nonpolyposis colorectal cancer. Gastroenterology 2000;118:829–34.

70. Daniels MS, Lu KH. Clearer picture of PMS2-associated Lynch syndrome is emerging. J Clin Oncol 2015;33(4):299–300.

71. Parry S, Win AK, Parry B, et al. Metachronous colorectal cancer risk for mismatch repair gene mutation carriers: the advantage of more extensive colon surgery. Gut 2011;60(7):950–7.

72. Burn J, Gerdes AM, Macrae F, et al. Long-term effect of aspirin on cancer risk in carriers of hereditary colorectal cancer: an analysis from the CAPP2 randomised controlled trial. Lancet 2011;378(9809):2081–7.

73. Burn J, Bishop DT, Mecklin JP, et al. Effect of aspirin or resistant starch on colorectal neoplasia in the Lynch syndrome. N Engl J Med 2008;359(24):2567–78.

74. Burn J, Mathers JC, Bishop DT. Chemoprevention in Lynch syndrome. Fam Cancer 2013;12(4):707–18.

75. Hernegger GS, Moore HG, Guillem JG. Attenuated familial adenomatous polyposis: an evolving and poorly understood entity. Dis Colon Rectum 2002;45(1): 127–34 [discussion: 134–6].

76. Knudsen AL, Bisgaard ML, Bulow S. Attenuated familial adenomatous polyposis (AFAP). A review of the literature. Fam Cancer 2003;2(1):43–55.

77. Bussey HJ. Familial polyposis coli. Family studies, histopathology, differential diagnosis and results of treatment. Baltimore (MD): Johns Hopkins University Press; 1975.

78. Jarvinen HJ. Epidemiology of familial adenomatous polyposis in Finland: impact of family screening on the colorectal cancer rate and survival. Gut 1992;33(3): 357–60.

79. Bulow S, Faurschou Nielsen T, Bulow C, et al. The incidence rate of familial adenomatous polyposis. Results from the Danish Polyposis Register. Int J Colorectal Dis 1996;11(2):88–91.

80. Bisgaard ML, Fenger K, Bulow S, et al. Familial adenomatous polyposis (FAP): frequency, penetrance, and mutation rate. Hum Mutat 1994;3(2):121–5.
81. Bjork J, Akerbrant H, Iselius L, et al. Epidemiology of familial adenomatous polyposis in Sweden: changes over time and differences in phenotype between males and females. Scand J Gastroenterol 1999;34(12):1230–5.
82. Iwama T, Tamura K, Morita T, et al. A clinical overview of familial adenomatous polyposis derived from the database of the Polyposis Registry of Japan. Int J Clin Oncol 2004;9(4):308–16.
83. Scheuner MT, McNeel TS, Freedman AN. Population prevalence of familial cancer and common hereditary cancer syndromes. The 2005 California Health Interview Survey. Genet Med 2010;12(11):726–35.
84. Neklason DW, Stevens J, Boucher KM, et al. American founder mutation for attenuated familial adenomatous polyposis. Clin Gastroenterol Hepatol 2008; 6:46–52.
85. Groves C, Lamlum H, Crabtree M, et al. Mutation cluster region, association between germline and somatic mutations and genotype-phenotype correlation in upper gastrointestinal familial adenomatous polyposis. Am J Pathol 2002; 160(6):2055–61.
86. Burt RW. Gastric fundic gland polyps. Gastroenterology 2003;125(5):1462–9.
87. Bulow S, Bjork J, Christensen IJ, et al. Duodenal adenomatosis in familial adenomatous polyposis. Gut 2004;53(3):381–6.
88. Jasperson KW, Tuohy TM, Neklason DW, et al. Hereditary and familial colon cancer. Gastroenterology 2010;138(6):2044–58.
89. Lopez-Ceron M, van den Broek FJ, Mathus-Vliegen EM, et al. The role of high-resolution endoscopy and narrow-band imaging in the evaluation of upper GI neoplasia in familial adenomatous polyposis. Gastrointest Endosc 2013;77(4): 542–50.
90. Bjork J, Akerbrant H, Iselius L, et al. Periampullary adenomas and adenocarcinomas in familial adenomatous polyposis: cumulative risks and APC gene mutations. Gastroenterology 2001;121(5):1127–35.
91. Vasen HF, Moslein G, Alonso A, et al. Guidelines for the clinical management of familial adenomatous polyposis (FAP). Gut 2008;57(5):704–13.
92. Clark SK, Neale KF, Landgrebe JC, et al. Desmoid tumours complicating familial adenomatous polyposis. Br J Surg 1999;86(9):1185–9.
93. Farmer KCR, Hawley PR, Phillips RK. Desmoid disease. In: Phillips RK, Spigelman AD, Thomason JPS, editors. Familial adenomatous polyposis and other polyposis syndromes. London: Edward Arnold; 1994. p. 128.
94. Heiskanen I, Jarvinen HJ. Occurrence of desmoid tumours in familial adenomatous polyposis and results of treatment. Int J Colorectal Dis 1996;11(4):157–62.
95. Sturt NJ, Gallagher MC, Bassett P, et al. Evidence for genetic predisposition to desmoid tumours in familial adenomatous polyposis independent of the germline APC mutation. Gut 2004;53(12):1832–6.
96. Durno C, Monga N, Bapat B, et al. Does early colectomy increase desmoid risk in familial adenomatous polyposis? Clin Gastroenterol Hepatol 2007;5(10): 1190–4.
97. Latchford AR, Sturt NJ, Neale K, et al. A 10-year review of surgery for desmoid disease associated with familial adenomatous polyposis. Br J Surg 2006;93(10): 1258–64.
98. Sinha A, Tekkis PP, Gibbons DC, et al. Risk factors predicting desmoid occurrence in patients with familial adenomatous polyposis: a meta-analysis. Colorectal Dis 2010;13(11):1222–9.

99. Gardner EJ. Follow-up study of a family group exhibiting dominant inheritance for a syndrome including intestinal polyps, osteomas, fibromas and epidermoid cysts. Am J Hum Genet 1962;14:376.

100. Nieuwenhuis MH, Mathus-Vliegen EM, Baeten CG, et al. Evaluation of management of desmoid tumours associated with familial adenomatous polyposis in Dutch patients. Br J Cancer 2011;104(1):37–42.

101. Aretz S, Koch A, Uhlhaas S, et al. Should children at risk for familial adenomatous polyposis be screened for hepatoblastoma and children with apparently sporadic hepatoblastoma be screened for APC germline mutations? Pediatr Blood Cancer 2006;47(6):811–8.

102. Hirschman BA, Pollock BH, Tomlinson GE. The spectrum of APC mutations in children with hepatoblastoma from familial adenomatous polyposis kindreds. J Pediatr 2005;147(2):263–6.

103. Sanders RP, Furman WL. Familial adenomatous polyposis in two brothers with hepatoblastoma: implications for diagnosis and screening. Pediatr Blood Cancer 2006;47(6):851–4.

104. Coffin CM, Hornick JL, Zhou H, et al. Gardner fibroma: a clinicopathologic and immunohistochemical analysis of 45 patients with 57 fibromas. Am J Surg Pathol 2007;31(3):410–6.

105. Hes FJ, Nielsen M, Bik EC, et al. Somatic APC mosaicism: an underestimated cause of polyposis coli. Gut 2008;57(1):71–6.

106. Jasperson KW, Burt RW. APC-associated polyposis conditions. In: Pagon RA, Bird TD, Dolan CR, et al, editors. GeneReviews. Seattle (WA): 1998. p. 1993–2015.

107. Groves CJ, Saunders BP, Spigelman AD, et al. Duodenal cancer in patients with familial adenomatous polyposis (FAP): results of a 10 year prospective study. Gut 2002;50(5):636–41.

108. Al-Tassan N, Chmiel NH, Maynard J, et al. Inherited variants of MYH associated with Somatic G:C–>T:A mutations in colorectal tumors. Nat Genet 2002;30(2):227–32.

109. Cleary SP, Cotterchio M, Jenkins MA, et al. Germline MutY human homologue mutations and colorectal cancer: a multisite case-control study. Gastroenterology 2009;136(4):1251–60.

110. Enholm S, Hienonen T, Suomalainen A, et al. Proportion and phenotype of MYH-associated colorectal neoplasia in a population-based series of Finnish colorectal cancer patients. Am J Pathol 2003;163(3):827–32.

111. Nielsen M, Morreau H, Vasen HF, et al. MUTYH-associated polyposis (MAP). Crit Rev Oncol Hematol 2010;79(1):1–16.

112. Filipe B, Baltazar C, Albuquerque C, et al. APC or MUTYH mutations account for the majority of clinically well-characterized families with FAP and AFAP phenotype and patients with more than 30 adenomas. Clin Genet 2009;76(3):242–55.

113. Boparai KS, Dekker E, Van Eeden S, et al. Hyperplastic polyps and sessile serrated adenomas as a phenotypic expression of MYH-associated polyposis. Gastroenterology 2008;135(6):2014–8.

114. Jenkins MA, Croitoru ME, Monga N, et al. Risk of colorectal cancer in monoallelic and biallelic carriers of MYH mutations: a population-based case-family study. Cancer Epidemiol Biomarkers Prev 2006;15(2):312–4.

115. Lubbe SJ, Di Bernardo MC, Chandler IP, et al. Clinical implications of the colorectal cancer risk associated with MUTYH mutation. J Clin Oncol 2009;27(24):3975–80.

116. Vogt S, Jones N, Christian D, et al. Expanded extracolonic tumor spectrum in MUTYH-associated polyposis. Gastroenterology 2009;137(6):1976–85.e1–10.

117. Giardiello FM, Trimbath JD. Peutz-Jeghers syndrome and management recommendations. Clin Gastroenterol Hepatol 2006;4(4):408–15.
118. Latchford AR, Neale K, Phillips RK, et al. Juvenile polyposis syndrome: a study of genotype, phenotype, and long-term outcome. Dis Colon Rectum 2012; 55(10):1038–43.
119. McGarrity TJ, Kulin HE, Zaino RJ. Peutz-Jeghers syndrome. Am J Gastroenterol 2000;95:596–604.
120. Schreibman IR, Baker M, Amos C, et al. The hamartomatous polyposis syndromes: a clinical and molecular review. Am J Gastroenterol 2005;100(2): 476–90.
121. Chow E, Macrae F. A review of juvenile polyposis syndrome. J Gastroenterol Hepatol 2005;20(11):1634–40.
122. Boardman LA. Heritable colorectal cancer syndromes: recognition and preventive management. Gastroenterol Clin North Am 2002;31(4):1107–31.
123. Beggs AD, Latchford AR, Vasen HF, et al. Peutz-Jeghers syndrome: a systematic review and recommendations for management. Gut 2010;59(7):975–86.
124. Hearle N, Schumacher V, Menko FH, et al. Frequency and spectrum of cancers in the Peutz-Jeghers syndrome. Clin Cancer Res 2006;12(10):3209–15.
125. Gammon A, Jasperson K, Kohlmann W, et al. Hamartomatous polyposis syndromes. Best Pract Res Clin Gastroenterol 2009;23(2):219–31.
126. Aretz S, Stienen D, Uhlhaas S, et al. High proportion of large genomic deletions and a genotype phenotype update in 80 unrelated families with juvenile polyposis syndrome. J Med Genet 2007;44(11):702–9.
127. Aretz S, Stienen D, Uhlhaas S, et al. High proportion of large genomic STK11 deletions in Peutz-Jeghers syndrome. Hum Mutat 2005;26(6):513–9.
128. Volikos E, Robinson J, Aittomaki K, et al. LKB1 exonic and whole gene deletions are a common cause of Peutz-Jeghers syndrome. J Med Genet 2006;43(5):e18.
129. Sweet K, Willis J, Zhou XP, et al. Molecular classification of patients with unexplained hamartomatous and hyperplastic polyposis. JAMA 2005;294(19): 2465–73.
130. Nikitakis NG, Koumaki D. Laugier-Hunziker syndrome: case report and review of the literature. Oral Surg Oral Med Oral Pathol Oral Radiol 2013;116(1):e52–8.
131. Rangwala S, Doherty CB, Katta R. Laugier-Hunziker syndrome: a case report and review of the literature. Dermatol Online J 2010;16(12):9.
132. Pilarski R, Burt R, Kohlman W, et al. Cowden syndrome and the PTEN hamartoma tumor syndrome: systematic review and revised diagnostic criteria. J Natl Cancer Inst 2013;105(21):1607–16.
133. Malkin D. Li-fraumeni syndrome. Genes Cancer 2011;2(4):475–84.
134. Church JM. Polymerase proofreading-associated polyposis: a new, dominantly inherited syndrome of hereditary colorectal cancer predisposition. Dis Colon Rectum 2014;57(3):396–7.
135. Jaeger E, Leedham S, Lewis A, et al. Hereditary mixed polyposis syndrome is caused by a 40-kb upstream duplication that leads to increased and ectopic expression of the BMP antagonist GREM1. Nat Genet 2012;44(6):699–703.
136. Whitelaw SC, Murday VA, Tomlinson IP, et al. Clinical and molecular features of the hereditary mixed polyposis syndrome. Gastroenterology 1997;112(2): 327–34.
137. Wimmer K, Kratz CP, Vasen HF, et al. Diagnostic criteria for constitutional mismatch repair deficiency syndrome: suggestions of the European consortium 'care for CMMRD' (C4CMMRD). J Med Genet 2014;51(6):355–65.

The Genetics of Breast Cancer

What the Surgical Oncologist Needs to Know

Jeffrey N. Weitzel, MD

KEYWORDS

- BRCA1 • Genetics • TP53 • Breast cancer • Ovarian cancer

KEY POINTS

- Surgeons need to understand the implications of germline predisposition to breast cancer, as revealed by increasingly more complicated next-generation sequencing–based tests.
- The rapid pace of change will continue to challenge paradigms for genetic cancer risk assessment (GCRA).
- Germline predisposition to breast cancer and GCRA can influence the medical and surgical management of breast cancer risk as well as strategies for screening and for risk reduction.

INTRODUCTION

Genetic cancer risk assessment (GCRA) is an established multidisciplinary practice that can be applied to the recognition/detection of hereditary forms of breast and ovarian cancer, to enable enhanced surveillance, risk-appropriate surgical management, and targeted therapy for metastatic disease.[1,2] Most breast cancer is hormone receptor positive, diagnosed after the age of 50 years old, and multifactorial in cause.[3]

Distinguishing features that suggest the subset of breast cancers associated with inherited predisposition include:

- Early age at onset
- Increased prevalence of bilateral breast cancer
- Association with ovarian cancer
- Family history of breast or ovarian cancer

Inheritance plays a role in the development of all human cancers to varying degrees. Hereditary forms of breast cancer constitute only 5% to 7% of breast cancer cases

The author has nothing to disclose.
Division of Clinical Cancer Genetics, City of Hope Comprehensive Cancer Center, 1500 East Duarte Road, Duarte, CA 91010, USA
E-mail address: JWeitzel@coh.org

http://dx.doi.org/10.1016/j.soc.2015.06.011
1055-3207/15/$ – see front matter © 2015 Elsevier Inc. All rights reserved.
surgonc.theclinics.com

overall. However, the magnitude of the risk that a woman will develop cancer if she inherits a highly penetrant cancer gene mutation (up to 85% lifetime risk for *BRCA1*) justifies the intense interest in predictive testing. There is a growing roster of identified breast cancer susceptibility genes, and next-generation sequencing (NGS) technologies have enabled diagnostic testing for an ever broader spectrum of relatively rare and incompletely understood causal variants.[4] Although less common than breast cancer, ovarian cancer is relatively more lethal, and several breast cancer associated genes are also associated with elevated ovarian cancer risk.[5] In addition, breast cancer can be a minor component of other genetic syndromes such as diffuse hereditary gastric cancer.[6,7] This article summarizes germline predisposition to breast cancer and how GCRA can influence the medical and surgical management of breast cancer risk as well as strategies for screening and for risk reduction.

THE PRIME EXEMPLAR: HEREDITARY BREAST AND OVARIAN CANCER ASSOCIATED WITH *BRCA1* AND *BRCA2* MUTATIONS

Consider the following clinical scenario illustrated in **Fig. 1**. The consultand (indicated by an *arrow*) was 45 years old and unaffected at the time of consultation, although she was certain she would develop cancer. She was contemplating both prophylactic mastectomy and oophorectomy because her mother and 2 of her sisters died of breast or ovarian cancer. She was also concerned about her own daughter's risk. A mutation in *BRCA1* (4184del4) had been found in her sister just before her death from breast cancer at age 50. After extensive counseling, the consultand decided to pursue genetic testing for the familial mutation. Fortunately, testing revealed that she did not carry the mutation. She canceled the surgical procedures after being told that her risk for breast or ovarian cancer was no more than that of the general population (11% and 1.6%, respectively). Moreover, she was relieved to learn that her daughter was not at increased risk either, because she had not inherited the familial mutation and thus could not pass it on to her. Other family members also came forward for testing. Her 47-year-old sister was found to carry the familial mutation (indicated by + in the **Fig. 1**). Before counseling and testing, she was so anxious about her cancer risk that she was unable to examine her own breasts. However, despite the bad news about her carrier status, she was empowered to pursue appropriate interventions from the surveillance and preventive surgery options presented. Genetic testing had a real impact on health care decisions in this carefully counseled high-risk family and presumably reassured some individuals and spared them from unnecessary procedures.

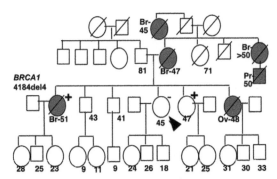

Fig. 1. Pedigree for family with hereditary breast and ovarian cancer.

BACKGROUND

The extent of the hereditary breast and ovarian cancer phenotype associated with *BRCA1* started to emerge from initial linkage studies in 1990.[8–10] The cumulative risk for developing breast cancer in hereditary breast ovarian cancer (HBOC) families exceeds 50% by age 50 years and is up to 85% by age 70 years.[11] The cloning of the *BRCA1* gene on chromosome 17 in 1994,[12] and of a second high-risk locus on chromosome 13 (*BRCA2*) in 1995,[13] ushered in an era with increasing appreciation of the potential for oncogenetics to influence breast cancer screening, treatment, and prevention.[2] The subsequent decades have been marked by an ever higher resolution understanding of gene-specific pathology, overall and age-specific risk for *BRCA*-associated breast cancers,[14–20] as well as a growing understanding of hormonal[21–33] and genetic[34–38] modifiers of risk.

GENETIC TESTING AND *BRCA* MUTATIONS

Commercial testing in a CLIA (Clinical Laboratory Improvement Amendments)-approved laboratory (http://wwwn.cdc.gov/CLIA/) became available for *BRCA1* and *BRCA2* in 1996 in the United States, and professional society policy statements affirmed the value of their use in GCRA.[39–41] *BRCA* testing has long been offered (through regional or national laboratories) in most of Europe, Australia, Israel, and Iceland (for specific founder mutations). The National Comprehensive Cancer Network (NCCN)[42] publishes testing guidelines that are updated annually and largely adopted by most insurers. Notable exceptions include Medicare (which does not cover testing for unaffected patients, even if a *BRCA* mutation is known in the family) and Medicaid, wherein coverage varies among different states. **Box 1** includes the top-level NCCN indicators for genetic testing,[42] most of which should be well known by surgeons involved in the care of women with breast cancer. A deeper appreciation of the more complicated combinations of family history indications for GCRA is helpful.

Specialized training is often warranted to achieve practitioner level competence in the application of GCRA[2,43–45] and knowledgeable interpretation of molecular genetic test results, including variants of uncertain significance (VUS). (Please see the article in this issue by Marc S. Greenblatt.) If a patient with a strong personal or family history of breast cancer is tested and *no* deleterious or pathogenic (pathogenic is another term increasingly used on genetic test reports) mutation is identified, they are grouped as "negative" test results as well as all VUS in the same clinical category, described as uninformative, because they are essentially uninformative and ambiguous findings in most cases.

Box 1
Key single case indicators[a] for genetic susceptibility testing

- Breast cancer diagnosis $\leq$ age 45 years
- Triple-negative breast cancer < age 60 years
- Bilateral breast cancer (with 1st diagnosis $\leq$ age 50 years)
- Male breast cancer
- Epithelial ovarian cancer

[a]Most apply to individual or close relative; see NCCN guidelines for additional family history–dependent indications.[42]

There are reasonable concerns that VUS results can be confusing to patients and providers alike. However, a longitudinal study of patients receiving a VUS result at an academic health center employing an experienced multidisciplinary team that includes certified genetic counselors as well as medical doctors suggested there was no evidence of patients choosing risk-inappropriate follow-up care.[46] Although a challenge, especially for a consultative practice, it is important that reclassifications of VUS results by genetic testing vendors, which may occur years later, be shared with patients and incorporated in to their record. (Please see articles in this issue by Vickie L. Venne and Maren T. Scheuner as well as by Amanda Gammon and Deborah W. Neklason.) The same concepts apply to VUS results from multigene panel tests, albeit with much less supportive evidence for the clinical implications of even pathogenic changes in the respective genes (see later discussion).[4]

A separate important issue is that testing is most informative when it is initiated with the youngest affected individual in a given family. Even if one is convinced that a family has hereditary cancers based on clinical criteria, there is only a 50% chance that an offspring or sibling of an affected patient will have inherited the familial mutation. Therefore, only a positive test result (detection of a known or likely deleterious mutation) is truly informative. Until the familial mutation is known, a negative test result could mean: (1) that the unaffected person being tested did not inherit the cancer susceptibility mutation; (2) that the person inherited the disease-associated gene, but the mutation was not detectable by the methods used; or (3) that the familial mutation is in an entirely different gene that has not yet been tested. Thus, there is a limit to how much reassurance (negative predictive value) is clinically appropriate and can be offered in the context of negative/uninformative testing for one or even for a comprehensive panel of multiple cancer predisposition genes. Low- to moderate-risk genes on such gene panels are even more problematic, because there seems to be a significant residual risk even after informative negative test results.[4] The residual risk is likely multifactorial, reflecting shared environmental factors as well as minor genetic determinants (such as single-nucleotide polymorphism [SNP] risk variants) that are not assessed in any panels and individually may convey miniscule (1%–2%) risk.

Despite the discovery of large genomic rearrangements (LGR) in the BRCA genes in 1999,[47,48] the approach to variant analysis remained limited to Sanger sequencing of translated exons and adjacent intronic regions for many subsequent years. This discovery was followed by the addition of targeted assays for the 5 most frequently identified recurrent LGRs (associated with apparent European origin).[49] More comprehensive screening for LGRs was offered by the commercial vendor in 2006, shortly after a publication from Dr Mary-Claire King's laboratory documented a 12% rate of LGRs among 300 multicase families with negative (uninformative) Sanger sequencing.[50] A clinic-based series suggested that LGRs represented greater than 10% of BRCA1 mutations detected among women meeting NCCN criteria for testing.[51] The author reported the discovery of a frequent LGR (BRCA1 ex9-12del) among Hispanic patients of Mexican ancestry in 2007.[52] In a study of 746 US Hispanic patients, 21 of 189 detected mutations were LGRs, and 13 of 21 (62%) LGRs were the BRCA1 ex9-12del. A recent study of the prevalence of BRCA LGRs among 48,456 patients tested by a commercial laboratory confirmed that approximately 10% of carriers had an LGR, and a 21% rate was reported for Latin American/Caribbean Islanders.[53] Notably, one-third of LGRs were the BRCA1 ex9-12del mutation in this latter group. Thus, BRCA1 ex9-12del is clinically significant and one of the most frequent population-specific large rearrangement mutations in the world as well as the first reported Mexican founder mutation. The bottom line for clinicians is that testing is not complete for given susceptibility genes unless complete sequencing and rearrangement screening are performed.

BRCA MUTATIONS AND FOUNDER POPULATIONS

Although thousands of different *BRCA* mutations have been documented, the spectrum of mutations among certain populations that are geographically or culturally isolated may be limited and characterized by the presence of specific founder mutations.[54–64] Perhaps the most extensively studied founder effects are the 3 *BRCA* mutations associated with Jewish ancestry, which are thought to account for up to 95% of *BRCA*-associated breast or ovarian cancers among Jews. The Ashkenazi Jewish population frequency of the *BRCA1* 185delAG (187delAG) is ~1%, and *BRCA2* 6174delT variants is about 1.5%. The *BRCA1* 5382insC (5385insC) variant is thought to be of Baltic origin and is detected in both Jewish (0.3%) and non-Jewish populations from that region. *BRCA1* 185delAG is present in Sephardic and Middle Eastern Jewish populations, although at a lower frequency, and has been reported among populations from Latin America as well, presumably from colonial Hispanic influences and the flight from the Spanish Inquisition in the fifteenth century.[65–67] There are founder mutations in most world populations, although few (eg, *BRCA2* 999del5 in Iceland) that account for most observed *BRCA* mutations in a given population as observed in the specific populations described above.[68]

TESTING STRATEGIES AND LIMITATIONS FOR PATIENTS WITHOUT CANCER

In some cases, no affected family members are available for testing. In that case, one may proceed with genetic testing of an unaffected person, but only after that individual has been thoroughly counseled regarding its risks, benefits, and limitations. Similarly and most important for this volume, unless there is a suggestive family history, cancer susceptibility testing is not considered appropriate for screening unaffected individuals in the general population. However, a recent study of population-based genetic testing for Jewish founder mutations, using unaffected men in Israel as a less biased reference population and then testing female relatives,[69] prompted Mary-Claire King in her 2014 Lasker Award address to call for population-based testing of women who are 30 years in age or older.[70] Although generally sympathetic to aspects of such an approach, careful consideration highlights unresolved issues: "There are some difficult questions that come up, centered around who is the right target, what is the right test, to whom should it be delivered, should it be full sequencing or should it just be looking for mutations in target populations, and what information do people need to be able to decide whether or not they want to participate?".[71] Nonetheless, it may be reasonable to test unaffected persons who are members of an ethnic group in which specific ancestral mutations are prevalent and whose family structure is limited (ie, the family is small, with few female relatives or no information due to premature death from noncancerous causes).[72]

BRCA-ASSOCIATED RISK, VARIABLE PENETRANCE, AND THE INDICATIONS FOR PROPHYLACTIC SURGERY

Among high-risk clinic populations, a woman with a *BRCA1* mutation faces a breast cancer risk of nearly 6% by the age of 30 years, 20% by the age of 40 years, and up to 85% lifetime.[11] Although *BRCA2* is often associated with a later age at onset than for *BRCA1*, the cumulative lifetime risk is similar. In contrast to high-risk clinic studies, population-based studies suggest a lower breast cancer penetrance (as low as 36% for carriers of BRCA2 999del5 in Iceland).[17,73–76] However, most patients are identified via clinic-based services, so adjustment of risk estimation is rarely necessary in that setting. A large study of cancer risk by mutation site/type, by the Consortium of Investigators of Modifiers of BRCA, confirmed previous observations of positional effects, such as a relatively greater risk for ovarian cancer with BRCA2 mutations in the middle third (ovarian cancer cluster region) of the gene.[77–79] In practice, even the lowest ovarian cancer risk associated with BRCA2 is still enough to warrant risk reduction salpingo-oophorectomy (RRSO), although one may consider it after age 40 years old if preferred by the patient, and in any event, as soon as practicable after menopause. There are a growing number of genetic modifiers of BRCA-associated breast and ovarian cancer risk.[80,81] It is known that family history confers risk beyond the BRCA gene status. There is controversy as to the negative predictive value of an informative negative test result (a close relative wherein a known family BRCA mutation was not detected).[82] However, most clinicians consider that almost all the familial risk tracks with a deleterious familial BRCA mutation. There is less negative predictive value of diagnostic testing for moderate risk genes (eg, CHEK2, ATM); that is, there is often still enough empiric risk to warrant enhanced surveillance for a CHEK2-negative daughter of a CHEK2-positive woman with breast cancer (see later discussion).

Expert opinion suggests it is important to calibrate risk estimation and management recommendations to be age and clinical scenario appropriate. That is, an unaffected 30-year-old woman with a BRCA1 mutation has the most to gain from risk reduction mastectomy (RRM) as measured by quality-adjusted years of life gained, compared with a 58-year-old woman with a recently diagnosed stage III BRCA-associated breast cancer, who may be better served by a unilateral therapeutic mastectomy alone.[83,84] That is, the latter woman would not be expected to benefit significantly from contralateral RRM with regard to reduced mortality, and she may suffer pain and complications of surgery.

Nonetheless, it is the extraordinary risk of BRCA-associated new primary breast cancers[85] that has driven the application of GCRA in the initial evaluation and management of young women with breast cancer. The author and others demonstrated that GCRA could be integrated into busy oncologic practices,[86,87] wherein most women chose risk-appropriate surgery. That is, they were more likely to choose unilateral (therapeutic) breast surgery if they were determined to have sporadic breast cancer and counseled about the respective, modest new primary breast cancer risk, and those with high (genetic) risk were more likely to choose therapeutic ipsilateral and risk reduction contralateral mastectomies.

It has been suggested that the best timeframe for GCRA was during adjuvant therapy after definitive resection of the tumor, but before adjuvant radiation therapy necessary to complete breast-conserving treatment.[86,88]

This window of opportunity for GCRA has increasingly shifted to immediately after biopsy, especially with increasing use of neoadjuvant chemotherapy. This shift represents a time when the cancer risk counseling service can be engaged to support a risk-informed approach for the patient and surgeon to decide about surgery appropriate to the circumstance. Most younger (<age 50) women with limited stage (I–II) BRCA-associated breast cancer will choose bilateral mastectomy if they understand the elevated risks for new primary ipsilateral and contralateral breast cancer. There is no compulsory approach, because conservative therapy is as effective for breast cancer treatment. The 2 issues driving decision-making for women is a strong desire to "never face this circumstance again" and limitation of options for reconstruction if a previously irradiated breast requires a mastectomy for treatment of ipsilateral breast tumor recurrence (most would require a tissue-based approach).

There are numerous counseling and support challenges for these newly diagnosed women, who are often overwhelmed with fear and information overload as they contemplate options for adjuvant chemotherapy and primary surgical management of the breast, which could include RRM.[89,90] Other potential intervention points for GCRA include survivors of early onset (≤45 years old) breast cancer, often at the behest of at-risk relatives, or when considering revision of breast reconstruction. Although breast-conserving therapy is efficacious with respect to treatment of BRCA-associated breast cancer,[91,92] there is an elevated risk for both ipsilateral and contralateral new primary breast cancers.[93]

Nuances of cancer risk counseling for newly diagnosed patients with breast cancer contemplating breast-conserving therapy include how to secure accurate GCRA to determine risks for ipsilateral breast tumor recurrence (local recurrence and ipsilateral new primary breast cancer risk) and contralateral new primary breast cancer risk moving forward. When counseling about the risk of future ipsilateral or contralateral breast cancer following breast-conserving therapy for invasive breast cancer, one approach is to consider annualized rather than cumulative lifetime risk estimates. This depends on menopausal status, regardless of whether premature due to RRSO or due to natural menopause. The BRCA-associated annualized risk for breast cancer is about 3% to 5% per year while premenopausal, and 1% to 2% per year when postmenopausal.[85] The risk of new primary cancers over 10 years after initial BRCA-associated breast cancer is listed as follows[85,94]:

- BRCA2—34% for breast cancer; 6% for ovarian cancer
- BRCA1—43% for breast cancer; 12% for ovarian cancer

Modifiers of risk:

- BRCA2 mutation is associated with less risk than BRCA1
- Less risk if first cancer diagnosis was age 50 years or older
- Tamoxifen reduced the risk of new primary breast cancers
- Oophorectomy reduced new primary breast cancer risk

Furthermore, premenopausal RRSO reduces ovarian cancer, breast cancer, and all-cause mortality (hazard ratio [HR] = 0.40 [0.26–0.61]), with the greatest breast cancer risk reduction (HR: 0.15 [95% confidence interval [CI] 0.04–0.63]) among BRCA1 mutation carriers without a prior diagnosis of breast cancer.[95]

Elevated risk for new primary breast cancer drives surgeons' opinions and patient preferences regarding both ipsilateral and contralateral mastectomy recommendations. The concept of considering options for the surgical approach as compared with recommendations may be a challenge for patients and surgeons alike, but shared decision-making is important for long-term satisfaction.

RRM is associated with greater than 95% reduction in new primary breast cancer risk among BRCA pathogenic mutation carriers, whether performed prophylactically bilaterally in an unaffected woman or as risk reduction for the contralateral breast in a woman treated for breast cancer.[96] The uptake of RRM among unaffected women varies by age, parity, marital status, and country of residence.[97–99] Quality-of-life issues associated with RRM include altered self-body image, and multiple studies suggest the potential for disruption in personal relationships following RRM.[100–104] The most frequently reported changes were in sexual attractiveness (55%), feeling less physically attractive (53%), and self-consciousness about appearance (53%). A minority of women had more serious psychological or body image concerns, usually in relation to surgical complications, and required psychiatric intervention.[105] Most concerns regarding RRM pertained to subsequent cosmetic options, including reconstruction. These concerns include the look and feel of implants, pain, numbness, scarring, and the details of some complex, multistep reconstruction options the technical aspects of which are well described in the literature, and beyond the scope of this article.[106] Although skin-sparing approaches would be considered standard of care, one key controversy is whether preservation of the nipple and areolar complex is safe.[107–110] Neoplastic involvement of the nipple was noted in 21% of 232 therapeutic mastectomies and none of 84 risk reduction procedures in one study.[107] The authors concluded that nipple-sparing mastectomy may be suitable for selected cases of breast carcinoma with low probability of nipple involvement by carcinoma; a retroareolar en-face margin may be used to test for occult involvement. Where this practice has been systematically studied, the nipple may retain erectile function, and the rate of neoplasia in the nipple is quite low and usually considered salvageable. However, there is usually significant anesthesia of the reconstructed breast. So, on balance, the absolute safest procedure includes removal of the nipple and subareolar complex, although a well-informed patient (and surgeon) may choose a nipple-sparing procedure if they prioritize a possibly better cosmetic outcome over the very modest risk of locally recurrent disease. Clearly, careful attention should be paid to the information needs of women undergoing RRM. However, despite the concerns, limitations, and challenges described above, most studies suggest satisfaction with risk reduction surgery decisions, especially if the woman feels that the locus of control was hers, rather than driven mostly by physician recommendation.[111]

BRCA-ASSOCIATED BREAST CANCER PATHOLOGY

BRCA1-associated breast cancer has relatively distinct pathologic characteristics, including a prevalence of estrogen receptor negative (ER-), progesterone receptor negative (PR-) HER2/neu-negative breast cancer (triple-negative breast cancer; TNBC).[112–115] There is usually a high histologic grade, and medullary histology is more common. TNBC tumors can be further subdivided into the basal subset, which is particularly associated with *BRCA1* status. Somatic *TP53* mutations are evident in greater than 80% of *BRCA*-associated breast cancers. There is a high level of pathology concordance between first and second primary *BRCA*-associated breast cancers; the 2 tumors are concordant more often than expected for ER status (P<.0001) and for grade (P<.0001), but not for histology (P = .55). The ER status of the first tumor was highly predictive of the ER status of the second tumor (odds ratio [OR], 8.7; 95% CI, 3.5–21.5; P<.0001). Neither age, menopausal status, oophorectomy, nor tamoxifen use was predictive of the ER status of the second tumor. Thus, there is strong concordance in ER status and tumor grade between independent primary breast tumors in women with a *BRCA* mutation.[116] Interestingly, tamoxifen seems to reduce new primary breast cancer risk regardless of receptor status or which *BRCA* gene is associated with the disease.[23,27,117]

THE ISSUE OF IONIZING RADIATION EXPOSURE: AGE-SPECIFIC WINDOW OF VULNERABILITY

Similar to the effect noted in survivors of Hodgkin disease treated with mantle radiation during the pubertal years,[118] there seems to be an increased breast cancer risk with medical radiation exposure, with important implications for the use of radiographic imaging in young *BRCA* carriers.[119,120] A study of chest radiographic exposures before age 30 among patients with breast cancer in a Polish registry also suggested early radiation exposure may be a risk factor for breast cancer in *BRCA1* carriers.[121] On the other hand, a large case-control study did not lend support to the idea that exposure to ionizing radiation through routine screening mammography contributes substantially to the burden of breast cancer in *BRCA1* and *BRCA2* mutation carriers.[122] Although the latter study was reassuring regarding the safety of mammography, it is common practice among oncogenetic services to use annual MRI alone for surveillance up to the age of 30 years.[42]

BRCA-ASSOCIATED RISK FOR OVARIAN CANCER: THE CLEAREST MEDICAL NECESSITY

Although virtually all breast surgery decisions based on genetic status are considered options for care (ultimately at the discretion of the patient, albeit with varying degrees of encouragement/support by the surgeon), RRSO is considered a recommendation for care and thus a medical necessity. Given the documented lack of efficacy of clinical screening surveillance for ovarian cancer,[123,124] advanced stage at diagnosis, and associated morbidity and mortality, RRSO upon completion of childbearing is a recommendation for women with a *BRCA* mutation (NCCN guidelines; Society of Gynecologic Oncology, and others).[42,125,126] Studies suggest that although women who choose to have RRSO have a good overall quality of life and significant decrease in risk perception as a result of surgery, they do experience menopausal symptoms and in some cases compromised sexual function.[127–129]

Observations from careful pathologic examination of RRSO specimens have revealed a 2% to 6% incidence of occult cancer, often in the fimbriated end of the fallopian tube at the time of risk reduction surgery.[130–133] There is an age trend, with the finding rare in women less than the age of 40 years and increasing frequency thereafter. Thus, recommendations for high-risk populations are that the fallopian tubes and ovaries should be submitted entirely, along with peritoneal washing for cytologic evaluation, and be evaluated by a pathologist with expertise in gynecologic malignances in serial sections, and that the laparoscopic surgeon should examine the peritoneal surfaces thoroughly at the time of prophylactic salpingo-oophorectomy.[134,135] Based on the high frequency of the tubal origin, some investigators have suggested salpingectomy alone as a risk reduction procedure among premenopausal *BRCA* carriers.[136] However, the residual possibility of ovarian cancer (at least 20% of the occult cancers are ovarian in origin) necessitates oophorectomy in any event. The author thinks the number of women, properly advised, who would choose salpingectomy alone, preserving the ovaries to preserve childbearing options in their 40s, would be very low. With recent technical advances, egg preservation is an increasingly viable (and preferable) solution (fertility preservation is an important issue in the management of young patients with breast cancer, but beyond the scope of this article). Thus, although possibly imperfect in terms of hormonal balance, RRSO coupled with hormone therapy at the lowest dose that preserves quality of life (eg, freedom from vasomotor symptoms, preservation of libido, and healthy vaginal mucosa) is preferable as it obviates a second surgical procedure. Despite evidence from the Women's Health Initiative trial suggesting modestly increased breast cancer risk associated with postmenopausal combination hormone (estrogen plus progesterone) therapy, monotherapy with conjugated estrogens appeared safe.[137] Furthermore, monotherapy with estrogen, possible if the uterus is absent (obviating the risk of uterine cancer in the face of either tamoxifen or estrogen monotherapy), is likely neutral with respect to breast cancer risk among *BRCA* carriers. Thus, salpingectomy alone as a risk reduction procedure should be considered an investigational risk management option of unproven usefulness, and questionable safety given that delay in oophorectomy could result in the development of lethal ovarian cancer as well as reduce the protective effect against breast cancer risk that has been documented in women who have undergone RRSO.[136] The increased proportion of the papillary serous uterine cancer subtype among *BRCA* carriers, albeit without measurable increased risk of uterine cancer, has prompted discussion about whether to consider hysterectomy concomitant with RRSO.[138,139] Although there is no consensus on this point, the other rationale for the latter approach is that it may enable post-RRSO monotherapy with estrogen for unaffected *BRCA* carriers, with associated enhanced quality of life.

Oral contraceptives seem to reduce the risk (adjusted OR, 0.5 [95% CI = 0.3–0.8]) for ovarian cancer among *BRCA* (both *BRCA1* and *BRCA2*) carriers, with a trend for more decreased risk with increasing duration of use (P for trend, <.001).[140] Additional studies confirm that oral contraceptives, number of full-term pregnancies, and tubal ligation are associated with ovarian cancer risk in *BRCA1* carriers, similar to that observed in the general population.[141]

The NCCN guidelines (NCCN.com) are updated annually and describe referral and testing criteria as well as evidence-based management guidelines.[42] **Box 2** presents a summary of current options and recommendations for care of the *BRCA* carrier.

MRI SCREENING FOR WOMEN AT HIGH RISK OF BREAST CANCER

Given the limited efficacy of mammography among young high-risk patients with significant breast density, one of the biggest advances in breast cancer screening was the validation of high sensitivity for contrast-enhanced breast MRI.[142] **Table 1** summarizes several studies demonstrating the superiority of MRI compared with mammography and firmly establishes the use of breast MRI as the standard of high-risk care.[142–145] The American Cancer Society guidelines suggest that women with high risk (eg, >20% empiric risk or carriers of genetic susceptibility mutations) would benefit from the addition of MRI to their surveillance regimen.[146]

Importantly, a prospective study of annual surveillance with breast MRI demonstrated a significant reduction in the incidence of advanced-stage breast cancer in

---

Box 2
Risk management options for *BRCA* mutation carriers*

Recommended for breast cancer detection:

Monthly self-examination of the breast beginning in late teen years

Beginning at age 25 (or 5–10 years before the earliest onset cancer in the family):

Clinician breast examination every 6 months, with alternating imaging procedures

Annual mammography, and

Annual breast MRI

Discussed as options:

Bilateral risk reduction mastectomy

Participation in clinical trials for chemoprevention

Recommended for ovarian cancer prevention or BC risk reduction:

Risk reduction salpingo-oophorectomy recommended on completion of childbearing

Considered from age 30 years to completion of childbearing:

Serum CA-125 every 6 months

Transvaginal ultrasonography every 6 months

*Also offered to women at increased risk because of a positive family history of hereditary breast and ovarian cancers but for whom genotypic information is not available.

Table 1
Efficacy of MRI versus mammography for the detection of breast cancer in *BRCA* carriers

	N with Mutations	Invasive Cancers	% by MRI	% by Mammogram
Warner et al,[143] 2004	236	16	81	31
Kriege et al,[147] 2004	358	20	80	33
MARIBS,[145] 2005	120	12	92	23
Total	714	48	83	30

BRCA carriers.[144] Given the data and practice guidelines indicating the use of MRI as standard of care,[42] a randomized trial with a mortality endpoint will not be forthcoming. Nonetheless, the evidence from these studies provides a measure of confidence for women who prefer not to pursue RRM.

OTHER GENETIC SYNDROMES ASSOCIATED WITH BREAST CANCER

Syndromes that have long been recognized as having a strong association with breast cancer susceptibility include Li-Fraumeni syndrome (LFS), associated with *TP53* mutations, Cowden disease (CD), associated with *PTEN* mutations, and diffuse hereditary gastric cancer and lobular breast cancer, associated with *CDH1* mutations. Each of these syndromes is quite rare. However, when faced with a young adult patient with breast cancer and no evidence of *BRCA* involvement, it is important to consider these other syndromes. Therefore, this article has included information regarding the clinical phenotypes for each. Efforts to define optimal clinical practice with regard to breast cancer screening, RRM, and optimal surgical management for first breast cancer diagnosis for these are hampered by relatively small numbers and the confounding effects of the other serious pathologies associated with each syndrome. However, recognition of the specific syndromic phenotypes described should serve as a prompt to secure focused diagnostic germline genetic testing because knowledge of carrier status greatly assists families and their providers in management decision-making. Importantly, the genes associated with predisposition to each of these syndromes are increasingly included on multigene testing panels. These genes include *TP53*, *PTEN CDH1*, *PALB2*, *CHEK2*, and *ATM*. Information regarding each of these genes as well as others increasingly included in breast cancer gene panel testing are summarized in later discussion (**Table 2**).[140–142]

Li-Fraumeni Syndrome (LFS)

LFS is one of the most severe breast cancer susceptibility phenotypes (50% cancer incidence in women with a *TP53* mutation by age 30, 90% lifetime) seen among the additional rare syndromes associated with breast cancer risk.[171] Associated with germline *TP53* mutations, LFS family members are at significant risk for the development of several tumor types, particularly sarcomas, breast cancer, brain tumors, and adrenocorticocarcinomas.[172,173] The incidence of de novo *TP53* mutations is approximately 10%,[174] which means that providers may encounter patients carrying de novo *TP53* mutations with no family history suggestive of the LFS. *BRCA*-negative women with breast cancer onset before age 36 years and association with other core Li-Fraumeni cancers in the family should prompt consideration of directed *TP53* testing.[42] The inclusion of *TP53* in multigene testing panels is yielding an ever greater number of cases (see later discussion). The phenotype of breast cancer in LFS is unique beyond markedly early onset disease with median age at diagnosis of 32 years (range 22–46). In the largest study to date, 43 tumors from 39 women demonstrated exclusively ductal

Table 2
Genes with established breast cancer risk

Gene	Magnitude of Relative Risk	Estimated Relative Risk (90% CI)	Absolute Risk by 80 y of Age (%)	Comments	Other Associated Cancers	References
BRCA1 / BRCA2	High	11.4–11.7	75	Estimates are based on the BOADICEA model for a woman born in 1960	Ovarian (18%–50%) Prostate (16%–34%) Pancreatic (5%–7%)	4,20,148–150
TP53	High	105 (62–165)		Risk estimates are subject to ascertainment bias	Childhood sarcoma, adrenocortical carcinoma, brain tumors (cumulative risk 73%–99%)	151,152
PTEN	High	Uncertain		Risk estimates are subject to ascertainment bias	Breast (25%–50%) Thyroid (10%) Endometrial (10%)	153,154
CDH1	High	6.6 (2.2–19.9)	53	Specific to lobular breast cancer	Gastric (40%–50%) Lobular breast cancer (40%–80%)	6,7
STK11	High	Uncertain	26	Risk estimates are subject to ascertainment bias	Breast (30%–50%) Colon (40%) Gastric (30%) Pancreatic (11%–36%) Ovarian (20%)	155
PALB2	High/moderate	5.3 (3.0–9.4)	27–58	Risk estimates are based on a meta-analysis of published case-control and family studies	Pancreas (<5%)	4,156–159
ATM	Moderate	2.8 (2.2–3.7)	~25	Certain missense variants are associated with higher risk than truncating variants	Pancreas (<5%)	4,160–163
CHEK2	Moderate	3.0 (2.6–3.5)	29	Most data refer to c.1100delC; p.Ile157Thr is associated with an increase in risk that is 1.3 times as high as in the general population	Colon (~8%)	4,164–167
NBN	Low	2.7 (1.9–3.7)	23	Most data pertain to the c.657del5 variant in Slavic populations	Unknown	168
NF1	Moderate	2.6 (2.1–3.2)	26	Estimates are based on cohort studies of patients with neurofibromatosis type 1	Malignant tumors of peripheral nerve sheath, brain, central nervous system	4,169,170

histology. Of the invasive cancers, 84% were positive for ER or PR; 81% were high grade. Sixty-three percent of invasive and 73% of in situ carcinomas were positive for HER2/neu (IHC 3+ or fluorescence in situ hybridization amplified).[175] These findings suggest that modern HER2-directed treatments may result in improved outcomes for women with LFS-associated breast cancer. In a landmark paper, David Malkin's group[172] documented decreased mortality for LFS patients participating in an intense multimodality surveillance protocol, albeit predominantly in a pediatric population.[176] A pilot project with PET-computed tomography detected several asymptomatic neoplasms, although there are reasonable concerns about potential morbidity from cumulative exposure to ionizing radiation exposure.[177] However, beyond a recommendation for annual contrast-enhanced breast MRI and colonoscopy,[178] there is less uniformity in the regimens being offered to adults with LFS, and the efficacy of surveillance programs for the diverse malignancies seen in LFS is uncertain.[42] Recommendations for management of the adult woman with LFS include monthly self-examination, clinical examination every 6 months, annual breast MRI from age 20 years of age on (or 5 years before earliest breast cancer in family, whichever is earlier). Concerns about ionizing radiation exposure prompt consideration of omission of mammograms until after 30 years old. The most common approach given the extraordinary risk for breast cancer is consideration of RRM.

Cowden disease (CD)

CD (multiple hamartoma syndrome) is a cancer-associated autosomal-dominant genodermatosis with characteristic mucocutaneous findings including multiple smooth facial papules (cutaneous tricholemmomas), acral keratosis, and multiple oral papillomas, associated with mutations in the PTEN gene.[179] Central nervous system manifestations of CD may include macrocephaly, epilepsy, and dysplastic gangliocytomas of the cerebellum (Lhermitte Duclos disease).[180] Other associated lesions include benign and malignant disease of the thyroid, intestinal polyps, and genitourinary abnormalities. Expression of the disease is variable and penetrance of the dermatologic lesions is thought to be complete by age 20. The incidence of breast cancer in affected women classically ranges from 22% to greater than 50%.[154,181–183] The risk for new primary breast cancers among women with PTEN-associated breast cancer is increased, although there are significant limitations of the available data. In one study, 11 of 51 (22%) PTEN mutation-positive patients with breast cancer had a subsequent new primary breast cancer and 10-year second breast cancer cumulative risk of 29% (95% CI, 15.3–43.7).[184] Although RRM may be considered, the risk of new primary breast cancers is more moderate than BRCA or TP53, and less well characterized. The major associated risks that prompt changes in care include thyroid cancer (10%–30%; annual thyroid ultrasound) and endometrium (10%–28%; annual transvaginal ultrasound and option for hysterectomy).[154] CD is one of the few cancer-associated syndromes wherein physical examination (eg, head circumference >58 cm; multinodular goiter, mucocutaneous findings) may have as much or more clinical sensitivity than molecular testing. The NCCN guidelines would support high-risk breast cancer surveillance, following essentially the same approach as for BRCA.

Hereditary Diffuse Gastric Cancer and Lobular Breast Cancer (HDGC)

HDGC and lobular breast cancer were first noted for autosomal-dominant high risk for diffuse, signet ring gastric cancer.[185,186] Later, it became clear that there was also a relatively high risk (30%–60%) for lobular breast cancer, and that some families presented with lobular breast cancer alone.[6,7,187] Thus, management of women with CDH1 mutations warrants MRI screening at the least.[188]

Partner and localizer of BRCA2 (PALB2)

Biallelic mutations in *PALB2* cause Fanconi anemia type N, characterized by growth retardation, developmental disabilities, and a high risk for pediatric solid tumors.[189] Monoallelic (heterozygous) mutations in *PALB2* cause an increased risk for breast cancer that seems to be modified by family history.[156,158,190] The largest study of *PALB2* mutation carriers to date indicated that the cumulative risk of breast cancer to age 70 was 35% regardless of family history, whereas those with 2 first-degree relatives diagnosed with breast cancer before age 50 had an absolute risk of 58% by age 70.[156] Thus, most clinicians now group *PALB2* with the other high-penetrance genes with regard to actionability (eg, high-risk surveillance and consideration, albeit less compelling, for RRM).

PALB2 founder mutations exist in Polish, Danish, and Russian HBOC cohorts.[159,191,192] Although there seems to be an increased ovarian cancer risk for *PALB2* carriers, findings did not reach statistical significance in the most recent study.[156] *PALB2* mutations have also been identified in a small proportion of hereditary pancreatic cancer families.[193,194] The magnitude of pancreatic cancer risk conferred by *PALB2* mutations remains unclear (likely <5% absolute risk), but it may be near the level observed in *BRCA2* mutation carriers.[195]

Ataxia-Telangiectasia Mutated (ATM) gene

Modest increased risk (relative risk, RR = 3.9–6.4) may be seen in women who are heterozygous for a mutation in ataxia telangiectasia mutated (*ATM*),[196,197] which is associated with the recessive disease ataxia-telangiectasia in the homozygous state. Carrier frequency is estimated at 1%. Although most studies suggest that female carriers have a moderately elevated risk of breast cancer (2–3 times), 2 *ATM* mutations found in families with multiple cases of breast cancer in Australia (T7271G, IVS10-6T > G) demonstrated 15.7-fold elevated risk of breast cancer in carriers.[198,199] Unfortunately, despite the relative rarity of these specific high-risk variants and the fact that the vast majority of variants seem to confer a risk of ~25% lifetime, test reports from genetic testing vendors often cite the high risk in the range of risk, raising concern about inappropriate application of RRM as part of management.

Genomic studies linked *ATM* to modestly elevated risk for pancreatic cancer (<5% absolute lifetime risk).[200] Given the frequency of *ATM* mutations on multigene panel test results, clarification of breast (and other) cancer risks will be important. There is no evidence to date suggesting a hazardous effect of screening mammography or therapeutic radiation.

Checkpoint kinase 2 (CHEK2)

CHEK2 is a moderate-risk tumor suppressor gene that encodes the checkpoint kinase 2 protein. Germline mutations in the *CHEK2* gene have been associated with a moderate risk for breast cancer, with an OR of 2.7 for unselected breast cancer cases.[201] Despite concerns about limited clinical utility[202,203] that have limited application of single gene testing for *CHEK2* mutations, emerging data on associated risk for bilateral breast cancer and breast cancer–related mortality,[166] as well as inclusion on multigene panels, have increased the clinical relevance of *CHEK2*. Evidence suggests there is an approximately 2-fold risk for CRC in *CHEK2* mutation carriers.[204,205] Currently, the breast cancer risk for *CHEK2* mutation carriers does not seem elevated enough to warrant consideration of risk-reducing bilateral mastectomy, but heightened surveillance with additional annual breast MRI is recommended.[42] In breast cancer families found to have a *CHEK2* mutation, empiric risk estimates (eg, Tyrer-Cuzick empiric risk model) may match the genetic risk, so that the impact on management may be modest.

MULTIGENE PANELS: THE "SHOTGUN" APPROACH

The introduction of multigene panels represents an important new and rapidly evolving genomic technology. Traditional genetic counseling and testing driven by syndromic features, with testing focused on one or a few high penetrance cancer predisposition genes, has been the standard of care for decades. However, recent technical advances, including NGS, have upended these well-established paradigms. (See the article by John Burn in this issue.) National guidelines now include discussion of hereditary cancer panels inclusive of multiple genes as a potentially cost- and time-effective alternative to sequentially test more than 2 to 3 single genes associated with a given phenotype, or when atypical family presentations or limited family structure make it difficult to use family history alone to determine the most appropriate gene or genes to test.[42] Moving beyond single-gene testing has unveiled new challenges to the clinician involved in providing GCRAs.[206] Since the implementation of multi-gene panels, significant gaps in the gene-specific phenotypic knowledge base have been identified. The prevalence of VUS (see article by Marc S. Greenblatt in this issue) and unexpected findings, such as off-phenotypic-target (gene mutation does not match or account for any of the clinical picture) gene mutations, challenge the counseling repertoire.[207]

Risk management guidelines, with varying degrees of supportive evidence, have been articulated for the high-penetrance genes and the associated syndromes.[42] However, absolute cancer risk estimates and management guidelines are largely lacking for identified intermediate- and low-risk genes. A recent review summarized the state of knowledge about many of the genes on the panels (see **Table 2**), limitations in absolute risk estimates, gaps and variations in management guidelines and outlined possible study designs for determining risks for the moderate-risk genes.[4] The practicing surgical oncologist needs to know about these trends as she or he is increasingly likely to come under pressure from commercial interests and patients to use these technologies when traditional genetic testing approaches fail to meet genetic diagnostic expectations. The problem for the clinician and their patient is the interpretation, clinical implementation, and medicolegal implications of results that lack evidence-based validation. These challenging issues underscore the value and professional importance of consulting a certified genetic counselor or clinical genetics service when confronted by these situations. (See the article in this issue by Zohra Ali-Khan Catts and Heather Hampel).

CANCER RISK AND MUTATION PROBABILITY MODELS

There are several models available to estimate the probability of an individual carrying a *BRCA* mutation, and these include Couch,[208] Penn 2,[209] and Myriad[210] models. Both mutation probability and empiric risk can be estimated by BRCAPRO,[211–213] Tyrer-Cuzick,[214] and BOADICEA.[215,216] The interested reader is directed to literature wherein these models have been reviewed.[217–220] For concerned patients with a low probability of a mutation, the numeric presentation may provide substantial reassurance supporting recommendations based on empiric cancer risks in lieu of or after uninformative genetic testing. Because most women who participate in GCRA receive uninformative (negative) test results, the art of breast cancer risk management depends on accurate estimation of empiric risk, and each of the models incorporates different factors, used selectively based on the characteristics of the patient's personal and family history. Claus and colleagues[221] determined useful age-specific risk estimates, based on the number and age of first- and second-degree relatives with breast cancer, from analysis of epidemiologic data from the Cancer and Steroid Hormone study. The author adapted the published tables to a free, easy-to-use application for the iPhone and iPad (BRisk; Breast Cancer Risk Assessment Application). All of these models may serve as a basis for determining applicability of breast MRI screening (see discussion above).[146] Although less applicable to women wherein family history of early onset breast or ovarian cancer is present, the Gail model,[222] based on age at menarche, age at first live birth, number of previous breast biopsies ($\pm$ atypical ductal hyperplasia), and number of first-degree relatives with breast cancer, has been validated in several ethnic populations and is the primary tool for determining eligibility for chemoprevention with tamoxifen or raloxifene.[223,224] For additional information regarding breast cancer risk probability models, please see the article by Zohra Ali-Khan Catts and Heather Hampel in this issue.

SUMMARY

This article summarizes the surgical implications of germline predisposition to breast cancer as it pertains to the application of increasingly more complicated NGS-based tests. The rapid pace of change will continue to challenge paradigms for GCRA, including contemplation of the interface between somatic (tumor) and germline genomic profiles.[2] This is a complex, rapidly changing field. Keep this issue with you at all times and please tell your colleagues to do the same.

REFERENCES

1. The National Comprehensive Cancer Network. NCCN clinical practice guidelines in oncology V.1.2014: colorectal cancer screening. NCCN Clinical Practice Guidelines. Fort Washington (PA): The National Comprehensive Cancer Network, Inc; 2014.
2. Weitzel JN, Blazer KR, MacDonald DJ, et al. Genetics, genomics and cancer risk assessment: state of the art and future directions in the era of personalized medicine. CA Cancer J Clin 2011;61(5):327–59.
3. Howlader N, et al. SEER Cancer Statistics Review, 1975-2011. 2014 April 2014. Available at: http://seer.cancer.gov/csr/1975_2011/. Accessed June 01, 2015.
4. Easton DF, Pharoah PD, Antoniou AC, et al. Gene-panel sequencing and the prediction of breast-cancer risk. N Engl J Med 2015;372(23):2243–57.
5. Walsh T, Lee MK, Casadei S, et al. Detection of inherited mutations for breast and ovarian cancer using genomic capture and massively parallel sequencing. Proc Natl Acad Sci U S A 2010;107(28):12629–33.
6. Pharoah PDP, Parry G, Carlos C. Incidence of gastric cancer and breast cancer in CDH1 (E-cadherin) mutation carriers from hereditary diffuse gastric cancer families. Gastroenterology 2001;121(6):1348–53.
7. Xie ZM, Li LS, Laquet C, et al. Germline mutations of the E-cadherin gene in families with inherited invasive lobular breast carcinoma but no diffuse gastric cancer. Cancer 2011;117(14):3112–7.
8. Hall JM, Lee MK, Newman B, et al. Linkage of early-onset familial breast cancer to chromosome 17q21. Science 1990;250(4988):1684–9.
9. Narod SA, Feunteun J, Lynch HT, et al. Familial breast-ovarian cancer locus on chromosome 17q12-23. Lancet 1991;338:82–3.

10. Lynch HT, Watson P, Conway TA, et al. DNA screening for breast/ovarian cancer susceptibility based on linked markers: a family study. Arch Intern Med 1993; 153:1979–87.
11. Ford D, Easton DF, Bishop DT, et al. Risks of cancer in BRCA1-mutation carriers. Lancet 1994;343:692–5.
12. Miki Y, Swensen J, Shattuck-Eidens D, et al. A strong candidate for the breast and ovarian susceptibility gene BRCA1. Science 1994;266:66–71.
13. Wooster R, Bignell G, Lancaster J, et al. Identification of the breast cancer susceptibility gene BRCA2. Nature 1995;378:789–92.
14. Struewing JP, Hartge P, Wacholder S, et al. The risk of cancer associated with specific mutations of BRCA1 and BRCA2 among Ashkenazi Jews. N Engl J Med 1997;336(20):1401–8.
15. Hopper JL, Southey MC, Dite GS, et al. Population-based estimate of the average age-specific cumulative risk of breast cancer for a defined set of protein-truncating mutations in BRCA1 and BRCA2. Cancer Epidemiol Biomarkers Prev 1999;8:741–7.
16. Brose MS, Rebbeck TR, Calzone KA, et al. Cancer risk estimates for BRCA1 mutation carriers identified in a risk evaluation program. J Natl Cancer Inst 2002; 94(18):1365–72.
17. Tryggvadottir L, Sigvaldason H, Olafsdottir GH, et al. Population-based study of changing breast cancer risk in Icelandic BRCA2 mutation carriers, 1920-2000. J Natl Cancer Inst 2006;98(2):116–22.
18. Tai YC, Domchek S, Parmigiani G, et al. Breast cancer risk among male BRCA1 and BRCA2 mutation carriers. J Natl Cancer Inst 2007;99(23):1811–4.
19. Metcalfe K, Lubinski J, Lynch HT, et al. Family history of cancer and cancer risks in women with BRCA1 or BRCA2 mutations. J Natl Cancer Inst 2010;102(24): 1874–8.
20. Antoniou A, Pharoah PD, Narod S, et al. Average risks of breast and ovarian cancer associated with BRCA1 or BRCA2 mutations detected in case series unselected for family history: a combined analysis of 22 studies. Am J Hum Genet 2003;72(5):1117–30.
21. Cullinane CA, Lubinski J, Neuhausen SL, et al. The effect of pregnancy as a risk factor for breast cancer in BRCA1/BRCA2 mutation carriers. Int J Cancer 2005; 117(6):988–91.
22. Finch AP, Lubinski J, Møller P, et al. Impact of oophorectomy on cancer incidence and mortality in women with a BRCA1 or BRCA2 mutation. J Clin Oncol 2014;32(15):1547–53.
23. Gronwald J, Tung N, Foulkes WD, et al. Tamoxifen and contralateral breast cancer in BRCA1 and BRCA2 carriers: an update. Int J Cancer 2006;118(9):2281–4.
24. Jernstrom H, Lubinski J, Lynch HT, et al. Breast-feeding and the risk of breast cancer in BRCA1 and BRCA2 mutation carriers. J Natl Cancer Inst 2004; 96(14):1094–8.
25. Kotsopoulos J, Lubinski J, Neuhausen SL, et al. Hormone replacement therapy and the risk of ovarian cancer in BRCA1 and BRCA2 mutation carriers. Gynecol Oncol 2006;100(1):83–8.
26. McLaughlin JR, Risch HA, Lubinski J, et al. Reproductive risk factors for ovarian cancer in carriers of BRCA1 or BRCA2 mutations: a case-control study. Lancet Oncol 2007;8(1):26–34.
27. Narod SA, Brunet JS, Ghadirian P, et al. Tamoxifen and risk of contralateral breast cancer in BRCA1 and BRCA2 mutation carriers: a case-control study. Lancet 2000;356:1876–81.

28. Narod SA, Dubé MP, Klijn J, et al. Oral contraceptives and the risk of breast cancer in BRCA1 and BRCA2 mutation carriers. J Natl Cancer Inst 2002;94(23): 1773–9.

29. Narod SA, Goldgar D, Cannon-Albright L, et al. Risk modifiers in carriers of BRCA1 mutations. Int J Cancer 1995;64:394–8.

30. Narod SA, Sun P. Ovarian cancer, oral contraceptives, and BRCA mutations. N Engl J Med 2001;345:1706.

31. Rebbeck TR, Friebel T, Wagner T, et al. Effect of short-term hormone replacement therapy on breast cancer risk reduction after bilateral prophylactic oophorectomy in BRCA1 and BRCA2 mutation carriers: the PROSE study group. J Clin Oncol 2005;23:7804–10.

32. Rebbeck TR, Lynch HT, Neuhausen SL, et al. Prophylactic oophorectomy in carriers of BRCA1 or BRCA2 mutations. N Engl J Med 2002;346(21): 1616–22.

33. Valentini A, Lubinski J, Byrski T, et al. The impact of pregnancy on breast cancer survival in women who carry a BRCA1 or BRCA2 mutation. Breast Cancer Res Treat 2013;142(1):177–85.

34. Antoniou AC, Sinilnikova OM, Simard J, et al. RAD51 135G−>C modifies breast cancer risk among BRCA2 mutation carriers: results from a combined analysis of 19 studies. Am J Hum Genet 2007;81(6):1186–200.

35. Antoniou AC, Wang X, Fredericksen ZS, et al. A locus on 19p13 modifies risk of breast cancer in BRCA1 mutation carriers and is associated with hormone receptor-negative breast cancer in the general population. Nat Genet 2010; 42(10):885–92.

36. Couch FJ, Wang X, McGuffog L, et al. Genome-wide association study in BRCA1 mutation carriers identifies novel loci associated with breast and ovarian cancer risk. PLoS Genet 2013;9(3):e1003212.

37. Gaudet MM, Kirchhoff T, Green T, et al. Common genetic variants and modification of penetrance of BRCA2-associated breast cancer. PLoS Genet 2010;6(10): e1001183.

38. Rebbeck TR, Mitra N, Domchek SM, et al. Modification of ovarian cancer risk by BRCA1/2-interacting genes in a multicenter cohort of BRCA1/2 mutation carriers. Cancer Res 2009;69(14):5801–10.

39. Clinical practice guidelines for the use of tumor markers in breast and colorectal cancer. Adopted on May 17, 1996 by the American Society of Clinical Oncology. J Clin Oncol 1996;14(10):2843–77.

40. Robson ME, Storm CD, Weitzel J, et al. American Society of Clinical Oncology Policy Statement Update: genetic and genomic testing for cancer susceptibility. J Clin Oncol 2010;28(5):893–901.

41. Statement of The American Society of Human Genetics on genetic testing for breast and ovarian cancer predisposition. Am J Hum Genet 1994;55: 22–5.

42. The National Comprehensive Cancer Network. NCCN clinical practice guidelines in oncology V.1.2015: genetic/familial high-risk assessment: breast and ovarian. NCCN Clinical Practice Guidelines. Fort Washington (PA): The National Comprehensive Cancer Network, Inc; 2015.

43. Blazer KR, Grant M, Sand SR, et al. Effects of a cancer genetics education programme on clinician knowledge and practice. J Med Genet 2004;41(7):518–22.

44. Blazer KR, Macdonald DJ, Culver JO, et al. Personalized cancer genetics training for personalized medicine: improving community-based healthcare through a genetically literate workforce. Genet Med 2011;13(9):832–40.

45. Blazer KR, MacDonald DJ, Ricker C, et al. Outcomes from intensive training in genetic cancer risk counseling for clinicians. Genet Med 2005;7(1):40–7.
46. Culver JO, Brinkerhoff CD, Clague J, et al. Variants of uncertain significance in BRCA testing: evaluation of surgical decisions, risk perception, and cancer distress. Clin Genet 2013;84(5):464–72.
47. Puget N, Stoppa-Lyonnet D, Sinilnikova OM, et al. Screening for germ-line rearrangements and regulatory mutations in BRCA1 led to the identification of four new deletions. Cancer Res 1999;59(2):455–61.
48. Mazoyer S. Genomic rearrangements in the BRCA1 and BRCA2 genes. Hum Mutat 2005;25(5):415–22.
49. Hendrickson BC, Judkins T, Ward BD, et al. Prevalence of five previously reported and recurrent BRCA1 genetic rearrangement mutations in 20,000 patients from hereditary breast/ovarian cancer families. Genes Chromosomes Cancer 2005;43(3):309–13.
50. Walsh T, Casadei S, Coats KH, et al. Spectrum of mutations in BRCA1, BRCA2, CHEK2, and TP53 in families at high risk of breast cancer. JAMA 2006;295(12): 1379–88.
51. Palma MD, Domchek SM, Stopfer J, et al. The relative contribution of point mutations and genomic rearrangements in BRCA1 and BRCA2 in high-risk breast cancer families. Cancer Res 2008;68(17):7006–14.
52. Weitzel JN, Lagos VI, Herzog JS, et al. Evidence for common ancestral origin of a recurring BRCA1 genomic rearrangement identified in high-risk Hispanic families. Cancer Epidemiol Biomarkers Prev 2007;16(8):1615–20.
53. Judkins T, Rosenthal E, Arnell C, et al. Clinical significance of large rearrangements in BRCA1 and BRCA2. Cancer 2012;118(21):5210–6.
54. Abrahamson J, Moslehi R, Vesprini D, et al. No association of the I1307K APC allele with ovarian cancer risk in Ashkenzi Jews. Cancer Res 1998;58:2919–22.
55. Donenberg T, Lunn J, Curling D, et al. A high prevalence of BRCA1 mutations among breast cancer patients from the Bahamas. Breast Cancer Res Treat 2011;125:591–6.
56. Elsakov P, Kurtinaitis J, Petraitis S, et al. The contribution of founder mutations in BRCA1 to breast and ovarian cancer in Lithuania. Clin Genet 2010; 78(4):373–6.
57. Gorski B, Jakubowska A, Huzarski T, et al. A high proportion of founder BRCA1 mutations in Polish breast cancer families. Int J Cancer 2004;110(5):683–6.
58. Hamel N, Feng BJ, Foretova L, et al. On the origin and diffusion of BRCA1 c.5266dupC (5382insC) in European populations. Eur J Hum Genet 2011; 19(3):300–6.
59. Metcalfe KA, Poll A, Royer R, et al. Screening for founder mutations in BRCA1 and BRCA2 in unselected Jewish women. J Clin Oncol 2010;28(3):387–91.
60. Neuhausen SL, Godwin AK, Gershoni-Baruch R, et al. Haplotype and phenotype analysis of nine recurrent BRCA2 mutations in 111 families: results of an international study. Am J Hum Genet 1998;62:1381–8.
61. Rodríguez AO, Llacuachaqui M, Pardo GG, et al. BRCA1 and BRCA2 mutations among ovarian cancer patients from Colombia. Gynecol Oncol 2012;124(2): 236–43.
62. Simard J, Tonin P, Durocher F, et al. Common origins of BRCA1 mutations in Canadian breast and ovarian cancer families. Nat Genet 1994;8:392–8.
63. Tonin P, Mes-Masson AM, Futreal PA, et al. Founder BRCA1 and BRCA2 mutations in French Canadian breast and ovarian cancer families. Am J Hum Genet 1998;63:1341–51.

64. Villarreal-Garza CM, Weitzel JN, Llacuachaqui M, et al. The prevalence of BRCA1 and BRCA2 mutations among young Mexican women with triple-negative breast cancer. Breast Cancer Res Treat 2015;150(2):389–94.
65. Laitman Y, Feng BJ, Zamir IM, et al. Haplotype analysis of the 185delAG BRCA1 mutation in ethnically diverse populations. Eur J Hum Genet 2013; 21(2):212–6.
66. Bar-Sade RB, Kruglikova A, Modan B, et al. The 185delAG BRCA1 mutation originated before the dispersion of Jews in the diaspora and is not limited to Ashkenazim. Hum Mol Genet 1998;7(5):801–5.
67. Weitzel JN, Clague J, Martir-Negron A, et al. Prevalence and type of BRCA mutations in Hispanics undergoing genetic cancer risk assessment in the southwestern United States: a report from the Clinical Cancer Genetics Community Research Network. J Clin Oncol 2013;31(2):210–6.
68. Thorlacius S, Olafsdottir G, Tryggvadottir L, et al. A single BRCA2 mutation in male and female breast cancer families from Iceland with varied cancer phenotypes. Nat Genet 1996;13:117–9.
69. Gabai-Kapara E, Lahad A, Kaufman B, et al. Population-based screening for breast and ovarian cancer risk due to BRCA1 and BRCA2. Proc Natl Acad Sci U S A 2014;111(39):14205–10.
70. King MC, Levy-Lahad E, Lahad A. Population-based screening for BRCA1 and BRCA2: 2014 Lasker Award. JAMA 2014;312(11):1091–2.
71. Hagen T. Broad BRCA Screening is Becoming a Thorny Public Health Issue. OncLive [Online Article] 2015; Available at: http://www.onclive.com/publications/Oncology-live/2015/April-2015/Broad-BRCA-Screening-is-Becoming-a-Thorny-Public-Health-Issue. Accessed June 01, 2015.
72. Weitzel JN, Lagos VI, Cullinane CA, et al. Limited family structure and BRCA gene mutation status in single cases of breast cancer. J Am Med Assoc 2007;297(23):2587–95.
73. Prevalence and penetrance of BRCA1 and BRCA2 mutations in a population-based series of breast cancer cases. Anglian Breast Cancer Study Group. Br J Cancer 2000;83(10):1301–8.
74. Langston AA, Malone KE, Thompson JD, et al. BRCA1 mutations in a population-based sample of young women with breast cancer. N Engl J Med 1996;334(3):137–42.
75. Risch HA, McLaughlin JR, Cole DE, et al. Prevalence and penetrance of germline BRCA1 and BRCA2 mutations in a population series of 649 women with ovarian cancer. Am J Hum Genet 2001;68(3):700–10.
76. Thorlacius S, Struewing JP, Hartge P, et al. Population-based study of risk of breast cancer in carriers of BRCA2 mutation. Lancet 1998;352(9137): 1337–9.
77. Gayther SA, Mangion J, Russell P, et al. Variation of risks of breast and ovarian cancer associated with different germline mutations of the BRCA2 gene. Nat Genet 1996;15:103–5.
78. Lubinski J, Phelan CM, Ghadirian P, et al. Cancer variation associated with the position of the mutation in the BRCA2 gene. Fam Cancer 2004;3(1):1–10.
79. Rebbeck TR, Mitra N, Wan F, et al. Association of type and location of BRCA1 and BRCA2 mutations with risk of breast and ovarian cancer. JAMA 2015; 313(13):1347–61.
80. Jakubowska A, Gronwald J, Menkiszak J, et al. The RAD51 135 G>C polymorphism modifies breast cancer and ovarian cancer risk in Polish BRCA1 mutation carriers. Cancer Epidemiol Biomarkers Prev 2007;16(2):270–5.

81. Wang X, Pankratz VS, Fredericksen Z, et al. Common variants associated with breast cancer in genome-wide association studies are modifiers of breast cancer risk in BRCA1 and BRCA2 mutation carriers. Hum Mol Genet 2010;19(14):2886–97.

82. Smith A, Moran A, Boyd MC, et al. Phenocopies in BRCA1 and BRCA2 families: evidence for modifier genes and implications for screening? J Med Genet 2007; 44(1):10–5.

83. Grann VR, Jacobson JS, Thomason D, et al. Effect of prevention strategies on survival and quality-adjusted survival of women with BRCA1/2 mutations: an updated decision analysis. J Clin Oncol 2002;20(10):2520–9.

84. Grann VR, Panageas KS, Whang W, et al. Decision analysis of prophylactic mastectomy and oophorectomy in BRCA1-positive or BRCA2-positive patients. J Clin Oncol 1998;16(3):979–85.

85. Metcalfe K, Lynch HT, Ghadirian P, et al. Contralateral breast cancer in BRCA1 and BRCA2 mutation carriers. J Clin Oncol 2004;22(12):2328–35.

86. Weitzel JN, McCaffrey SM, Nedelcu R, et al. Effect of genetic cancer risk assessment on surgical decisions at breast cancer diagnosis. Arch Surg 2003;138(12):1323–9.

87. Schwartz MD, Lerman C, Brogan B, et al. Impact of BRCA1/BRCA2 counseling and testing on newly diagnosed breast cancer patients. J Clin Oncol 2004; 22(10):1823–9.

88. Palomares MR, Paz IB, Weitzel JN. Genetic cancer risk assessment in the newly diagnosed breast cancer patient is useful and possible in practice. J Clin Oncol 2005;23(13):3165–6 [author reply: 3166–7].

89. Protheroe D, Turvey K, Horgan K, et al. Stressful life events and difficulties and onset of breast cancer: case-control study. Br Med J 1999;319:1027–30.

90. Trask PC, Paterson AG, Wang C, et al. Cancer-specific worry interference in women attending a breast and ovarian cancer risk evaluation program: impact on emotional distress and health functioning. Psychooncology 2001;10:349–60.

91. Pierce LJ, Haffty BG. Radiotherapy in the treatment of hereditary breast cancer. Semin Radiat Oncol 2011;21(1):43–50.

92. Pierce LJ, Levin AM, Rebbeck TR, et al. Ten-year multi-institutional results of breast-conserving surgery and radiotherapy in BRCA1/2-associated stage I/II breast cancer. J Clin Oncol 2006;24(16):2437–43.

93. Haffty BG, Harrold E, Khan AJ, et al. Outcome of conservatively managed early-onset breast cancer by BRCA1/2 status. Lancet 2002;359(9316):1471–7.

94. Metcalfe KA, Lynch HT, Ghadirian P, et al. The risk of ovarian cancer after breast cancer in BRCA1 and BRCA2 carriers. Gynecol Oncol 2005;96(1):222–6.

95. Domchek SM, Friebel TM, Singer CF, et al. Association of risk-reducing surgery in BRCA1 or BRCA2 mutation carriers with cancer risk and mortality. J Am Med Assoc 2010;304(9):967–75.

96. Rebbeck TR, Friebel T, Lynch HT, et al. Bilateral prophylactic mastectomy reduces breast cancer risk in BRCA1 and BRCA2 mutation carriers: the PROSE study group. J Clin Oncol 2004;22(6):1055–62.

97. Friebel TM, Domchek SM, Neuhausen SL, et al. Bilateral prophylactic oophorectomy and bilateral prophylactic mastectomy in a prospective cohort of unaffected BRCA1 and BRCA2 mutation carriers. Clin Breast Cancer 2007;7(11):875–82.

98. Metcalfe KA, Birenbaum-Carmeli D, Lubinski J, et al. International variation in rates of uptake of preventive options in BRCA1 and BRCA2 mutation carriers. Int J Cancer 2008;122(9):2017–22.

99. Metcalfe KA, Lubinski J, Ghadirian P, et al. Predictors of contralateral prophylactic mastectomy in women with a BRCA1 or BRCA2 mutation: the

Hereditary Breast Cancer Clinical Study Group. J Clin Oncol 2008;26(7): 1093–7.

100. Bluman LG, Rimer BK, Regan Sterba K, et al. Attitudes, knowledge, risk perceptions and decision-making among women with breast and/or ovarian cancer considering testing for BRCA1 and BRCA2 and their spouses. Psychooncology 2003;12(5):410–27.

101. Brandberg Y, Sandelin K, Erikson S, et al. Psychological reactions, quality of life, and body image after bilateral prophylactic mastectomy in women at high risk for breast cancer: a prospective 1-Year follow-up study. J Clin Oncol 2008; 26(24):3943–9.

102. Bresser PJ, Seynaeve C, Van Gool AR, et al. Satisfaction with prophylactic mastectomy and breast reconstruction in genetically predisposed women. Plast Reconstr Surg 2006;117(6):1675–82 [discussion: 1683–4].

103. Altschuler A, Nekhlyudov L, Rolnick SJ, et al. Positive, negative, and disparate–women's differing long-term psychosocial experiences of bilateral or contralateral prophylactic mastectomy. Breast J 2008;14(1):25–32.

104. Frost MH, Schaid DJ, Sellers TA, et al. Long-term satisfaction and psychological and social function following bilateral prophylactic mastectomy. J Am Med Assoc 2000;284(3):319–24.

105. Hopwood P, Lee A, Shenton A, et al. Clinical follow-up after bilateral risk reducing ('prophylactic') mastectomy: mental health and body image outcomes. Psychooncology 2000;9(6):462–72.

106. Rolnick SJ, Altschuler A, Nekhlyudov L, et al. What women wish they knew before prophylactic mastectomy. Cancer Nurs 2007;30(4):285–91 [quiz: 292–3].

107. Brachtel EF, Rusby JE, Michaelson JS, et al. Occult nipple involvement in breast cancer: clinicopathologic findings in 316 consecutive mastectomy specimens. J Clin Oncol 2009;27(30):4948–54.

108. Edge SB. Nipple-sparing mastectomy: how often is the nipple involved? J Clin Oncol 2009;27(30):4930–2.

109. Schecter AK, Freeman MB, Giri D, et al. Applicability of the nipple-areola complex-sparing mastectomy: a prediction model using mammography to estimate risk of nipple-areola complex involvement in breast cancer patients. Ann Plast Surg 2006;56(5):498–504 [discussion: 504].

110. Gerber B, Krause A, Reimer T, et al. Skin-sparing mastectomy with conservation of the nipple-areola complex and autologous reconstruction is an oncologically safe procedure. Ann Surg 2003;238(1):120–7.

111. Janz NK, Wren PA, Copeland LA, et al. Patient-physician concordance: preferences, perceptions, and factors influencing the breast cancer surgical decision. J Clin Oncol 2004;22(15):3091–8.

112. Lynch BJ, Holden JA, Buys SS, et al. Pathobiologic characteristics of hereditary breast cancer. Hum Pathol 1998;29(10):1140–4.

113. Foulkes WD, Metcalfe K, Sun P, et al. Estrogen receptor status in BRCA1- and BRCA2-related breast cancer: the influence of age, grade, and histological type. Clin Cancer Res 2004;10(6):2029–34.

114. Chappuis PO, Nethercot V, Foulkes WD. Clinico-pathological characteristics of BRCA1- and BRCA2-related breast cancer. Semin Surg Oncol 2000;18(4): 287–95.

115. Mavaddat N, Barrowdale D, Andrulis IL, et al. Pathology of breast and ovarian cancers among BRCA1 and BRCA2 mutation carriers: results from the Consortium of Investigators of Modifiers of BRCA1/2 (CIMBA). Cancer Epidemiol Biomarkers Prev 2012;21(1):134–47.

116. Weitzel JN, Robson M, Pasini B, et al. A comparison of bilateral breast cancers in BRCA carriers. Cancer Epidemiol Biomarkers Prev 2005;14(6):1534–8.
117. Gronwald J, Robidoux A, Kim-Sing C, et al. Duration of tamoxifen use and the risk of contralateral breast cancer in BRCA1 and BRCA2 mutation carriers. Breast Cancer Res Treat 2014;146(2):421–7.
118. Bhatia S, Robison LL, Oberlin O, et al. Breast cancer and other second neoplasms after childhood Hodgkin's disease. N Engl J Med 1996;334: 745–51.
119. Bernstein JL, Haile RW, Stovall M, et al. Radiation exposure, the ATM gene, and contralateral breast cancer in the women's environmental cancer and radiation epidemiology study. J Natl Cancer Inst 2010;102(7):475–83.
120. Andrieu N, Easton DF, Chang-Claude J, et al. Effect of chest X-rays on the risk of breast cancer among BRCA1/2 mutation carriers in the international BRCA1/2 carrier cohort study: a report from the EMBRACE, GENEPSO, GEO-HEBON, and IBCCS Collaborators' Group. J Clin Oncol 2006;24(21): 3361–6.
121. Gronwald J, Pijpe A, Byrski T, et al. Early radiation exposures and BRCA1-associated breast cancer in young women from Poland. Breast Cancer Res Treat 2008;112(3):581–4.
122. Narod SA, Lubinski J, Ghadirian P, et al. Screening mammography and risk of breast cancer in BRCA1 and BRCA2 mutation carriers: a case-control study. Lancet Oncol 2006;7(5):402–6.
123. Buys SS, Partridge E, Black A, et al. Effect of screening on ovarian cancer mortality: the Prostate, Lung, Colorectal and Ovarian (PLCO) Cancer Screening Randomized Controlled Trial. JAMA 2011;305(22):2295–303.
124. Olivier RI, Lubsen-Brandsma MA, Verhoef S, et al. CA125 and transvaginal ultrasound monitoring in high-risk women cannot prevent the diagnosis of advanced ovarian cancer. Gynecol Oncol 2006;100(1):20–6.
125. Society of Gynecologic Oncologists Clinical Practice Committee Statement on Prophylactic Salpingo-oophorectomy. Gynecol Oncol 2005;98(2):179–81.
126. Walker JL, Powell CB, Chen LM, et al. Society of gynecologic oncology recommendations for the prevention of ovarian cancer. Cancer 2015. Commentary. [Epub ahead of print].
127. Elit L, Esplen MJ, Butler K, et al. Quality of life and psychosexual adjustment after prophylactic oophorectomy for a family history of ovarian cancer. Fam Cancer 2001;1(3–4):149–56.
128. Finch A, Metcalfe KA, Chiang JK, et al. The impact of prophylactic salpingo-oophorectomy on menopausal symptoms and sexual function in women who carry a BRCA mutation. Gynecol Oncol 2011;121(1):163–8.
129. Robson M, Hensley M, Barakat R, et al. Quality of life in women at risk for ovarian cancer who have undergone risk-reducing oophorectomy. Gynecol Oncol 2003; 89(2):281–7.
130. Finch A, Shaw P, Rosen B, et al. Clinical and pathologic findings of prophylactic salpingo-oophorectomies in 159 BRCA1 and BRCA2 carriers. Gynecol Oncol 2006;100(1):58–64.
131. Sherman ME, Piedmonte M, Mai PL, et al. Pathologic findings at risk-reducing salpingo-oophorectomy: primary results from gynecologic oncology group trial GOG-0199. J Clin Oncol 2014;32(29):3275–83.
132. Callahan MJ, Crum CP, Medeiros F, et al. Primary fallopian tube malignancies in BRCA-positive women undergoing surgery for ovarian cancer risk reduction. J Clin Oncol 2007;25(25):3985–90.

133. Domchek SM, Friebel TM, Garber JE, et al. Occult ovarian cancers identified at risk-reducing salpingo-oophorectomy in a prospective cohort of BRCA1/2 mutation carriers. Breast Cancer Res Treat 2010;124(1):195–203.

134. Leeper K, Garcia R, Swisher E, et al. Pathologic findings in prophylactic oophorectomy specimens in high-risk women. Gynecol Oncol 2002;87(1):52–6.

135. Powell CB, Kenley E, Chen LM, et al. Risk-reducing salpingo-oophorectomy in BRCA mutation carriers: role of serial sectioning in the detection of occult malignancy. J Clin Oncol 2005;23(1):127–32.

136. Greene MH, Mai PL, Schwartz PE. Does bilateral salpingectomy with ovarian retention warrant consideration as a temporary bridge to risk-reducing bilateral oophorectomy in BRCA1/2 mutation carriers? Am J Obstet Gynecol 2011;204(1): 19.e1–6.

137. Anderson GL, Chlebowski RT, Aragaki AK, et al. Conjugated equine oestrogen and breast cancer incidence and mortality in postmenopausal women with hysterectomy: extended follow-up of the Women's Health Initiative randomised placebo-controlled trial. Lancet Oncol 2012;13(5):476–86.

138. Goshen R, Chu W, Elit L, et al. Is uterine papillary serous adenocarcinoma a manifestation of the hereditary breast-ovarian cancer syndrome? Gynecol Oncol 2000;79(3):477–81.

139. Lavie O, Ben-Arie A, Gemer O. Possible association between BRCA-1 carriers and incidence of uterine papillary serous carcinoma (UPSC). Int J Gynecol Cancer 2008;18(5):1150.

140. Narod SA, Risch H, Moslehi R, et al. Oral contraceptives and the risk of hereditary ovarian cancer. N Engl J Med 1998;339:424–8.

141. Antoniou AC, Rookus M, Andrieu N, et al. Reproductive and hormonal factors, and ovarian cancer risk for BRCA1 and BRCA2 mutation carriers: results from the International BRCA1/2 Carrier Cohort Study. Cancer Epidemiol Biomarkers Prev 2009; 18(2):601–10.

142. Warner E, Plewes DB, Shumak RS, et al. Comparison of breast magnetic resonance imaging, mammography, and ultrasound for surveillance of women at high risk for hereditary breast cancer. J Clin Oncol 2001;19: 3524–31.

143. Warner E, Plewes DB, Hill KA, et al. Surveillance of BRCA1 and BRCA2 mutation carriers with magnetic resonance imaging, ultrasound, mammography, and clinical breast examination. JAMA 2004;292(11):1317–25.

144. Warner E, Hill K, Causer P, et al. Prospective study of breast cancer incidence in women with a BRCA1 or BRCA2 mutation under surveillance with and without magnetic resonance imaging. J Clin Oncol 2011;29(13):1664–9.

145. Leach MO, Boggis CR, Dixon AK, et al. Screening with magnetic resonance imaging and mammography of a UK population at high familial risk of breast cancer: a prospective multicentre cohort study (MARIBS). Lancet 2005; 365(9473):1769–78.

146. Saslow D, Boetes C, Burke W, et al. American Cancer Society guidelines for breast screening with MRI as an adjunct to mammography. CA Cancer J Clin 2007;57(2):75–89.

147. Kriege M, Brekelmans CT, Boetes C, et al. Efficacy of MRI and mammography for breast-cancer screening in women with a familial or genetic predisposition. N Engl J Med 2004;351(5):427–37.

148. Lee AJ, Cunningham AP, Kuchenbaecker KB, et al. BOADICEA breast cancer risk prediction model: updates to cancer incidences, tumour pathology and web interface. Br J Cancer 2014;110(2):535–45.

149. Chen S, Parmigiani G. Meta-analysis of BRCA1 and BRCA2 penetrance. J Clin Oncol 2007;25(11):1329–33.

150. Mavaddat N, Peock S, Frost D, et al. Cancer risks for BRCA1 and BRCA2 mutation carriers: results from prospective analysis of EMBRACE. J Natl Cancer Inst 2013;105(11):812–22.

151. Hisada M, Garber JE, Fung CY, et al. Multiple primary cancers in families with Li-Fraumeni syndrome. J Natl Cancer Inst 1998;90(8):606–11.

152. Hwang SJ, Lozano G, Amos CI, et al. Germline p53 mutations in a cohort with childhood sarcoma: sex differences in cancer risk. Am J Hum Genet 2003; 72(4):975–83.

153. Bubien V, Bonnet F, Brouste V, et al. High cumulative risks of cancer in patients with PTEN hamartoma tumour syndrome. J Med Genet 2013;50(4):255–63.

154. Tan M-H, Mester JL, Ngeow J, et al. Lifetime cancer risks in individuals with germline PTEN mutations. Clin Cancer Res 2012;18(2):400–7.

155. Hearle N, Schumacher V, Menko FH, et al. Frequency and spectrum of cancers in the Peutz-Jeghers syndrome. Clin Cancer Res 2006;12(10):3209–15.

156. Antoniou AC, Casadei S, Heikkinen T, et al. Breast-cancer risk in families with mutations in PALB2. N Engl J Med 2014;371(6):497–506.

157. Heikkinen T, Kärkkäinen H, Aaltonen K, et al. The breast cancer susceptibility mutation PALB2 1592delT is associated with an aggressive tumor phenotype. Clin Cancer Res 2009;15(9):3214–22.

158. Rahman N, Seal S, Thompson D, et al. PALB2, which encodes a BRCA2-interacting protein, is a breast cancer susceptibility gene. Nat Genet 2007; 39(2):165–7.

159. Erkko H, Xia B, Nikkilä J, et al. A recurrent mutation in PALB2 in Finnish cancer families. Nature 2007;446(7133):316–9.

160. Renwick A, Thompson D, Seal S, et al. ATM mutations that cause ataxia-telangiectasia are breast cancer susceptibility alleles. Nat Genet 2006;38(8):873–5.

161. Thompson D, Duedal S, Kirner J, et al. Cancer risks and mortality in heterozygous ATM mutation carriers. J Natl Cancer Inst 2005;97(11):813–22.

162. Janin N, Andrieu N, Ossian K, et al. Breast cancer risk in ataxia telangietasia (AT) heterozygotes: haplotype study in French AT families. Br J Cancer 1999; 80:1042–5.

163. Olsen JH, Hahnemann JM, Børresen-Dale AL, et al. Breast and other cancers in 1445 blood relatives of 75 Nordic patients with ataxia telangiectasia. Br J Cancer 2005;93(2):260–5.

164. Meijers-Heijboer H, van den Ouweland A, Klijn J, et al. Low-penetrance susceptibility to breast cancer due to CHEK2(*)1100delC in noncarriers of BRCA1 or BRCA2 mutations. Nat Genet 2002;31(1):55–9.

165. CHEK2 Breast Cancer Case-Control Consortium. CHEK2*1100delC and susceptibility to breast cancer: a collaborative analysis involving 10,860 breast cancer cases and 9,065 controls from 10 studies. Am J Hum Genet 2004;74(6):1175–82.

166. Weischer M, Nordestgaard BG, Pharoah P, et al. CHEK2*1100delC heterozygosity in women with breast cancer associated with early death, breast cancer–specific death, and increased risk of a second breast cancer. J Clin Oncol 2012;30(35):4308–16.

167. Kilpivaara O, Vahteristo P, Falck J, et al. CHEK2 variant I157T may be associated with increased breast cancer risk. Int J Cancer 2004;111(4):543–7.

168. Zhang G, Zeng Y, Liu Z, et al. Significant association between Nijmegen breakage syndrome 1 657del5 polymorphism and breast cancer risk. Tumour Biol 2013;34(5):2753–7.

169. Madanikia SA, Bergner A, Ye X, et al. Increased risk of breast cancer in women with NF1. Am J Med Genet A 2012;158A(12):3056–60.
170. Seminog OO, Goldacre MJ. Age-specific risk of breast cancer in women with neurofibromatosis type 1. Br J Cancer 2015;112(9):1546–8.
171. Li FP, Garber JE, Friend SH, et al. Recommendations on predictive testing for germline p53 mutations among cancer-prone individuals. J Natl Cancer Inst 1992;84:1156–60.
172. Malkin D, Li FP, Strong LC, et al. Germ line p53 mutations in a familial syndrome of breast cancer, sarcomas, and other neoplasms. Science 1990;250:1233–7.
173. Gonzalez KD, Noltner KA, Buzin CH, et al. Beyond Li Fraumeni Syndrome: clinical characteristics of families with p53 germline mutations. J Clin Oncol 2009; 27(8):1250–6.
174. Gonzalez KD, Buzin CH, Noltner KA, et al. High frequency of de novo mutations in Li-Fraumeni syndrome. J Med Genet 2009;46(10):689–93.
175. Masciari S, Dillon DA, Rath M, et al. Breast cancer phenotype in women with TP53 germline mutations: a Li-Fraumeni syndrome consortium effort. Breast Cancer Res Treat 2012;133(3):1125–30.
176. Villani A, Tabori U, Schiffman J, et al. Biochemical and imaging surveillance in germline TP53 mutation carriers with Li-Fraumeni syndrome: a prospective observational study. Lancet Oncol 2011;12(6):559–67.
177. Masciari S, Van den Abbeele AD, Diller LR, et al. F18-fluorodeoxyglucose-positron emission tomography/computed tomography screening in Li-Fraumeni syndrome. JAMA 2008;299(11):1315–9.
178. Wong P, Verselis SJ, Garber JE, et al. Prevalence of early onset colorectal cancer in 397 patients with classic Li-Fraumeni syndrome. Gastroenterology 2006;130(1): 73–9.
179. Nelen MR, Padberg GW, Peeters EA, et al. Localization of the gene for Cowden disease to chromosome 10q22-23. Nat Genet 1996;13:114–6.
180. Albrecht S, Haber RM, Goodman JC, et al. Cowden syndrome and Lhermitte-Duclos disease. Cancer 1992;70:869–76.
181. Starink TM, van der Veen JP, Arwert F, et al. The Cowden syndrome: a clinical and genetic study in 21 patients. Clin Genet 1986;29:222–33.
182. Walton BJ, Morain WD, Baughman RD, et al. Cowden's disease: a further indication for prophylactic mastectomy. Surgery 1986;99:82–6.
183. Brownstein MH, Wolf M, Bikowski JB. Cowden's disease: a cutaneous marker of breast cancer. Cancer 1978;41:2393–8.
184. Ngeow J, Stanuch K, Mester JL, et al. Second malignant neoplasms in patients with Cowden syndrome with underlying germline PTEN mutations. J Clin Oncol 2014;32(17):1818–24.
185. Richards FM, McKee SA, Rajpar MH, et al. Germline E-cadherin gene (CDH1) mutations predispose to familial gastric cancer and colorectal cancer. Hum Mol Genet 1999;8:607–10.
186. Huntsman DG, Carneiro F, Lewis FR, et al. Early gastric cancer in young, asymptomatic carriers of germ-line E-cadherin mutations. N Engl J Med 2001;344: 1904–9.
187. Kaurah P, Huntsman D. Hereditary diffuse gastric cancer [Internet]. In: Pagon RA, Adam MP, Ardinger HH, et al, editors. GeneReviews. Seattle (WA): University of Washington; 2011.
188. Fitzgerald RC, Hardwick R, Huntsman D, et al. Hereditary diffuse gastric cancer: updated consensus guidelines for clinical management and directions for future research. J Med Genet 2010;47(7):436–44.

189. Reid S, Schindler D, Hanenberg H, et al. Biallelic mutations in PALB2 cause Fanconi anemia subtype FA-N and predispose to childhood cancer. Nat Genet 2007;39(2):162–4.
190. Casadei S, Norquist BM, Walsh T, et al. Contribution of inherited mutations in the BRCA2-interacting protein PALB2 to familial breast cancer. Cancer Res 2011; 71(6):2222–9.
191. Dansonka-Mieszkowska A, Kluska A, Moes J, et al. A novel germline PALB2 deletion in Polish breast and ovarian cancer patients. BMC Med Genet 2010; 11:20.
192. Prokofyeva D, Bogdanova N, Bermisheva M, et al. Rare occurrence of PALB2 mutations in ovarian cancer patients from the Volga-Ural region. Clin Genet 2012;82(1):100–1.
193. Jones S, Hruban RH, Kamiyama M, et al. Exomic sequencing identifies PALB2 as a pancreatic cancer susceptibility gene. Science 2009;324(5924):217.
194. Slater EP, Langer P, Niemczyk E, et al. PALB2 mutations in European familial pancreatic cancer families. Clin Genet 2010;78(5):490–4.
195. Holter S, Borgida A, Dodd A, et al. Germline BRCA mutations in a large clinic-based cohort of patients with pancreatic adenocarcinoma. J Clin Oncol 2015. [Epub ahead of print].
196. Swift M, Reitnauer PJ, Morrell D, et al. Breast and other cancers in families with ataxia-telangiectasia. N Engl J Med 1987;316:1289–94.
197. Swift M, Morrell D, Massey RB, et al. Incidence of cancer in 161 families affected by ataxia-telangiectasia. N Engl J Med 1991;325:1831–6.
198. Bernstein JL, Teraoka S, Southey MC, et al. Population-based estimates of breast cancer risks associated with ATM gene variants c.7271T>G and c.1066-6T>G (IVS10-6T>G) from the Breast Cancer Family Registry. Hum Mutat 2006;27(11):1122–8.
199. Goldgar DE, Healey S, Dowty JG, et al. Rare variants in the ATM gene and risk of breast cancer. Breast Cancer Res 2011;13(4):R73.
200. Roberts NJ, Jiao Y, Yu J, et al. ATM mutations in patients with hereditary pancreatic cancer. Cancer Discov 2012;2(1):41–6.
201. Weischer M, Bojesen SE, Ellervik C, et al. CHEK2*1100delC genotyping for clinical assessment of breast cancer risk: meta-analyses of 26,000 patient cases and 27,000 controls. J Clin Oncol 2008;26(4):542–8.
202. Narod SA. Testing for CHEK2 in the cancer genetics clinic: ready for prime time? Clin Genet 2010;78(1):1–7.
203. Robson M. CHEK2, breast cancer, and the understanding of clinical utility. Clin Genet 2010;78(1):8–10.
204. Suchy J, Cybulski C, Wokołorczyk D, et al. CHEK2 mutations and HNPCC-related colorectal cancer. Int J Cancer 2010;126(12):3005–9.
205. Xiang HP, Geng XP, Ge WW, et al. Meta-analysis of CHEK2 1100delC variant and colorectal cancer susceptibility. Eur J Cancer 2011;47(17):2546–51.
206. Domchek SM, Bradbury A, Garber JE, et al. Multiplex genetic testing for cancer susceptibility: out on the high wire without a net? J Clin Oncol 2013;31(10): 1267–70.
207. Blazer KR, et al. Next-generation testing for cancer risk: perceptions, experiences and needs among early adopters in community healthcare settings. Genetic Testing and Molecular Biomarkers, in press.
208. Couch F, DeShano ML, Blackwood MA, et al. BRCA1 mutations in women attending clinics that evaluate the risk of breast cancer. N Engl J Med 1997; 336:1409–15.

209. The Penn II BRCA1 and BRCA2 Mutation Risk Evaluation Model Official Web Site. 2011. Available at: http://www.afcri.upenn.edu/itacc/penn2/. Accessed March 1, 2011.

210. Frank TS, Deffenbaugh AM, Reid JE, et al. Clinical characteristics of individuals with germline mutations in BRCA1 and BRCA2: analysis of 10,000 individuals. J Clin Oncol 2002;20(6):1480–90.

211. Berry DA, Iversen ES Jr, Gudbjartsson DF, et al. BRCAPRO validation, sensitivity of genetic testing of BRCA1/BRCA2, and prevalence of other breast cancer susceptibility genes. J Clin Oncol 2002;20(11):2701–12.

212. Berry DA, Parmigiani G, Sanchez J, et al. Probability of carrying a mutation of breast-ovarian cancer gene BRCA1 based on family history. J Natl Cancer Inst 1997;89:227–38.

213. Parmigiani G, Berry D, Aguilar O. Determining carrier probabilities for breast cancer-susceptibility genes BRCA1 and BRCA2. Am J Hum Genet 1998;62:145–58.

214. Tyrer J, Duffy SW, Cuzick J. A breast cancer prediction model incorporating familial and personal risk factors. Stat Med 2004;23(7):1111–30.

215. Antoniou AC, Pharoah PP, Smith P, et al. The BOADICEA model of genetic susceptibility to breast and ovarian cancer. Br J Cancer 2004;91(8):1580–90.

216. Antoniou AC, Cunningham AP, Peto J, et al. The BOADICEA model of genetic susceptibility to breast and ovarian cancers: updates and extensions. Br J Cancer 2008;98(8):1457–66.

217. Culver JO, Lowstuter K, Bowling L. Assessing breast cancer risk and BRCA1/2 carrier probability. Breast Dis 2007;27:5–20.

218. Amir E, Freedman OC, Seruga B, et al. Assessing women at high risk of breast cancer: a review of risk assessment models. J Natl Cancer Inst 2010;102(10):680–91.

219. Evans DG, Howell A. Breast cancer risk-assessment models. Breast Cancer Res 2007;9(5):213.

220. Jacobi C, de Bock GH, Siegerink B, et al. Differences and similarities in breast cancer risk assessment models in clinical practice: which model to choose? Breast Cancer Res Treat 2009;115(2):381–90.

221. Claus EB, Risch N, Thompson WD. Autosomal dominant inheritance of early-onset breast cancer. Implications for risk prediction. Cancer 1994;73:643–51.

222. Gail MH, Brinton LA, Byar DP, et al. Projecting individualized probabilities of developing breast cancer for white females who are being examined annually. J Natl Cancer Inst 1989;81:1879–86.

223. Vogel VG, Costantino JP, Wickerham DL, et al. Update of the National Surgical Adjuvant Breast and Bowel Project Study of Tamoxifen and Raloxifene (STAR) P-2 Trial: preventing breast cancer. Cancer Prev Res (Phila) 2010;3(6):696–706.

224. Fisher B, Costantino JP, Wickerham DL, et al. Tamoxifen for prevention of breast cancer: report of the national surgical adjuvant breast and bowel project P-1 study. J Natl Cancer Inst 1998;90(18):1371–88.

Hereditary Pancreatic Cancer Syndromes

Ashton A. Connor, MD, Steven Gallinger, MD, MSc*

KEYWORDS

- Hereditary • Familial • Syndrome • Pancreas • Cancer • Exocrine
- Adenocarcinoma • Genetics

KEY POINTS

- Up to 10% of patients with pancreatic ductal adenocarcinoma (PDAC) have an affected first-degree relative, implying inherited predisposition.
- In approximately 10% of these patients, a pathogenic germline variant in a hereditary pancreatic cancer (HPC) syndrome gene can be identified.
- Taking a detailed family history is key identifying patients who may have pathogenic germline variants.
- A significant number of patients with germline predisposition will not have significant family history because of variable penetrance of some pathogenic variants. Strategies of universal testing for germline variants have not been explored in PDAC.
- Primary and secondary prevention programs are recommended for carriers of HPC syndromes, but there is little consensus on this subject. Screening for PDAC should be considered investigational.

INTRODUCTION

Pancreatic ductal adenocarcinoma (PDAC) remains among the most lethal malignancies despite more than 5 decades of research into its biology and epidemiology.[1] The high mortality from PDAC is attributable to several factors, including its inherently bad biology, that symptoms and signs are nonspecific and occur late in its natural history, the inability to screen for PDAC, and a dearth of knowledge regarding pathogenesis and evolution of PDAC.

Poor outcomes will be improved when standard of care for PDAC is similar to that of other malignancies, such as colon and breast cancer, by, foremost, screening that allows the detection of noninvasive precursors and nonmetastatic neoplasms, second,

The authors have nothing to disclose.

Division of General Surgery, Department of Surgery, Faculty of Medicine, University of Toronto, Toronto, Ontario, Canada

* Correspondiing author. Toronto General Hospital, 200 Elizabeth Street, Room EN10-206, Toronto, Ontario M5G 2C4, Canada.

E-mail address: steven.gallinger@uhn.ca

Surg Oncol Clin N Am 24 (2015) 733–764

http://dx.doi.org/10.1016/j.soc.2015.06.007

1055-3207/15/$ – see front matter © 2015 Elsevier Inc. All rights reserved.

surgonc.theclinics.com

by tumor subtyping with the rational use of immunohistochemistry and molecular testing; and finally, by more rational chemotherapy.

There is ample evidence that population-based primary and secondary prevention programs have ameliorated outcomes for more common malignancies, including colorectal[2] and breast,[3] and for malignancies with traditionally high mortality, including primary lung adenocarcinoma.[4] In the case of primary lung adenocarcinoma, this has been seen when screening is focused on those with elevated risk for the disease.[5] In the case of colorectal cancer, this has been seen when screening is tailored to those with hereditary predisposition.[6]

Epidemiologic risk factors for PDAC neither individually nor in aggregate greatly increase the risk of developing the disease.[7] Germline variants in any of 15 genes do significantly increase relative risk of developing PDAC, and these are collectively referred to as hereditary pancreatic cancer (HPC) syndromes.[7,8] Although much work has been done to investigate these syndromes, questions remain regarding their overall and individual prevalence, their penetrance, their impact on tumor biology, and the benefit of cancer screening in carriers of pathogenic germline variants.

Tumor subtyping has been advantageous in the management of other epithelial adenocarcinomas, including breast and colorectal cancer. With the latter, this has been informed by understanding unique high-risk cases with germline predisposition.[9] For example, Lynch syndrome (LS) cases are marked by somatic tumor microsatellite instability, which is both prognostic of outcome and predictive of chemotherapy response in both the germline and the sporadic microsatellite unstable colorectal cancers.[10] There is strong reason to suspect that PDAC patients with germline predisposition also represent subgroups informative for both those with inherited and those with sporadic defects in key driver genes, and that this grouping is predictive of chemotherapy response, as is described later.

Here, PDAC, including natural history and clinical risk factors, and the HPC syndromes, including strategies for their identification and management, are reviewed, and the importance that these syndromes have in improving the understanding and management of PDAC are relayed.

CLINICAL AND EPIDEMIOLOGIC OVERVIEW

The incidence of PDAC is approximately 4,700 per year in Canada and 46,400 in the United States, meaning that the lifetime risk of developing PDAC is roughly 1.5% in North America.[11]

The mortality of PDAC is nearly as high as its incidence, with an estimated 4,400 deaths per year in Canada and 39,600 deaths per year in the United States. Overall survival at 5 years is 7%, the lowest of all cancers and only double of what it was in 1990.[11] From these trends, it is estimated that PDAC will be the second leading cause of cancer death in North America within 10 years.[1]

For these aforementioned statistics to remain so dismal despite decades of research is testament to the inherent malevolence of PDAC biology. Symptoms and signs of PDAC are nonspecific and occur late in its natural history, with the exception of painless jaundice due to tumors in the head of the gland that fortuitously obstruct biliary drainage.[12,13] Only 15% to 20% of patients present with potentially curable disease, and often these are detected incidentally.[12,13] The time from invasion to metastasis was initially thought to be on the order of 10 to 15 years,[14] but more recent work suggests that it is much shorter,[15] possibly being acquired as soon as the tumor becomes invasive.[16] PDAC is also highly resistant to systemic therapies, including newer targeted agents.[17]

Staging investigations may include measurements of serum carcinoembryonic antigen (CEA) and CA 19-9, non-invasive imaging including computed tomography (CT), and MRI, and invasive modalities, including endoscopic ultrasound (EUS), endoscopic retrograde cholangiopancreatography (ERCP) with cytologic brushings and endoscopic or percutaneous fine-needle aspiration (FNA), or core biopsies.[12,13,18] Non-invasive imaging allows staging according to the American Joint Committee on Cancer TNM (AJCC) system[19] and by the less rigorously defined, 4-tiered system of potentially resectable, borderline resectable, locally advanced, and metastatic, the former 3 largely dictated by the extent of tumor invasion into adjacent vascular structures.[18] A rapid autopsy series from Johns Hopkins implies that 70% of patients develop miliary metastatic disease, 18% develop oligometastatic, and 12% remain locally advanced.[20] In those patients with potentially and borderline resectable disease, en bloc, oncologic resection by either Whipple, distal, or total pancreatectomy is usually attempted first, followed by adjuvant chemotherapy with either gemcitabine or 5-fluorouracil (5-FU)-based chemotherapy, although preoperative neoadjuvant therapy is used in some centers.[21–23] Patients with borderline resectable and locally advanced tumors are usually offered chemotherapy, sometimes in the context of a clinical trial, with rare downstaging to resectability.[23,24]

PDAC management should be in specialized centers, because surgical volume and perioperative mortality are strongly correlated.[25] Standard chemotherapy is gemcitabine, although recent trials suggest potentially greater (albeit slight) benefit with FOLFIRINOX[17,23,26,27] or the combination of gemcitabine with either nab-paclitaxel[28] or erlotinib[29] in the metastatic setting. The role of radiation therapy is less clear.[30] When patients are optimally managed, median survival for potentially resectable cases is 18 to 24 months, borderline resectable 14 to 20 months, locally advanced 6 to 12 months, and metastatic 3 to 9 months.[12,13]

RISK FACTORS

Risk factors for PDAC can be divided into 2 groups, namely environmental and genetic, the latter being either low penetrant, common variants, or more highly penetrant, rare variants.

Numerous putative associations of PDAC with lifestyle factors have been reported in older literature. More recently, 2 large groups, the Pancreatic Cancer Case-Control Consortium (PanC4) and the Pancreatic Cancer Cohort Consortium (PanScan), have carried out methodologically rigorous epidemiologic studies on PDAC risk, and their results are concordant. These studies have shown only a few consistent modifiable risk factors for PDAC (**Table 1**). These studies are briefly reviewed here, relying mostly on the results of the PanC4 analyses in which the authors' group was involved.

Table 1
Odds ratios for modifiable factors associated with pancreatic ductal adenocarcinoma risk

Factor	Condition	OR (95% CI)
Smoking	Current smokers	2.2 (1.7–2.8)
Pancreatitis	Diagnosed 2 or more years before PDAC diagnosis	2.71 (1.96–3.74)
Alcohol	>9 drinks/day	1.6 (1.2–2.2)
Obesity	BMI >35	1.55 (1.16–2.07)
DM2	Diagnosed 2 or more years before PDAC diagnosis	1.90 (1.72–2.09)
Allergies	Hay fever or animals	0.73 (0.64–0.84)

Smoking is the most established environmental risk factor, and smoking cessation is the only evidence-based PDAC preventative measure. Compared with never smokers, PanC4 found an odds ratio (OR) of 1.2 (95% confidence interval [CI] 1.0 to 1.3) for former smokers and 2.2 (95% CI 1.7–2.8) for current cigarette smokers, with increasing risk with increasing number of cigarettes smoked and increasing duration of cigarette smoking up to 40 years.[31,32] Risk decreased with increasing time since cigarette smoking cessation, returning to baseline 20 years after quitting.[31,32] There is also evidence that second-hand smoke exposure (OR 1.21 [95% CI 0.60–2.44])[33] and cigar smoking[34] also increases the risk of PDAC, although inconsistent associations have been found for pipe smoking and smokeless tobacco.[34]

Diabetes mellitus type 2 (DM2) is a risk factor for PDAC.[35] The association is strongest when DM2 is diagnosed within 2 years of PDAC but persists in those diagnosed 2 or more years before PDAC development. The risk is independent of other factors, including body mass index (BMI) and tobacco smoking. Interestingly, risk decreases with duration of diabetes but never reaches baseline, with an OR of 1.30 (95% CI 1.03–1.63) 20 or more years after diabetes diagnosis. Use of oral hypoglycemics for more than 15 years is protective (OR 0.31, 95% CI 0.14–0.69), while insulin use is associated with increased risk (OR 2.66, 95% CI 2.07–3.43), although not for 10 or more years' duration, implying reverse causation and strongly linked covariates in this association. Thus, although DM2 diagnosed within 2 years of a PDAC diagnosis may be a consequence of the growing neoplasm (so-called Type3c DM), there is little doubt that diabetics are at increased risk for PDAC, the biological mechanism of which may be increased circulating levels of mitogenic insulin due to peripheral insulin resistance.[36,37]

Pancreatitis and PDAC are associated conditions. The strength of the association is less at diagnostic intervals of greater than 2 years (OR: 2.71, 95% CI: 1.96–3.74) compared with intervals of less than 2 years (OR: 13.56, 95% CI: 8.72–21.90), probably due to both reverse causation and misdiagnosis of PDAC as pancreatitis. At intervals of greater than 2 years, the population attributable fraction is only 1.34% (95% CI: 0.612%–2.07%). Thus, while the inflammation of pancreatitis does likely predispose to PDAC, it accounts for only a small proportion of cases.[37]

There is no association between occasional (<1 drink per day) and moderate (≤4 drinks per day) alcohol consumption and PDAC risk. Heavy alcohol consumption (≥6 drinks per day) does increase risk, independently of type of drink, duration of drinking, tobacco smoking, history of pancreatitis, or race.[38,39]

Severe obesity (BMI >35) and risk of PDAC are positively associated according to a PanScan study (OR 1.55 [95% CI 1.16–2.07]). Although this effect may have been attenuated when controlling for DM2 status, there was nonetheless a significant trend for increasing PDAC risk with increasing BMI (adjusted OR for the highest vs lowest BMI quartile, 1.33; 95% CI, 1.12–1.58; P (trend) <.001).[40] A separate meta-analysis has shown that the estimated summary relative risk of PDAC per 5 point increase in BMI was 1.12 (95% CI 1.06–1.17), and that this was essentially independent of gender.[41]

Previous associations of PDAC with peptic ulcer disease and recent surgery, especially gastrectomy and cholecystectomy, have been disproved by PanC4 analyses.[42] The associations were strongest within 2 years of PDAC diagnosis with no significantly increased risk observed beyond 2 years, strongly suggesting that the previously observed associations were due to increased cancer detection during investigation, misdiagnosis of symptoms caused by PDAC, and treatment of those other conditions.

The authors' group and others have recently provided evidence for a protective association between allergies and PDAC risk.[43,44] Respiratory allergies, especially hay fever (OR = 0.74, 95% CI: 0.56, 0.96), and allergies to animals (OR = 0.62, 95% CI: 0.41, 0.94) are most related to lower risk, while other allergies and asthma may not be protective. Older age at onset of allergies is also slightly more protective than earlier age. However, the mechanism for these associations is unknown, and they do not suggest clinical actionability. Allergy association studies also suffer from recall bias, as most allergies occur in childhood, whereas PDAC occurs in adults.

A hereditary component is implied in up to 10% of PDAC cases given the family history of an affected first-degree relative.[8,45,46] Highly penetrant alleles in known cancer susceptibility genes account for 10% to 15% of familial cases.[8] Characterized genetic conditions are associated with these high penetrance alleles, including the hereditary breast and ovarian cancer syndrome (HBOC), LS, familial adenomatous polyposis (FAP), Peutz-Jeghers syndrome (PJS), familial atypical multiple mole melanoma syndrome (FAMMM), hereditary pancreatitis (HP), cystic fibrosis (CF), and ataxia-telangiectasia (AT) (**Fig. 1**).[7,8] These genetic conditions have been shown to increase the risk of PDAC anywhere from 2- to 132-fold (**Table 2**). The remaining 85% to 90% of cases with strong family histories lack mutations in these aforementioned syndromic cancer genes. These are referred to as familial pancreatic cancer (FPC). Genetic models point toward autosomal-dominant transmission of fairly high penetrant mutations.[9] The syndromes are discussed later.

There are several common, low-penetrant alleles that mediate genetic risk for PDAC in the general population, identified through both genome-wide association studies (GWAS) and candidate gene studies. There have been 8 GWAS for PDAC[47–54] that have identified 43 alleles mapped to 35 genes associated with PDAC risk at genome-wide significance, the ORs of which range from 1.19 (95% CI 1.11–1.27) to 3.73 (95% CI 2.24–6.21). The populations studied include those of European, Chinese, and Japanese ancestry. The most interesting finding has been the rs505922 SNP, an intron in the ABO gene on chromosome 9, with an alternate allele frequency of 0.35. Carriers have an OR of 1.2 (95% CI 1.12–1.28) for PDAC. Subsequent studies have genotyped blood groups in large numbers of cases and controls demonstrating

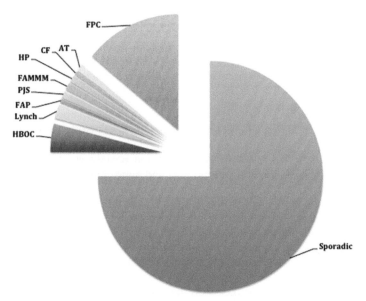

Fig. 1. Pie chart showing approximate attributable fraction of each HPC syndrome to PDAC.

Table 2
Summary of hereditary pancreatic cancer syndromes, including genes, relative risks, and additional cancers associated with each syndrome

Syndrome	Genes	RR for PDAC	Other Associated Cancers
HBOC	BRCA1	2–3	Breast, ovarian, prostate, testicular, melanoma
	BRCA2	3.5	
	PALB2	6	
LS	MLH1, MSH2, MSH6, PMS2, EPCAM	8.5	Colon, endometrium, ovary, stomach, small intestine, urinary tract, brain, cutaneous sebaceous glands
FAP	APC	4.5	Colon, desmoid, duodenum, thyroid, brain, ampullary, hepatoblastoma
PJ	STK11/LKB1	130	Esophagus, stomach, small intestine, colon, lung, breast, uterus, ovary
FAMMM	CDKN2A	13–65	Melanoma
HP	PRSS1, SPINK1	50–70	NA
CF	CFTR biallelic	5.3	NA
	CFTR monoallelic	1.4	
AT	ATM biallelic	NA	Leukemia, lymphoma
	ATM monoallelic	5	
FPC	Unknown	1.8–32	NA

Abbreviations: NA, not applicable; RR, relative risk.

that, compared with blood type O, the ORs for PDAC in subjects with types A, AB, and B blood types were 1.38 (95% CI 1.18–1.62), 1.47 (95% CI 1.07–2.02), and 1.53 (95% CI 1.21–1.92), respectively.[55,56] The population attributable fraction for non-O blood type is 19.5%, remarkably. The mechanism for this association is unknown, though, and does not seem to involve chronic pancreatitis.[57]

Based on epidemiologic studies on environmental and dietary risk factors for PDAC, several candidate gene studies have sequenced polymorphisms in genes involved in carcinogen metabolism, insulin signaling, inflammation, DNA repair, and metabolism of alcohol, folate, and Vitamin D, but these have not yielded consistent results of alleles associated with PDAC risk and outcome.[58] A thorough review of these is beyond the scope of this article, but a good resource is found in the references.[58]

PATHOLOGY

Greater than 90% of invasive tumors of the pancreas arise from the exocrine component of the gland.[59,60] These invasive tumors comprise many different histologic types, including typical PDAC, serous cystadenocarcinoma, acinar cell carcinoma, pancreatoblastoma, solid pseudopapillary carcinoma, and many rarer types. Of these, PDAC is the most common, comprising more than 80% of cases, and the one which is discussed further here.[59,60]

The anatomic site of disease is relevant to management, and tumors are divided into those arising in the head and uncinate process (ie, to the right of the superior mesenteric vein), those arising in the body (ie, between the superior mesenteric vein and the aorta), and those arising in the tail of the pancreas (between the aorta and the hilum of the spleen).[61,62]

Histologic grade is assigned based on the extent of glandular differentiation, with grade 1 composed of greater than 95% glands, grade 2 composed of 50% to 95%

glands, grade 3 composed of 49% or less glands, and grade 4 only in rare, tiny glandular foci.[61] Separate groups have shown that higher grades are prognostic for worse outcomes,[63–67] although the definitions used to grade tumors were not consistent across their studies.

Pathologic staging is most commonly done according to the AJCC TNM.[61,62] The T stage is based on tumor size and on involvement of the arterial celiac axis, because both are prognostic factors.[67–71] The N stage is based only on the presence or absence of regional lymph node metastases, as these are prognostic factors, although most studies have shown that the absolute number and the ratio of positive to total lymph nodes are more informative for outcome than a dichotomous N stage.[67,70–76] The M stage is based on distant metastases, including peritoneal seeding and malignant ascitic fluid.[61,62] The aggregate of T, N, and M scores determines overall stage.

Pancreatic intraepithelial neoplasias (PanIN) are noninvasive, dysplastic lesions often present in PDAC resection specimens that sometimes blend with the tumor, and hence, they are presumed to be precursor lesions. They have been classed into types 1A, 1B, 2, and 3 (ie, carcinoma in situ) according to their degree of dysplasia and papillary architecture and are presumed to progress linearly through these stages from normal epithelium to invasive malignancy.[60,77] There is evidence that worsening PanIN morphology is associated with increasing numbers of somatic mutations in cancer-associated genes in the PanIN itself.[78] Two other precursor lesions for PDAC have also been proposed, namely, intraductal papillary mucinous neoplasms (IPMN) and mucinous cystadenomas (MCA), which presumably progress to invasive disease by distinct pathways from PanINs, the details of which are beyond the scope of this review.[59–62]

PDAC arising in HPC syndrome carriers may be associated with distinct pathologic abnormalities.

Two series have shown that resected PDAC in FPC cases have greater numbers of PanIN lesions relative to sporadic cases,[79] particularly PanIN 3.[45]

No unique histologic features are strongly associated with PDAC in the setting of HBOC. Cases of acinar cell carcinoma have been reported in BRCA1 variant carriers.[80,81]

PDAC in LS patients may have characteristic histologic features. Case series have shown that PDAC with microsatellite instability are more often poorly differentiated with expanding borders and a syncytial growth pattern, so-called medullary phenotype by some authors.[60,82–84] In contrast with microsatellite unstable colorectal cancers, neither Crohn-like lymphoid infiltrate nor extracellular mucin production is prominent in these PDAC.[83] Molecular descriptions of microsatellite unstable PDAC compared with sporadic tumors are lacking, although they have been noted in small series to be KRAS wild type with diploid genomes.[82,83] Not all PDAC with medullary histology are microsatellite unstable,[60,83] however, and, due to their rarity, the yield of germline testing for germline mismatch repair genes in a large sample of medullary cases is unknown. Also, cases of acinar cell carcinoma have been reported in LS patients as well.[81]

PDAC in PJS and FAP patients may arise via IPMN precursors[85] rather than via PanIN precursors. There are sparse clinical and molecular reports that suggest an association between PJS and IPMN[86,87] and FAP and IPMN,[88–90] including some by the authors' institution, but this has unfortunately not been studied in large PJS or FAP cohorts due to the compounded rarities of PJS, FAP, and IPMN. Targeted sequencing of IPMN specimens has not revealed a high frequency of STK11 or APC somatic mutations.[91–94]

HEREDITARY SYNDROMES ASSOCIATED WITH PANCREATIC DUCTAL ADENOCARCINOMA
Overall

Most studies find familial clustering in up to 10% of PDAC cases, defined as having 2 affected first-degree relatives,[8,45,95] although multicenter, population-based series[96,97] that considered only medically proven PDAC diagnoses have shown familial clustering in only 1% to 3% and a meta-analysis of 9 studies places the population attributable fraction at approximately 1%.[98] In up to 15% of these, a known cancer susceptibility gene cosegregates with the disease, and those are reviewed here (see **Fig. 1**), collectively referred to as HPC syndromes. The cause in the remaining 85% to 90% of families is unknown, and these are referred to as FPC. The clustering in these families may be due to shared genetic factors, common environmental factors, or random chance,[99] although an inherited genetic factor is thought to be the primary cause[99] based on family, twin, case-control, and cohort studies.[95,100] Segregation analysis of 287 PDAC families estimated that 3 in every 500 individuals carry a predisposing germline allele with high penetrance for PDAC, with corresponding 32% risk of PDAC by age 85.[95]

Most studies of the prevalence, penetrance, and clinicopathologic features of HPC syndrome germline variants in PDAC focus on specific subsets of PDAC patients, based on ethnicity or particular family histories, and consider only one or several syndromes given the limits of sample size and cost of genetic testing. It is from such studies that nearly all of the information presented herein is derived, summarized in **Table 2**.

With the maturity of high-risk registries, biorepositories, and next-generation sequencing technologies, multigene testing by targeted panels of large PDAC cohorts is now possible, allowing better estimates of the role of HPC syndromes in PDAC. The authors recently published a study on PDAC using stratified random sampling to select 290 probands and found a prevalence of 3.8% (95% CI 2.1–5.6) of HPC syndrome variants in their population-based registry in the province of Ontario, Canada.[101] Although the stratification was designed to minimize the variance estimate of BRCA1 and BRCA2 prevalence, they were surprised to find a prevalence of LS nearly as high as that of HBOC in their study.

The authors have subsequently completed BRCA testing on an unselected, consecutively, and prospectively collected cohort of 306 clinic-based patients[102] showing that 4.6% of PDAC patients have pathogenic BRCA1 or BRCA2 germline variants.

As the current knowledge of each syndrome is reviewed, it is worth emphasizing that with increased adoption of next-generation sequencing by clinical laboratories and increased recognition of the value of genetic testing for those with cancer diagnoses, the currently accepted, well-established phenotypes of hereditary cancer syndromes described in later discussion will likely expand, and prevalence and penetrance estimates will change.

Hereditary Breast and Ovarian Cancer Syndrome

HBOC syndrome is caused by germline heterozygous inactivation of BRCA1, BRCA2, or PALB2 genes. These tumor suppressor genes code for proteins involved in double-stranded DNA break repair.

Pathogenic BRCA1 and BRCA2 alleles have a high penetrance for ovarian cancers in women (24% and 8.4% by age 80 for BRCA1 and BRCA2, respectively), breast cancers in women (90% and 41% by age 80 for BRCA1 and BRCA2, respectively), and breast cancers in men (1.2% and 6.8% for BRCA1 and BRCA2, respectively).[103] An example of a BRCA2 pedigree is provided in **Fig. 2**. Germline PALB2 variants have also been associated with increased relative risk of breast cancer.[104]

The prevalence of pathogenic germline BRCA1 and BRCA2 variants in the general population is 1 in 400[105,106] combined, two-thirds of which is BRCA2 and one-third of which is BRCA1, while in the Ashkenazi Jewish (AJ) population, it is 1 in 40[107,108] combined. Those Ashkenazi founder mutations include the BRCA1 185delAG,[109,110] the BRCA1 5382ins,[111] and the BRCA2 6174delT.[107,110,111]

Prevalence estimates in PDAC patients vary widely in the literature due to small sample sizes, retrospective cohorts, selective inclusion criteria (eg, by race), and limited genetic testing (eg, only specific alleles). The reported prevalence of deleterious BRCA2 germline mutations ranges from 5% to 20% in FPC kindreds[112–114] and 7% in sporadic PDAC.[115] The prevalence of the BRCA1 and BRCA2 founder mutations in a series of AJ with PDAC was found to range from 1% to 8% and 4% to 12%, respectively.[116,117] As stated above, the authors found a prevalence of 4.6% for BRCA1 and BRCA2 germline pathogenic variants in 306 unselected, consecutive, clinic-based PDAC patients (1% BRCA1, 3.6% BRCA2).[102] Although this is lower than previous estimates, it is likely more accurate given the larger sample size and unbiased study design.

BRCA1/2 are also part of the Fanconi anemia gene family, and thus, biallelic defects give rise to the recessive Fanconi anemia phenotype described in later discussion.

Some series have shown that heterozygous BRCA1 germline carriers have 2 to 3 times the risk of PDAC relative to the general population,[118,119] whereas other studies have not shown an increased relative risk.[120,121]

There is no disagreement in the literature that BRCA2 heterozygous germline carriers are at increased risk for PDAC, with a roughly 3.5 relative risk (range 2.3–7 across studies).[103,122–125] Given its high prevalence, BRCA2 is the most frequent inherited risk factor for PDAC.[112,114]

Age of PDAC onset has not been consistently shown to be earlier in BRCA1 and BRCA2 carriers compared with the general population.[101,126]

Pathogenic germline variants in PALB2 were recently found to increase risk of PDAC,[127] and this has been validated by some other groups[127,128,130] but not by all.[131] The prevalence of PALB2 in PDAC is likely quite low, as these studies have shown, estimated at less than 3% of FPC kindreds.[127–130] Notably, no deleterious PALB2 variants were found in the authors' targeted sequencing study.[101] The relative risk of PDAC in PALB2 carriers may be as high as 6 times[132] according to one study.

Because BRCA2 and PALB2 are Fanconi anemia genes, germline variants in other Fanconi anemia genes have been investigated in familial PDAC. The largest efforts

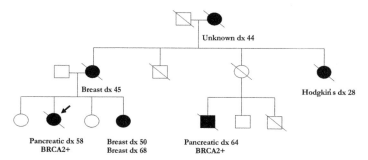

Fig. 2. Pedigree of family with BRCA2 variant cosegregating with HBOC syndrome spectrum malignancies. Arrow, proband. BRCA2+, confirmed germline carriers; breast, breast cancer; dx, age at diagnosis; Hodgkin's, Hodgkin lymphoma; Pancreatic, pancreatic ductal adenocarcinomas.

have been in FANCA, FANCC, and FANCG.[133–136] The current consensus is that there is not sufficient evidence to attribute increased PDAC risk to germline variants in these genes.

Lynch Syndrome

This syndrome is caused by heterozygous germline inactivation of any of 4 genes in the mismatch repair pathway, namely, MLH1, MSH2, MSH6, and PMS2, or by deletions of the EPCAM gene.[137] The latter results in hypermethylation of the MSH2 promoter, silencing one copy of MSH2.[138]

The penetrance of cancer phenotypes in LS patients varies considerably, but it is 50% to 80% for colorectal, 25% to 60% for endometrial, 5% to 15% for gastric, 5% to 10% for ovarian cancer, 3% to 6% for small bowel, 1% to 10% for dermatologic, and 1% to 4% for urothelial cancers, overall.[139] The variable penetrance is partly dependent on which specific gene is inactivated and also partly attributed to other germline variants that act as genetic modifiers of cancer risk.[140]

LS syndrome has a high population prevalence, estimated at 1:440.[141] The authors' retrospective study suggested that the prevalence of LS in PDAC was nearly as high as that of HBOC.[101] Before the retrospective study, only 2 studies had sequenced mismatch repair (MMR) genes in PDAC cohorts sampled for ethnicity[142] and family history,[143] and they are thus not directly comparable.

Biallelic MMR defects lead to constitutional mismatch repair deficiency syndrome (CMMRDS). Carriers develop primary tumors of the central nervous system and hematopoetic system in childhood. No cases of PDAC have been reported in CMMRDS.

LS carriers have up to 8.5 times the relative risk of PDAC,[144,145] although estimates in the literature do vary. Given their comparable relative risks and population-based prevalence, it is perhaps not surprising that the frequency of LS in the authors' randomly sampled cohort of PDAC patients was nearly equal to that of HBOC.[101] The relative risk for PDAC may depend on the inactivated MMR gene, as with other LS spectrum malignancies, but there is currently no evidence of this variability.

The age of onset of PDAC in LS patients has not been consistently shown to be earlier compared with sporadic PDAC cases.[101,145]

Germline variants in other MMR pathway genes have neither been consistently associated with LS in general nor with PDAC specifically.

Familial Adenomatous Polyposis

This syndrome is caused by heterozygous germline inactivation of the APC gene, which is responsible for β-catenin degradation and microtubule stability.[139]

The penetrance for colorectal cancer depends on the germline variant. The phenotype is divided into classic (∼90%) and attenuated (∼10%) depending on the number of colonic polyps detected, and the colonic phenotype is associated with germline variants in specific regions of the APC gene. In classic FAP, adenomas develop by the age of 20 and colorectal cancer by the age of 40 in 100% of carriers.[139] In attenuated FAP, median age at CRC diagnosis is ∼50 years, and the penetrance is estimated at 70% by age 80 years.[146] All carriers are also at risk for malignancies in extracolonic tissues, including soft tissue, duodenum, thyroid, brain, ampulla, and liver.[139]

The estimated prevalence of FAP is 2 to 3 per 100,000.[139,147]

FAP patients have roughly 4.5 times relative risk of periampullary malignancies, mostly duodenal or ampullary cancers, but also PDAC.[148] Increased risk of PDAC in attenuated FAP has not been shown, but presumably it is similar to classic FAP as with other extracolonic features, such as desmoid tumors and periampullary neoplasia.

The age of onset of PDAC in FAP has not been shown to be earlier compared with sporadic PDAC cases.

Although approximately 25% of patients with an FAP phenotype do not have known germline variants in APC, other genes have not been found to cause FAP.[139]

Peutz-Jeghers Syndrome

This syndrome is caused by heterozygous germline inactivation in the STK11/LKB1 gene, a serine-threonine kinase whose exact function is not well described but may have to do with mammalian target of rapamycin activity.[149]

The penetrance for all associated malignancies is 93% by the age of 64, including esophageal, stomach, small intestine, colon, pancreas, lung, breast, uterus, and ovarian cancers, and 100% penetrance for gastrointestinal hamartomas and mucocutaneous pigmentation.[150,151]

Population prevalence estimates range widely from 1:25,000 to 1:280,000. PJS occurs in all racial or ethnic groups.

PJS has a roughly 130 times relative risk of PDAC,[150,151] the highest of any predisposition syndrome, although its rarity makes its frequency in a randomly sampled PDAC cohort quite low. The lifetime risk of PDAC in PJS ranges from 11% to 32%.[151]

Pathogenic germline variants in STK11/LKB1 account for up to 80% of individuals with a clinical diagnosis of PJS.[152] However, no other predisposing genetic locus has been identified or associated with either PJS or PJS and PDAC specifically.

Familial Atypical Multiple Mole Melanoma Syndrome

It is estimated that 40% of cases of this syndrome are caused by heterozygous germline inactivation of the CDKN2A gene, which encodes the p16^{INK4A} protein that functions in cell-cycle regulation.[153,154]

The penetrance for malignant melanoma in p16 carriers is 60% to 90% by the age of 80 years.[154–156]

The prevalence of CDKN2A in PDAC is quite low and hence poorly estimated.[157] There is a Dutch founder mutation, named p16-Leiden, which is a 19-base-pair deletion in exon 2 of the CDKN2A gene.[155]

The relative risk for PDAC in FAMMM carriers has been reported in small series and ranges broadly from 13- to 65-fold.[155,158,159] Many series suggest that different CDKN2A variants have different penetrance for PDAC, explaining that only 60% develop PDAC.[160,161] There are reported CDKN2A kindreds with PDAC and no history of melanoma.[162] Those with the p16-Leiden founder allele have a 17% risk of developing PDAC by age 75.[155] The risk of PDAC is greater in smokers.[162]

FAMMM due to germline variants in other genes, including CDK4 and MITF, has not been associated with increased PDAC risk.

Hereditary Pancreatitis

This syndrome is caused by germline variants in PRSS1 and SPINK1 genes. PRSS1 encodes trypsinogen, and SPINK1 encodes a trypsin inhibitor. The pathogenic germline variants result in either premature activation or reduced inhibition of the digestive trypsin enzyme, leading to pancreatic injury.[163] Pathogenic PRSS1 alleles follow an autosomal-dominant mode of inheritance,[163] while SPINK1 alleles may follow autosomal-recessive inheritance.[164,165] The exact mechanisms of action are unclear, and germline variants in these genes interact with other genetic and environmental factors to precipitate pancreatitis in ways that are outside the scope of this review.[163,165]

As a result of these [epi]genetic and environmental modifiers, the penetrance of pancreatitis ranges from 40% to 90% in different studies.[166,167]

The population prevalence of HP has been estimated at 3 in 1,000,000,[167] and the frequency of PRSS1 and SPINK1 germline variants in unselected patients with chronic or idiopathic pancreatitis can be as high as 2% to 4%.[163]

HP patients have a 50 to 70 times relative risk for PDAC compared with the general population.[163,168,169] That risk has been shown to be as much as double in HP patients who are also current smokers.[170]

It is estimated that 30% to 40% of HP carriers develop PDAC by age 70 years.[163,169,170] The age of onset of PDAC in HP patients has been shown to be lower by as much as 20 years from the average in current smokers.[170]

Other genes have been associated with HP, but an associated risk of PDAC is not as well described.[163]

Cystic Fibrosis

This syndrome is caused by biallelic inactivating variants in the CFTR gene, which codes for a plasma membrane ion transporter. Its complete inactivation leads to thickened mucous that obstructs hollow viscera causing recurrent disease of the exocrine pancreas, intestine, respiratory tract, male genital tract, hepatobiliary system, and exocrine sweat glands. There is poor genotype-phenotype correlation, implying both modifier genes and environmental factors; these are poorly described.[171]

More than 2000 variants in CFTR have been described, of which less than 150 are likely to be pathogenic. Most of these alleles are fully penetrant.[172]

The carrier frequency for CFTR varies with ethnic group, being highest in Northern Europeans and AJ at roughly 1:30, resulting in a disease incidence of 1 in 3200 live births in these groups.[173,174]

The relative risk of PDAC in CF is 5.3 times that of the general population.[175] However, the prevalence of PDAC in CF is quite low given that the overall median survival in CF is only 36 years.[175] The relative risk of PDAC in CFTR variant carriers is 1.4 times that of the general population.[176] Other studies have failed to show an association between monoallelic CFTR variant carriers and PDAC risk.[177]

The age of onset of PDAC is much lower in CF patients, with a median of 35 years.[175] The age of onset in CFTR variant carriers is also lower, with a median of 62 years, or 60 years in those who are also smokers.[176]

Ataxia Telangiectasias

This syndrome is caused by biallelic germline inactivation of the ATM gene that codes for a serine/threonine kinase involved in repair of DNA double-stranded breaks.[178]

Biallelic inactivation is thought to be fully penetrant for the clinical phenotypes of neurologic disorders, blood vessel abnormalities, immune system dysfunction, sensitivity to ionizing radiation, and primary hematologic malignancies.[178] Monoallelic inactivation is associated with an increased risk of malignancy, especially breast cancer, for which the penetrance in carriers of ATM protein truncating variants has been reported at 60% by age 80 years.[179]

The prevalence of biallelic inactivation is 1 in 40,000 to 1 in 100,000 live births,[178] and this prevalence varies with the degree of consanguinity in a country. The prevalence of monoallelic inactivation is estimated at 0.5% to 1%.[178,180] The prevalence of monoallelic ATM inactivation in PDAC probands has been reported to be as high as 2.4%.[181]

The relative risk of PDAC in monoallelic carriers is twice that of the general population. The association of PDAC with monoallelic ATM inactivation carriers was first suspected in population and family-based studies[182–184] and then validated by a recent sequencing study in an FPC cohort.[181] The high frequency of monoallelic ATM inactivation and the low frequency of PDAC in the general population imply that the PDAC risk in monoallelic carriers is modified by either environmental or other genetic factors that remain to be discovered.

Familial Pancreatic Cancer

This syndrome is defined as pedigrees with 2 or more first-degree relatives with PDAC in the absence of a known genetic cause. An example of such a pedigree is provided in **Fig. 3**.

The syndrome is quite prevalent, accounting for as many as 90% of familial cases or up to 10% of all PDAC cases.[45,99]

One of the largest studies showed that the relative risk of PDAC for first-degree relatives of FPC cases is 9 times greater than it is among first-degree relatives of sporadic PDAC cases.[95] The risk is proportional to the number of first-degree relatives with PDAC, increasing with 1 (4.6; CI, 0.5–16.4), 2 (6.4; CI, 1.8–16.4), or 3 (32.0; 95% CI, 10.2–74.7) first-degree relatives with PDAC.[95] However, a meta-analysis[98] of 9 studies found a relative risk of 1.80 (95% CI: 1.48–2.12) regardless of the degree of relatedness, and 1.71 (1.37–2.05) when stratified for those with affected first-degree relatives, indicating that there is a range in observed risk in different studies and that shared, nongenetic factors may account for some of the risk. In fact, smoking has been shown to be an independent risk factor in FPC.[185]

Most series have not found a significant difference in age at diagnosis.[45,101,186,187] Nevertheless, some series have shown genetic anticipation of PDAC across generations of FPC pedigrees, with PDAC onset approximately 10 years earlier than in affected parents in roughly 70% of pedigrees.[45,128,187]

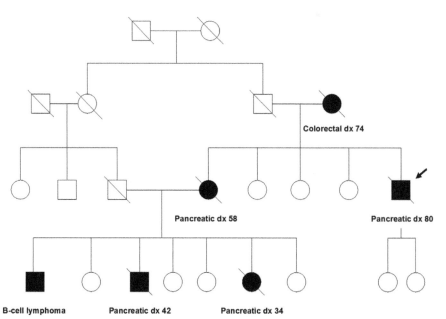

Fig. 3. Pedigree of a FPC family without known deleterious allele in a known germline PDAC predisposition gene. Arrow, proband. Colorectal, colorectal cancer; dx, age at diagnosis; Pancreatic, pancreatic ductal adenocarcinomas.

Genetic modeling suggests an autosomal-dominant, high-penetrant allele responsible for the syndrome.[99] The probability of extrapancreatic malignancies in relatives of FPC probands is greater than in relatives of sporadic PDAC probands, particularly melanoma and endometrial cancer in one study, although a personal history of malignancy is not.[45]

Linkage analysis of a large American FPC pedigree showed significant linkage (logarithm of odds score 5.36) in the region of chromosome 4q32-34.[188] A subsequent study identified a missense allele in the PALLD (palladin) gene as cosegregating with disease in this pedigree,[189] but neither this linkage result[190] nor this variant[191,192] has been validated by other groups. No other candidates have been put forward since, and all available unpublished and preliminary data point toward marked genetic heterogeneity in FPC, although non-coding variants and epigenetic effects have not been explored to date.

STRATEGIES FOR THE IDENTIFICATION OF MUTATION CARRIERS

The principal strategy for identifying HPC syndrome carriers is by taking a family history at the time of cancer diagnosis. PDAC is often managed in tertiary care centers[193] where physicians are acutely aware of the significance of HPC syndromes, and genetic counselors are available to coordinate testing and provide patient education.[194] In the United States, guidelines have recently been published by the American College of Medical Genetics and Genomics (ACMG) and the National Society of Genetic Counselors (NSGC) on indications for referral for cancer predisposition assessment based on history obtained at the time of PDAC diagnosis.[195] These guidelines are presented in **Table 3**. Genetic counseling and testing should be offered at the time of diagnosis because identification of an HPC syndrome may inform treatment (see later discussion) and is crucially important given the high overall mortality of PDAC.

Note that the ACMG guidelines apply to PDAC patients at any age of diagnosis. The conspicuous lack of an earlier age of diagnosis of PDAC in HPC syndrome carriers, despite their inherited predisposition, means that often the HPC syndrome is

Table 3
Indications for referral for cancer predisposition assessment at the time of pancreatic ductal adenocarcinoma diagnosis by the American College of Medical Genetics and Genomics and the National Society of Genetic Counselors

Criteria	Most Likely Syndrome
Two or more cases of PDAC in close relatives	HBOC
Two or more cases of breast, ovarian, or aggressive prostate cancer in close relatives	HBOC
AJ ancestry	HBOC
History of PJ polyp in the same patient	PJS
Two or more additional cases of LS-associated cancer (see **Table 2**) in the same patient or close relatives	LS
Three or more cases of PDAC or melanoma in close relatives	FAMMM
History of melanoma in the same patient	FAMMM

Adapted from Hampel H, Bennett RL, Buchanan A, et al, Guideline Development Group, American College of Medical Genetics and Genomics Professional Practice and Guidelines Committee and National Society of Genetic Counselors Practice Guidelines Committee. A practice guideline from the American College of Medical Genetics and Genomics and the National Society of Genetic Counselors: referral indications for cancer predisposition assessment. Genet Med 2015;17(1):70–87.

diagnosed in the patient or their family before PDAC. Characteristic family histories of malignancy imply specific inherited cancer syndromes, and criteria for testing based on these histories exist in various jurisdictions. Many HPC syndromes also involve distinct phenotypes that lead to their identification early in the life of the carrier.

The most notable exception to this with regards to PDAC is HBOC. It has been well documented that BRCA carriers may have no personal history of extrapancreatic malignancy, and that, despite not being de novo carriers, their family history is similarly not suspicious for BRCA deficiency,[112–115] even in high-risk groups like AJ.[196] It has been shown, in the authors' prospective, unselected series of 306 PDAC patients, that although having a significant cancer family history or self-reporting as AJ is significantly associated with BRCA mutation status in an unselected group of PDAC patients, most BRCA mutation-positive cases do not meet current genetic testing criteria.[102] The authors found that 12% of AJ PDAC patients had germline BRCA1 and 2 mutations, a rate consistent with previous series,[116,117] and that all of the mutations were known AJ founders. It is therefore suggested that all PDAC patients of AJ ancestry be offered BRCA1 and 2 testing for the founder mutations as discussed earlier. To identify BRCA carriers who are not AJ and lack significant family histories, the authors recommend HBOC testing in all PDAC patients with personal or family histories of breast cancer, as explained later. There is insufficient evidence at the current time to make recommendations when to test for PALB2, but it is reasonable to do so when family history strongly implies BRCA1 or 2 but no germline mutations are found.

In the authors' retrospective, stratified sample of 290 PDAC probands,[101] HPC syndrome carrier status was associated with breast cancer in the proband or first-degree relative and with colorectal cancer in the proband or first-degree relative, but not family history of PDAC, age, or stage at diagnosis. Roughly 10% of PDAC patients with a personal or family history of breast or colorectal cancer carried pathogenic HPC syndrome germline variants. These trends are statistically powered by the high prevalence of BRCA and MMR deficiency carriers in the cohort, and for this reason, it is suggested to test all PDAC patients with personal or family histories of breast and colorectal cancer for HBOC and LS, respectively. Notably, no patient with germline MMR deficiency in the authors' series met the Amsterdam II criteria for LS.[101] Less than half of those who tested positive for HPC syndromes in the study satisfied criteria for genetic testing.

Alternative approaches to germline testing include the use of scoring tools to risk stratify carrying HPC syndrome variants. One such tool is PancPRO, a Bayesian prediction model meant to estimate the probability of carrying a PDAC susceptibility gene and the absolute risk of PDAC in people with a family history of the disease.[197] PancPRO was validated in a cohort of more than 6000 individuals from 961 families.

The low prevalence of many of the HPC syndromes precludes their universal testing at the current time. As the cost of genetic sequencing declines, it may soon be cost-efficient to test all PDAC patients for germline mutations even if the yield is low, particularly if this impacts their care, as is discussed later. Although targeted sequencing using multigene panels currently seems to be the most attractive method, based on the authors' experience with these, they agree with current recommendations that gene panels only be used when the family history is consistent with more than one well-established hereditary cancer syndrome.[198] Otherwise, the current standard of care is to sequence individual genes as directed by the family history, known syndromic phenotypes, and guidelines.

The authors' stratified, retrospective gene panel study[101] also identified more than one hundred rare variants of uncertain significance in 13 HPC syndrome genes in their 290 PDAC probands. This study emphasizes the importance of rigorously reporting and annotating rare variants in cancer predisposition genes in publically accessible format, such as the ClinVar[199] and Insight[200] databases.

CLINICAL MANAGEMENT OPTIONS FOR UNAFFECTED MUTATION CARRIERS

The low incidence of PDAC in the general population precludes population-based screening strategies at the current time. Screening is only appropriate in high-risk cohorts in the context of investigational trials. The low relative risks and population attributable fractions associated with modifiable PDAC risk factors (see **Table 1**) make these inappropriate standards for defining high-risk cohorts, either individually or in aggregate. Unaffected HPC syndrome mutation carriers and at-risk members of FPC kindreds thus constitute the main cohort currently undergoing investigational PDAC screening, the goal of which is primary and secondary prevention—detection of precursor lesions or invasive lesions that have yet to gain metastatic potential.

A study of tumor evolution in PDAC suggested a long period of time, perhaps up to 15 years, between the first initiating carcinogenic event and usual clinical presentation of invasive PDAC with a resectable tumor, locally advanced unresectable disease, or metastatic disease.[14] This encouraged novel approaches to hopefully enable early detection and treatment of the disease. Several prospective observational studies have screened high-risk individuals using a combination of circulatory biomarkers, EUS, CT, MRI, or ERCP,[87,201–208] but no group has yet to definitively document that early detection and treatment results in an overall reduction in morbidity and mortality. As the screening modality, starting age, interval, and duration differed in most of these protocols, an attempt was made to arrive at consensus guidelines, as discussed later.

The guidelines by the International Cancer of the Pancreas Screening (CAPS) program suggest the following inclusion criteria for PDAC screening programs: (1) 2 first degree relatives (FDRs) with PDAC; (2) 2 blood relatives with PDAC and at least one FDR; (3) PJS; (4) BRCA2 carriers with one FDR with PDAC or 2 affected family members; (5) PALB2 mutation carriers with at least one FDR with PDAC; (6) p16 mutation carriers (FAMMM) with at least one FDR with PDAC; and (7) LS and one FDR with PDAC. No consensus was reached regarding when to start and stop screening or at what interval to screen.[209]

In the authors' local study, screening started at age 50 years or 10 years less than the youngest age of PDAC diagnosis in a family.[208] Most studies started screening at age 40 to 50 years,[87,201–208] although there is some evidence that diagnostic yield is highest when screening is applied to those aged 65 years or greater.[206]

The principal circulatory biomarker for PDAC is CA19-9, and it is the only one with US Food and Drug Administration approval in PDAC. Serum CA19-9 has a sensitivity of 70% to 80% and specificity of 80% to 90% for PDAC, lower than those of colonoscopy for colorectal cancer or mammography for breast cancer, and too low to endorse its use as a screening tool in either general or high-risk populations.[210,211] A multitude of other diagnostic biomarkers have been proposed, including gene expression profiles, circulating tumor DNA and microRNA, and serum proteins, but none are ready for clinical use.[210]

The principal imaging modalities are EUS and MRI; these have demonstrated the most accuracy for detecting small, cystic lesions.[207,209] However, the main PDAC precursor lesion, the PanIN, is not visible on imaging. One study showed that lobular parenchymal atrophy detected by EUS is associated with the presence of PanINs and IPMNs in the subsequent resection specimen, suggesting that this may act as a surrogate for PanIN detection by EUS.[212] CT subjects patients to radiation and has a suboptimal detection rate compared with EUS and MRI. ERCP is an invasive test with a significant risk of morbidity, particularly of pancreatitis, and is thus not suited for screening.[207,209] The CAPS program specified that EUS and MRI are the ideal screening modalities.[209]

The cost-effectiveness of PDAC screening in high-risk cohorts has been modeled. One study showed that screening was cost-effective if the prevalence of dysplasia was greater than 16% or if the sensitivity of EUS was greater than 84%.[213] Another study modeled strategies for managing 45 year old FDRs of PDAC probands with chronic pancreatitis, finding that "doing nothing" provided the greatest remaining years of life, the lowest cost, and the greatest remaining quality-adjusted life years (QALYs), whereas annual screening with EUS or prophylactic total pancreatectomies provided the fewest remaining years of life and the fewest remaining QALYs, assuming a lifetime risk of cancer of less than 46% in FDRs.[214] Such cost-effectiveness studies suffer from imperfect estimations of risk of dysplasia or invasive disease in high-risk cohorts, as described in earlier discussion, making their analyses dependent on inappropriate estimations.

One must also consider that recent studies have challenged the concept that metastatic spread is a late step in the natural history of PDAC, with both statistical[15] and animal models[215] suggesting early dissemination of disease. Early dissemination of disease may also explain why screening efforts have failed to demonstrate robust improvements in patient outcomes.

Discovery of an HPC syndrome germline variant in a proband also allows their family members the options of genetic counseling and testing for extrapancreatic disease. There are surveillance protocols and risk-reducing interventions appropriate to each syndrome that are beyond the scope of this review (eg, prophylactic mastectomy).

Another approach to primary prevention is total pancreatectomy with islet cell autotransplantation (TPIAT),[216] a procedure first described in 1977 for managing pain-stricken chronic pancreatitis patients. Although TPIAT has not been formally studied as a method to reduce risk of subsequent cancer, a recent expert consensus statement lists very high risk for PDAC as an indication for the procedure.[216] For several reasons, it has not acquired widespread adoption, including lack of evidence on the appropriate timing of surgery, postoperative endocrinopathies, and limited laboratory experience required for performing islet isolation.[216] The latter is quite important for and has been associated with post-operative insulin independence.[217] Although there is a hypothetical concern that occult dysplastic and invasive cells may be transplanted into the liver with this procedure, no post-TPIAT cases of cancer of pancreatic origin have been reported in the liver since the introduction of the procedure.

There have also been studies on dietary practices for primary prevention of PDAC. These studies have described risk reduction with diets high in fruits and vegetables,[218] risk reduction with high daily intake of Vitamin D,[219] and risk increase with diets high in red and processed meat.[220] These studies are generally small and not validated, but it is well established that BMI greater than 35 increases the relative risk of PDAC as discussed earlier.

CLINICAL MANAGEMENT OPTIONS FOR MUTATION CARRIERS DIAGNOSED WITH THE ASSOCIATED DISEASE PHENOTYPE

PDAC arising in HPC syndrome carriers has historically been managed in the same way as sporadic PDAC.

Powered by next-generation sequencing studies of PDAC,[221,222] it is hoped that PDAC associated with HPC syndromes will inform rational tumor subtyping.

BRCA and PALB2 germline pathogenic variants may inform PDAC management. DNA double-stranded break repair deficiency in BRCA- and PALB2-associated PDAC tumors results in characteristic genomic changes, the signature of which has been detected previously in breast and ovarian tumors.[222] In breast and ovarian cancer, deficiencies of double-stranded break repair have been shown to mediate sensitivity to platinum-based chemotherapy and PARP inhibitors in both cell lines[223,224] and clinical series.[225] Although initial, small studies[226,227] of combination therapies in PDAC did not show their superiority over gemcitabine or 5-FU monotherapy, subsequent larger trials[26,228] and meta-analyses[229–232] have shown significantly improved response rates, progression-free survival, and overall survival in unselected PDAC, albeit with increased toxicities. This has since been reported specifically in a BRCA2 germline mutation carrier,[233] in a PALB2 germline mutation carrier,[234] in a BRCA1 and BRCA2 germline deficient PDAC cohort,[235] and in PDAC with significant genomic instability and the double-stranded break repair deficiency signature.[221] Although still quite preliminary, it is hoped that the increased responses detected in meta-analyses of platinum-based chemotherapy were driven by the strength of the responses seen in the double-stranded break repair deficient subset. There is an ongoing trial investigating the addition of PARP inhibitors to maintenance chemotherapy in PDAC[236] as well, with case reports of exceptional responders with BRCA2 germline inactivation.[80,237]

Analysis of ICGC PDAC genome sequencing data has shown that roughly 20% of PDAC bears the double-stranded break repair deficiency signature, of which only half have a germline predisposition variant (Lincoln D. Stein, personal communication, 2015), implying that acquired, somatic processes can give rise to comparable double-stranded break-repair deficiency phenotypes. Analogous to colorectal cancer, then, tumors in germline carriers may be representative of larger subclasses of PDAC, giving hope to the hypothesis that therapies targeted to tumors in germline carriers will be effective in PDAC that acquire similar phenotypes somatically. It is still too early to translate PDAC tumor subtypes into the clinic by the rational use of immunohistochemistry or molecular tests, although it is hoped that this will follow closely.

Most interestingly, it has also been shown that patients with PDAC with MMR deficiency are long-term survivors,[82–84] albeit in small series, and this has also been the authors' anecdotal experience. One might hypothesize that the microsatellite instability phenotype may make this subset of PDAC tumors sensitive to therapies targeted to the defective MMR pathway,[238] such as irinotecan.

SUMMARY

The literature on risk factors for PDAC has been reviewed, showing that modifiable and common genetic risk factors have small effects on PDAC risk, whereas rare, highly penetrant alleles in a small number of genes greatly increase risk of PDAC in carriers. There are emerging strategies to improve screening, tumor subtyping, and targeted therapy for PDAC, all of which are informed by the study of HPC syndrome carriers. Although these strategies have yet to show definitive improvements in PDAC outcomes, there is much hope that they will in the foreseeable future, given the examples of similar successes with other solid organ tumors, including colorectal and breast cancers.

REFERENCES

1. Rahib L, Smith BD, Aizenberg R, et al. Projecting cancer incidence and deaths to 2030: the unexpected burden of thyroid, liver, and pancreas cancers in the United States. Cancer Res 2014;74(11):2913–21 [Erratum appears in Cancer Res 2014;74(14):4006].

2. Nishihara R, Wu K, Lochhead P, et al. Long-term colorectal-cancer incidence and mortality after lower endoscopy. N Engl J Med 2013;369(12): 1095–105.

3. US Preventive Services Task Force. Screening for breast cancer: U.S. Preventive Services Task Force recommendation statement. Ann Intern Med 2009; 151(10):716–26. W-236. [Erratum appears in Ann Intern Med 2010;152(10): 688; and Erratum appears in Ann Intern Med 2010;152(3):199–200].

4. National Lung Screening Trial Research Team, Church TR, Black WC, et al. Results of initial low-dose computed tomographic screening for lung cancer. N Engl J Med 2013;368(21):1980–91.

5. de Koning HJ, Meza R, Plevritis SK, et al. Benefits and harms of computed tomography lung cancer screening strategies: a comparative modeling study for the U.S. Preventive Services Task Force. Ann Intern Med 2014;160(5):311–20.

6. Jenkins MA, Dowty JG, Ait Ouakrim D, et al. Short-term risk of colorectal cancer in individuals with lynch syndrome: a meta-analysis. J Clin Oncol 2015;33(4): 326–31.

7. Becker AE, Hernandez YG, Frucht H, et al. Pancreatic ductal adenocarcinoma: risk factors, screening, and early detection. World J Gastroenterol 2014;20(32): 11182–98.

8. Roberts NJ, Klein AP. Genome-wide sequencing to identify the cause of hereditary cancer syndromes: with examples from familial pancreatic cancer. Cancer Lett 2013;340(2):227–33.

9. Arends MJ. Pathways of colorectal carcinogenesis. Appl Immunohistochem Mol Morphol 2013;21(2):97–102.

10. Ribic CM, Sargent DJ, Moore MJ, et al. Tumor microsatellite-instability status as a predictor of benefit from fluorouracil-based adjuvant chemotherapy for colon cancer. N Engl J Med 2003;349(3):247–57.

11. Siegel R, Ma J, Zou Z, et al. Cancer statistics, 2014. CA Cancer J Clin 2014; 64(1):9–29 [Erratum appears in CA Cancer J Clin 2014;64(5):364].

12. Kanji ZS, Gallinger S. Diagnosis and management of pancreatic cancer. CMAJ 2013;185(14):1219–26.

13. Ryan DP, Hong TS, Bardeesy N. Pancreatic adenocarcinoma. N Engl J Med 2014;371(11):1039–49.

14. Yachida S, Jones S, Bozic I, et al. Distant metastasis occurs late during the genetic evolution of pancreatic cancer. Nature 2010;467(7319):1114–7.

15. Haeno H, Gonen M, Davis MB, et al. Computational modeling of pancreatic cancer reveals kinetics of metastasis suggesting optimum treatment strategies. Cell 2012;148(1–2):362–75.

16. Rhim AD, Mirek ET, Aiello NM, et al. EMT and dissemination precede pancreatic tumor formation. Cell 2012;148(1–2):349–61.

17. Saif MW. Advanced stage pancreatic cancer: novel therapeutic options. Expert Rev Clin Pharmacol 2014;7(4):487–98.

18. McIntyre CA, Winter JM. Diagnostic evaluation and staging of pancreatic ductal adenocarcinoma. Semin Oncol 2015;42(1):19–27.

19. Edge S, Byrd DR, Compton CC, et al, editors. AJCC cancer staging manual. 7th edition. New York: Springer; 2010.

20. Iacobuzio-Donahue CA, Fu B, Yachida S, et al. DPC4 gene status of the primary carcinoma correlates with patterns of failure in patients with pancreatic cancer. J Clin Oncol 2009;27(11):1806–13.

21. Donahue TR, Reber HA. Surgical management of pancreatic cancer-pancreaticoduodenectomy. Semin Oncol 2015;42(1):98–109.

22. Parikh PY, Lillemoe KD. Surgical management of pancreatic cancer-distal pancreatectomy. Semin Oncol 2015;42(1):110–22.

23. Li D, O'Reilly EM. Adjuvant and neoadjuvant systemic therapy for pancreas adenocarcinoma. Semin Oncol 2015;42(1):134–43.

24. Winner M, Goff SL, Chabot JA. Neoadjuvant therapy for non-metastatic pancreatic ductal adenocarcinoma. Semin Oncol 2015;42(1):86–97.

25. Gooiker GA, van Gijn W, Wouters MW, et al, Signalling Committee Cancer of the Dutch Cancer Society. Systematic review and meta-analysis of the volume-outcome relationship in pancreatic surgery. Br J Surg 2011;98(4):485–94.

26. Conroy T, Desseigne F, Ychou M, et al, Groupe Tumeurs Digestives of Unicancer, PRODIGE Intergroup. FOLFIRINOX versus gemcitabine for metastatic pancreatic cancer. N Engl J Med 2011;364(19):1817–25.

27. Papadatos-Pastos D, Thillai K, Rabbie R, et al. FOLFIRINOX—a new paradigm in the treatment of pancreatic cancer. Expert Rev Anticancer Ther 2014;14(10): 1115–25.

28. Von Hoff DD, Ervin T, Arena FP, et al. Increased survival in pancreatic cancer with nab-paclitaxel plus gemcitabine. N Engl J Med 2013;369(18):1691–703.

29. Moore MJ, Goldstein D, Hamm J, et al, National Cancer Institute of Canada Clinical Trials Group. Erlotinib plus gemcitabine compared with gemcitabine alone in patients with advanced pancreatic cancer: a phase III trial of the National Cancer Institute of Canada Clinical Trials Group. J Clin Oncol 2007;25(15): 1960–6.

30. Chuong MD, Boggs DH, Patel KN, et al. Adjuvant chemoradiation for pancreatic cancer: what does the evidence tell us? J Gastrointest Oncol 2014;5(3):166–77.

31. Bosetti C, Lucenteforte E, Silverman DT, et al. Cigarette smoking and pancreatic cancer: an analysis from the International Pancreatic Cancer Case-Control Consortium (Panc4). Ann Oncol 2012;23(7):1880–8 [Erratum appears in Ann Oncol 2012;23(10):2773].

32. Lynch SM, Vrieling A, Lubin JH. Cigarette smoking and pancreatic cancer: a pooled analysis from the pancreatic cancer cohort consortium. Am J Epidemiol 2009;170(4):403–13.

33. Villeneuve PJ, Johnson KC, Mao Y, et al, Canadian Cancer Registries Research Group. Environmental tobacco smoke and the risk of pancreatic cancer: findings from a Canadian population-based case-control study. Can J Public Health 2004;95(1):32–7.

34. Bertuccio P, La Vecchia C, Silverman DT. Cigar and pipe smoking, smokeless tobacco use and pancreatic cancer: an analysis from the International Pancreatic Cancer Case-Control Consortium (PanC4). Ann Oncol 2011; 22(6):1420–6.

35. Bosetti C, Rosato V, Li D. Diabetes, antidiabetic medications, and pancreatic cancer risk: an analysis from the International Pancreatic Cancer Case-Control Consortium. Ann Oncol 2014;25(10):2065–72.

36. Elena JW, Steplowski E, Yu K. Diabetes and risk of pancreatic cancer: a pooled analysis from the pancreatic cancer cohort consortium. Cancer Causes Control 2013;24(1):13–25.

37. Duell EJ, Lucenteforte E, Olson SH. Pancreatitis and pancreatic cancer risk: a pooled analysis in the International Pancreatic Cancer Case-Control Consortium (PanC4). Ann Oncol 2012;23(11):2964–70.

38. Lucenteforte E, La Vecchia C, Silverman D, et al. Alcohol consumption and pancreatic cancer: a pooled analysis in the International Pancreatic Cancer Case-Control Consortium (PanC4). Ann Oncol 2012;23(2):374–82.

39. Michaud DS, Vrieling A, Jiao L, et al. Alcohol intake and pancreatic cancer: a pooled analysis from the pancreatic cancer cohort consortium (PanScan). Cancer Causes Control 2010;21(8):1213–25.

40. Arslan AA, Helzlsouer KJ, Kooperberg C, et al, Pancreatic Cancer Cohort Consortium (PanScan). Anthropometric measures, body mass index, and pancreatic cancer: a pooled analysis from the Pancreatic Cancer Cohort Consortium (PanScan). Arch Intern Med 2010;170(9):791–802.

41. Larsson SC, Orsini N, Wolk A. Body mass index and pancreatic cancer risk: a meta-analysis of prospective studies. Int J Cancer 2007;120(9):1993–8.

42. Bosetti C, Lucenteforte E, Bracci PM, et al. Ulcer, gastric surgery and pancreatic cancer risk: an analysis from the International Pancreatic Cancer Case-Control Consortium (PanC4). Ann Oncol 2013;24(11):2903–10.

43. Cotterchio M, Lowcock E, Hudson TJ, et al. Association between allergies and risk of pancreatic cancer. Cancer Epidemiol Biomarkers Prev 2014;23(3):469–80.

44. Olson SH, Hsu M, Satagopan JM, et al, Pancreatic Cancer Case-Control Consortium. Allergies and risk of pancreatic cancer: a pooled analysis from the Pancreatic Cancer Case-Control Consortium. Am J Epidemiol 2013;178(5): 691–700.

45. Humphris JL, Johns AL, Simpson SH, et al, Australian Pancreatic Cancer Genome Initiative. Clinical and pathologic features of familial pancreatic cancer. Cancer 2014;120(23):3669–75.

46. Klein AP, Beaty TH, Bailey-Wilson JE, et al. Evidence for a major gene influencing risk of pancreatic cancer. Genet Epidemiol 2002;23(2):133–49.

47. Amundadottir L, Kraft P, Stolzenberg-Solomon RZ, et al. Genome-wide association study identifies variants in the ABO locus associated with susceptibility to pancreatic cancer. Nat Genet 2009;41(9):986–90.

48. Petersen GM, Amundadottir L, Fuchs CS, et al. A genome-wide association study identifies pancreatic cancer susceptibility loci on chromosomes 13q22.1, 1q32.1 and 5p15.33. Nat Genet 2010;42(3):224–8.

49. Diergaarde B, Brand R, Lamb J, et al. Pooling-based genome-wide association study implicates gamma-glutamyltransferase 1 (GGT1) gene in pancreatic carcinogenesis. Pancreatology 2010;10(2–3):194–200.

50. Low SK, Kuchiba A, Zembutsu H, et al. Genome-wide association study of pancreatic cancer in Japanese population. PLoS One 2010;5(7):e11824.

51. Wu C, Miao X, Huang L, et al. Genome-wide association study identifies five loci associated with susceptibility to pancreatic cancer in Chinese populations. Nat Genet 2011;44(1):62–6.

52. Willis JA, Olson SH, Orlow I, et al. A replication study and genome-wide scan of single-nucleotide polymorphisms associated with pancreatic cancer risk and overall survival. Clin Cancer Res 2012;18(14):3942–51.

53. Wu C, Kraft P, Stolzenberg-Solomon R, et al. Genome-wide association study of survival in patients with pancreatic adenocarcinoma. Gut 2014;63(1):152–60.

54. Wolpin BM, Rizzato C, Kraft P, et al. Genome-wide association study identifies multiple susceptibility loci for pancreatic cancer. Nat Genet 2014;46(9): 994–1000.

55. Wolpin BM, Kraft P, Gross M, et al. Pancreatic cancer risk and ABO blood group alleles: results from the pancreatic cancer cohort consortium. Cancer Res 2010; 70(3):1015–23.

56. Wolpin BM, Kraft P, Xu M, et al. Variant ABO blood group alleles, secretor status, and risk of pancreatic cancer: results from the pancreatic cancer cohort consortium. Cancer Epidemiol Biomarkers Prev 2010;19(12):3140–9.

57. Greer JB, LaRusch J, Brand RE, et al, NAPS2 Study Group. ABO blood group and chronic pancreatitis risk in the NAPS2 cohort. Pancreas 2011;40(8):1188–94.
58. Lin Y, Yagyu K, Egawa N, et al. An overview of genetic polymorphisms and pancreatic cancer risk in molecular epidemiologic studies. J Epidemiol 2011; 21(1):2–12.
59. Bosman FT, Carneiro F, Hruban RH, et al, editors. World Health Organization, International Agency for Research on Cancer. WHO classification of tumours of the digestive system. 4th edition. Geneva (Switzerland): WHO Press; 2010.
60. Rishi A, Goggins M, Wood LD, et al. Pathological and molecular evaluation of pancreatic neoplasms. Semin Oncol 2015;42(1):28–39.
61. Edge SB, Byrd DR, Carducci MA, et al, editors. AJCC cancer staging manual. 7th edition. New York: Springer; 2009.
62. Compton CC, Byrd DR, Garcia-Aguilar J, et al, editors. AJCC cancer staging Atlas. New York: Springer; 2012.
63. Adsay NV, Basturk O, Bonnett M, et al. A proposal for a new and more practical grading scheme for pancreatic ductal adenocarcinoma. Am J Surg Pathol 2005; 29(6):724–33.
64. Giulianotti PC, Boggi U, Fornaciari G, et al. Prognostic value of histological grading in ductal adenocarcinoma of the pancreas. Klöppel vs TNM grading. Int J Pancreatol 1995;17(3):279–89.
65. Wasif N, Ko CY, Farrell J, et al. Impact of tumor grade on prognosis in pancreatic cancer: should we include grade in AJCC staging? Ann Surg Oncol 2010;17(9): 2312–20.
66. Rochefort MM, Ankeny JS, Kadera BE, et al. Impact of tumor grade on pancreatic cancer prognosis: validation of a novel TNMG staging system. Ann Surg Oncol 2013;20(13):4322–9.
67. Lim JE, Chien MW, Earle CC. Prognostic factors following curative resection for pancreatic adenocarcinoma: a population-based, linked database analysis of 396 patients. Ann Surg 2003;237(1):74–85.
68. Park H, An S, Eo SH, et al. Survival effect of tumor size and extrapancreatic extension in surgically resected pancreatic cancer: proposal for improved T classification. Hum Pathol 2014;45(11):2341–6.
69. Matsumoto G, Muta M, Tsuruta K, et al. Tumor size significantly correlates with postoperative liver metastases and COX-2 expression in patients with resectable pancreatic cancer. Pancreatology 2007;7(2–3):167–73.
70. Moon HJ, An JY, Heo JS, et al. Predicting survival after surgical resection for pancreatic ductal adenocarcinoma. Pancreas 2006;32(1):37–43.
71. Geer RJ, Brennan MF. Prognostic indicators for survival after resection of pancreatic adenocarcinoma. Am J Surg 1993;165(1):68–72 [discussion: 72–3].
72. Garcea G, Dennison AR, Ong SL, et al. Tumour characteristics predictive of survival following resection for ductal adenocarcinoma of the head of pancreas. Eur J Surg Oncol 2007;33(7):892–7.
73. House MG, Gönen M, Jarnagin WR, et al. Prognostic significance of pathologic nodal status in patients with resected pancreatic cancer. J Gastrointest Surg 2007;11(11):1549–55.
74. Pawlik TM, Gleisner AL, Cameron JL, et al. Prognostic relevance of lymph node ratio following pancreaticoduodenectomy for pancreatic cancer. Surgery 2007; 141(5):610–8.
75. Riediger H, Keck T, Wellner U, et al. The lymph node ratio is the strongest prognostic factor after resection of pancreatic cancer. J Gastrointest Surg 2009; 13(7):1337–44.

76. Dusch N, Weiss C, Ströbel P, et al. Factors predicting long-term survival following pancreatic resection for ductal adenocarcinoma of the pancreas: 40 years of experience. J Gastrointest Surg 2014;18(4):674–81.

77. Hruban RH, Adsay NV, Albores-Saavedra J, et al. Pancreatic intraepithelial neoplasia: a new nomenclature and classification system for pancreatic duct lesions. Am J Surg Pathol 2001;25(5):579–86.

78. Hruban RH, Goggins M, Parsons J, et al. Progression model for pancreatic cancer. Clin Cancer Res 2000;6(8):2969–72.

79. Shi C, Klein AP, Goggins M, et al. Increased prevalence of precursor lesions in familial pancreatic cancer patients. Clin Cancer Res 2009;15:7737–43.

80. Lowery MA, Kelsen DP, Stadler ZK, et al. An emerging entity: pancreatic adenocarcinoma associated with a known BRCA mutation: clinical descriptors, treatment implications, and future directions. Oncologist 2011;16(10):1397–402.

81. Lowery MA, Klimstra DS, Shia J, et al. Acinar cell carcinoma of the pancreas: new genetic and treatment insights into a rare malignancy. Oncologist 2011; 16(12):1714–20.

82. Banville N, Geraghty R, Fox E, et al. Medullary carcinoma of the pancreas in a man with hereditary nonpolyposis colorectal cancer due to a mutation of the MSH2 mismatch repair gene. Hum Pathol 2006;37(11):1498–502.

83. Goggins M, Offerhaus GJ, Hilgers W, et al. Pancreatic adenocarcinomas with DNA replication errors (RER+) are associated with wild-type K-ras and characteristic histopathology. Poor differentiation, a syncytial growth pattern, and pushing borders suggest RER+. Am J Pathol 1998;152(6):1501–7.

84. Wilentz RE, Goggins M, Redston M, et al. Genetic, immunohistochemical, and clinical features of medullary carcinoma of the pancreas: a newly described and characterized entity. Am J Pathol 2000;156(5):1641–51.

85. Denost Q, Chafai N, Arrive L, et al. Hereditary intraductal papillary mucinous neoplasm of the pancreas. Clin Res Hepatol Gastroenterol 2012;36(2): e23–5.

86. Sato N, Rosty C, Jansen M, et al. STK11/LKB1 Peutz-Jeghers gene inactivation in intraductal papillary-mucinous neoplasms of the pancreas. Am J Pathol 2001; 159(6):2017–22.

87. Canto MI, Goggins M, Hruban RH, et al. Screening for early pancreatic neoplasia in high-risk individuals: a prospective controlled study. Clin Gastroenterol Hepatol 2006;4(6):766–81 [quiz: 665].

88. Maire F, Hammel P, Terris B, et al. Intraductal papillary and mucinous pancreatic tumour: a new extracolonic tumour in familial adenomatous polyposis. Gut 2002; 51(3):446–9.

89. Chetty R, Salahshor S, Bapat B, et al. Intraductal papillary mucinous neoplasm of the pancreas in a patient with attenuated familial adenomatous polyposis. J Clin Pathol 2005;58(1):97–101.

90. Chetty R, Serra S, Salahshor S, et al. Expression of Wnt-signaling pathway proteins in intraductal papillary mucinous neoplasms of the pancreas: a tissue microarray analysis. Hum Pathol 2006;37(2):212–7.

91. Wu J, Matthaei H, Maitra A, et al. Recurrent GNAS mutations define an unexpected pathway for pancreatic cyst development. Sci Transl Med 2011;3(92):92ra66.

92. Furukawa T, Kuboki Y, Tanji E, et al. Whole-exome sequencing uncovers frequent GNAS mutations in intraductal papillary mucinous neoplasms of the pancreas. Sci Rep 2011;1:161.

93. Takano S, Fukasawa M, Maekawa S, et al. Deep sequencing of cancer-related genes revealed GNAS mutations to be associated with intraductal papillary

mucinous neoplasms and its main pancreatic duct dilation. PLoS One 2014; 9(6):e98718.

94. Amato E, Molin MD, Mafficini A, et al. Targeted next-generation sequencing of cancer genes dissects the molecular profiles of intraductal papillary neoplasms of the pancreas. J Pathol 2014;233(3):217–27.

95. Klein AP, Brune KA, Petersen GM, et al. Prospective risk of pancreatic cancer in familial pancreatic cancer kindreds. Cancer Res 2004;64(7):2634–8.

96. Bartsch DK, Kress R, Sina-Frey M, et al. Prevalence of familial pancreatic cancer in Germany. Int J Cancer 2004;110(6):902–6.

97. Hemminki K, Li X. Familial and second primary pancreatic cancers: a nationwide epidemiologic study from Sweden. Int J Cancer 2003;103(4):525–30.

98. Permuth-Wey J, Egan KM. Family history is a significant risk factor for pancreatic cancer: results from a systematic review and meta-analysis. Fam Cancer 2009;8(2):109–17.

99. Tomasetti C, Vogelstein B. Cancer etiology. Variation in cancer risk among tissues can be explained by the number of stem cell divisions. Science 2015;347(6217): 78–81.

100. Fernandez E, La Vecchia C, D'Avanzo B, et al. Family history and the risk of liver, gallbladder, and pancreatic cancer. Cancer Epidemiol Biomarkers Prev 1994; 3(3):209–12.

101. Grant RC, Selander I, Connor AA, et al. Prevalence of germline mutations in cancer predisposition genes in patients with pancreatic cancer. Gastroenterology 2015;148(3):556–64.

102. Holter S, Borgida A, Dodd A, et al. BRCA Mutations in a Large Clinic-Based Cohort of Patients With Pancreatic Adenocarcinoma. J Clin Oncol 2015. [Epub ahead of print].

103. Risch HA, McLaughlin JR, Cole DE, et al. Population BRCA1 and BRCA2 mutation frequencies and cancer penetrances: a kin-cohort study in Ontario, Canada. J Natl Cancer Inst 2006;98(23):1694–706.

104. Rahman N, Seal S, Thompson D, et al, Breast Cancer Susceptibility Collaboration (UK). PALB2, which encodes a BRCA2-interacting protein, is a breast cancer susceptibility gene. Nat Genet 2007;39(2):165–7.

105. Prevalence and penetrance of BRCA1 and BRCA2 mutations in a population-based series of breast cancer cases. Anglian Breast Cancer Study Group. Br J Cancer 2000;83(10):1301–8.

106. Whittemore AS, Gong G, John EM, et al. Prevalence of BRCA1 mutation carriers among U.S. non-Hispanic Whites. Cancer Epidemiol Biomarkers Prev 2004; 13(12):2078–83.

107. Struewing JP, Hartge P, Wacholder S, et al. The risk of cancer associated with specific mutations of BRCA1 and BRCA2 among Ashkenazi Jews. N Engl J Med 1997;336(20):1401–8.

108. King MC, Marks JH, Mandell JB, New York Breast Cancer Study Group. Breast and ovarian cancer risks due to inherited mutations in BRCA1 and BRCA2. Science 2003;302(5645):643–6.

109. John EM, Miron A, Gong G, et al. Prevalence of pathogenic BRCA1 mutation carriers in 5 US racial/ethnic groups. JAMA 2007;298(24):2869–76.

110. Struewing JP, Abeliovich D, Peretz T, et al. The carrier frequency of the BRCA1 185delAG mutation is approximately 1 percent in Ashkenazi Jewish individuals. Nat Genet 1995;11(2):198–200 [Erratum appears in Nat Genet 1996;12(1):110].

111. Roa BB, Boyd AA, Volcik K, et al. Ashkenazi Jewish population frequencies for common mutations in BRCA1 and BRCA2. Nat Genet 1996;14(2):185–7.

112. Murphy KM, Brune KA, Griffin C, et al. Evaluation of candidate genes MAP2K4, MADH4, ACVR1B, and BRCA2 in familial pancreatic cancer: deleterious BRCA2 mutations in 17%. Cancer Res 2002;62(13):3789–93.
113. Hahn SA, Greenhalf B, Ellis I, et al. BRCA2 germline mutations in familial pancreatic carcinoma. J Natl Cancer Inst 2003;95(3):214–21.
114. Couch FJ, Johnson MR, Rabe KG, et al. The prevalence of BRCA2 mutations in familial pancreatic cancer. Cancer Epidemiol Biomarkers Prev 2007;16(2): 342–6.
115. Goggins M, Schutte M, Lu J, et al. Germline BRCA2 gene mutations in patients with apparently sporadic pancreatic carcinomas. Cancer Res 1996;56(23): 5360–4.
116. Lucas AL, Shakya R, Lipsyc MD, et al. High prevalence of BRCA1 and BRCA2 germline mutations with loss of heterozygosity in a series of resected pancreatic adenocarcinoma and other neoplastic lesions. Clin Cancer Res 2013;19(13): 3396–403.
117. Ferrone CR, Levine DA, Tang LH, et al. BRCA germline mutations in Jewish patients with pancreatic adenocarcinoma. J Clin Oncol 2009;27(3):433–8.
118. Brose MS, Rebbeck TR, Calzone KA, et al. Cancer risk estimates for BRCA1 mutation carriers identified in a risk evaluation program. J Natl Cancer Inst 2002; 94(18):1365–72.
119. Thompson D, Easton DF, Breast Cancer Linkage Consortium. Cancer incidence in BRCA1 mutation carriers. J Natl Cancer Inst 2002;94(18):1358–65.
120. Axilbund JE, Argani P, Kamiyama M, et al. Absence of germline BRCA1 mutations in familial pancreatic cancer patients. Cancer Biol Ther 2009;8(2):131–5.
121. Moran A, O'Hara C, Khan S, et al. Risk of cancer other than breast or ovarian in individuals with BRCA1 and BRCA2 mutations. Fam Cancer 2012;11(2): 235–42.
122. Breast Cancer Linkage Consortium. Cancer risks in BRCA2 mutation carriers. J Natl Cancer Inst 1999;91(15):1310–6.
123. Mersch J, Jackson MA, Park M, et al. Cancers associated with BRCA1 and BRCA2 mutations other than breast and ovarian. Cancer 2015;121(2):269–75.
124. Iqbal J, Ragone A, Lubinski J, et al, Hereditary Breast Cancer Study Group. The incidence of pancreatic cancer in BRCA1 and BRCA2 mutation carriers. Br J Cancer 2012;107(12):2005–9.
125. van Asperen CJ, Brohet RM, Meijers-Heijboer EJ, et al, Netherlands Collaborative Group on Hereditary Breast Cancer (HEBON). Cancer risks in BRCA2 families: estimates for sites other than breast and ovary. J Med Genet 2005;42(9): 711–9.
126. Kim DH, Crawford B, Ziegler J, et al. Prevalence and characteristics of pancreatic cancer in families with BRCA1 and BRCA2 mutations. Fam Cancer 2009; 8(2):153–8.
127. Jones S, Hruban RH, Kamiyama M, et al. Exomic sequencing identifies PALB2 as a pancreatic cancer susceptibility gene. Science 2009;324(5924):217.
128. Slater EP, Langer P, Niemczyk E, et al. PALB2 mutations in European familial pancreatic cancer families. Clin Genet 2010;78(5):490–4.
129. Tischkowitz MD, Sabbaghian N, Hamel N, et al. Analysis of the gene coding for the BRCA2-interacting protein PALB2 in familial and sporadic pancreatic cancer. Gastroenterology 2009;137(3):1183–6.
130. Schneider R, Slater EP, Sina M, et al. German national case collection for familial pancreatic cancer (FaPaCa): ten years experience. Fam Cancer 2011;10(2): 323–30.

131. Harinck F, Kluijt I, van Mil SE, et al. Routine testing for PALB2 mutations in familial pancreatic cancer families and breast cancer families with pancreatic cancer is not indicated. Eur J Hum Genet 2012;20(5):577–9.

132. Casadei S, Norquist BM, Walsh T, et al. Contribution of inherited mutations in the BRCA2-interacting protein PALB2 to familial breast cancer. Cancer Res 2011; 71(6):2222–9.

133. Rogers CD, Couch FJ, Brune K, et al. Genetics of the FANCA gene in familial pancreatic cancer. J Med Genet 2004;41(12):e126.

134. van der Heijden MS, Yeo CJ, Hruban RH, et al. Fanconi anemia gene mutations in young-onset pancreatic cancer. Cancer Res 2003;63(10):2585–8.

135. Rogers CD, van der Heijden MS, Brune K, et al. The genetics of FANCC and FANCG in familial pancreatic cancer. Cancer Biol Ther 2004;3(2):167–9.

136. Couch FJ, Johnson MR, Rabe K, et al. Germ line Fanconi anemia complementation group C mutations and pancreatic cancer. Cancer Res 2005; 65(2):383–6.

137. Lynch HT, Snyder CL, Shaw TG, et al. Milestones of Lynch syndrome: 1895–2015. Nat Rev Cancer 2015;15(3):181–94.

138. Kuiper RP, Vissers LE, Venkatachalam R, et al. Recurrence and variability of germline EPCAM deletions in Lynch syndrome. Hum Mutat 2011;32(4): 407–14.

139. Al-Sukhni W, Aronson M, Gallinger S. Hereditary colorectal cancer syndromes: familial adenomatous polyposis and Lynch syndrome. Surg Clin North Am 2008; 88(4):819–44, vii.

140. Talseth-Palmer BA, Wijnen JT, Grice DM, et al. Genetic modifiers of cancer risk in Lynch syndrome: a review. Fam Cancer 2013;12(2):207–16.

141. Chen S, Wang W, Lee S, et al, Colon Cancer Family Registry. Prediction of germline mutations and cancer risk in the Lynch syndrome. JAMA 2006;296(12): 1479–87.

142. Laitman Y, Herskovitz L, Golan T, et al. The founder Ashkenazi Jewish mutations in the MSH2 and MSH6 genes in Israeli patients with gastric and pancreatic cancer. Fam Cancer 2012;11(2):243–7.

143. Gargiulo S, Torrini M, Ollila S, et al. Germline MLH1 and MSH2 mutations in Italian pancreatic cancer patients with suspected Lynch syndrome. Fam Cancer 2009;8(4):547–53.

144. Kastrinos F, Mukherjee B, Tayob N, et al. Risk of pancreatic cancer in families with Lynch syndrome. JAMA 2009;302(16):1790–5.

145. Geary J, Sasieni P, Houlston R, et al. Gene-related cancer spectrum in families with hereditary non-polyposis colorectal cancer (HNPCC). Fam Cancer 2008; 7(2):163–72.

146. Neklason DW, Stevens J, Boucher KM, et al. American founder mutation for attenuated familial adenomatous polyposis. Clin Gastroenterol Hepatol 2008; 6(1):46–52.

147. Green RC, Green JS, Buehler SK, et al. Very high incidence of familial colorectal cancer in Newfoundland: a comparison with Ontario and 13 other population-based studies. Fam Cancer 2007;6(1):53–62.

148. Giardiello FM, Offerhaus GJ, Lee DH, et al. Increased risk of thyroid and pancreatic carcinoma in familial adenomatous polyposis. Gut 1993;34(10):1394–6.

149. Korsse SE, Peppelenbosch MP, van Veelen W. Targeting LKB1 signaling in cancer. Biochim Biophys Acta 2013;1835(2):194–210.

150. Giardiello FM, Brensinger JD, Tersmette AC, et al. Very high risk of cancer in familial Peutz-Jeghers syndrome. Gastroenterology 2000;119(6):1447–53.

151. van Lier MG, Wagner A, Mathus-Vliegen EM, et al. High cancer risk in Peutz-Jeghers syndrome: a systematic review and surveillance recommendations. Am J Gastroenterol 2010;105(6):1258–64 [author reply: 1265].

152. Olschwang S, Boisson C, Thomas G. Peutz-Jeghers families unlinked to STK11/LKB1 gene mutations are highly predisposed to primitive biliary adenocarcinoma. J Med Genet 2001;38(6):356–60.

153. Foulkes WD, Flanders TY, Pollock PM, et al. The CDKN2A (p16) gene and human cancer. Mol Med 1997;3(1):5–20.

154. Aoude LG, Wadt KA, Pritchard AL, et al. Genetics of familial melanoma: 20 years after CDKN2A. Pigment Cell Melanoma Res 2015;28(2):148–60.

155. Vasen HF, Gruis NA, Frants RR, et al. Risk of developing pancreatic cancer in families with familial atypical multiple mole melanoma associated with a specific 19 deletion of p16 (p16-Leiden). Int J Cancer 2000;87(6):809–11.

156. Goldstein AM, Struewing JP, Chidambaram A, et al. Genotype-phenotype relationships in U.S. melanoma-prone families with CDKN2A and CDK4 mutations. J Natl Cancer Inst 2000;92(12):1006–10.

157. Lynch HT, Brand RE, Hogg D, et al. Phenotypic variation in eight extended CDKN2A germline mutation familial atypical multiple mole melanoma-pancreatic carcinoma-prone families: the familial atypical mole melanoma-pancreatic carcinoma syndrome. Cancer 2002;94(1):84–96.

158. Goldstein AM, Chan M, Harland M, et al, Melanoma Genetics Consortium (GenoMEL). High-risk melanoma susceptibility genes and pancreatic cancer, neural system tumors, and uveal melanoma across GenoMEL. Cancer Res 2006;66(20):9818–28.

159. Borg A, Sandberg T, Nilsson K, et al. High frequency of multiple melanomas and breast and pancreas carcinomas in CDKN2A mutation-positive melanoma families. J Natl Cancer Inst 2000;92(15):1260–6.

160. Goldstein AM, Fraser MC, Struewing JP, et al. Increased risk of pancreatic cancer in melanoma-prone kindreds with p16INK4 mutations. N Engl J Med 1995;333(15):970–4.

161. Bartsch DK, Sina-Frey M, Lang S, et al. CDKN2A germline mutations in familial pancreatic cancer. Ann Surg 2002;236(6):730–7.

162. McWilliams RR, Wieben ED, Rabe KG, et al. Prevalence of CDKN2A mutations in pancreatic cancer patients: implications for genetic counseling. Eur J Hum Genet 2011;19(4):472–8.

163. LaRusch J, Whitcomb DC. Genetics of pancreatitis. Curr Opin Gastroenterol 2011;27(5):467–74.

164. Witt H, Luck W, Hennies HC, et al. Mutations in the gene encoding the serine protease inhibitor, Kazal type 1 are associated with chronic pancreatitis. Nat Genet 2000;25(2):213–6.

165. Aoun E, Chang CC, Greer JB, et al. Pathways to injury in chronic pancreatitis: decoding the role of the high-risk SPINK1 N34S haplotype using meta-analysis. PLoS One 2008;3(4):e2003.

166. de las Heras-Castaño G, Castro-Senosiaín B, Fontalba A, et al. Hereditary pancreatitis: clinical features and inheritance characteristics of the R122C mutation in the cationic trypsinogen gene (PRSS1) in six Spanish families. JOP 2009;10(3):249–55.

167. Rebours V, Boutron-Ruault MC, Schnee M, et al. The natural history of hereditary pancreatitis: a national series. Gut 2009;58(1):97–103.

168. Raimondi S, Lowenfels AB, Morselli-Labate AM, et al. Pancreatic cancer in chronic pancreatitis; aetiology, incidence, and early detection. Best Pract Res Clin Gastroenterol 2010;24(3):349–58.

169. Lowenfels AB, Maisonneuve P, DiMagno EP, et al. Hereditary pancreatitis and the risk of pancreatic cancer. International Hereditary Pancreatitis Study Group. J Natl Cancer Inst 1997;89(6):442–6.

170. Lowenfels AB, Maisonneuve P, Whitcomb DC, et al. Cigarette smoking as a risk factor for pancreatic cancer in patients with hereditary pancreatitis. JAMA 2001; 286(2):169–70.

171. Guillot L, Beucher J, Tabary O, et al. Lung disease modifier genes in cystic fibrosis. Int J Biochem Cell Biol 2014I;52:83–93.

172. Sosnay PR, Siklosi KR, Van Goor F, et al. Defining the disease liability of variants in the cystic fibrosis transmembrane conductance regulator gene. Nat Genet 2013;45(10):1160–7.

173. Hamosh A, FitzSimmons SC, Macek M Jr, et al. Comparison of the clinical manifestations of cystic fibrosis in black and white patients. J Pediatr 1998;132(2): 255–9.

174. Kerem B, Chiba-Falek O, Kerem E. Cystic fibrosis in Jews: frequency and mutation distribution. Genet Test 1997;1(1):35–9.

175. Maisonneuve P, Marshall BC, Lowenfels AB. Risk of pancreatic cancer in patients with cystic fibrosis. Gut 2007;56(9):1327–8.

176. McWilliams RR, Petersen GM, Rabe KG, et al. Cystic fibrosis transmembrane conductance regulator (CFTR) gene mutations and risk for pancreatic adenocarcinoma. Cancer 2010;116(1):203–9.

177. Matsubayashi H, Fukushima N, Sato N, et al. Polymorphisms of SPINK1 N34S and CFTR in patients with sporadic and familial pancreatic cancer. Cancer Biol Ther 2003;2(6):652–5.

178. Mavrou A, Tsangaris GT, Roma E, et al. The ATM gene and ataxia telangiectasia. Anticancer Res 2008;28(1B):401–5.

179. Goldgar DE, Healey S, Dowty JG, et al, BCFR, kConFab. Rare variants in the ATM gene and risk of breast cancer. Breast Cancer Res 2011;13(4):R73.

180. Taylor AM, Byrd PJ. Molecular pathology of ataxia telangiectasia. J Clin Pathol 2005;58(10):1009–15.

181. Roberts NJ, Jiao Y, Yu J, et al. ATM mutations in patients with hereditary pancreatic cancer. Cancer Discov 2012;2(1):41–6.

182. Swift M, Sholman L, Perry M, et al. Malignant neoplasms in the families of patients with ataxia-telangiectasia. Cancer Res 1976;36(1):209–15.

183. Swift M, Reitnauer PJ, Morrell D, et al. Breast and other cancers in families with ataxia-telangiectasia. N Engl J Med 1987;316(21):1289–94.

184. Geoffroy-Perez B, Janin N, Ossian K, et al. Cancer risk in heterozygotes for ataxia-telangiectasia. Int J Cancer 2001;93(2):288–93.

185. Rulyak SJ, Lowenfels AB, Maisonneuve P, et al. Risk factors for the development of pancreatic cancer in familial pancreatic cancer kindreds. Gastroenterology 2003;124(5):1292–9.

186. Barton JG, Schnelldorfer T, Lohse CM, et al. Patterns of pancreatic resection differ between patients with familial and sporadic pancreatic cancer. J Gastrointest Surg 2011;15(5):836–42.

187. McFaul CD, Greenhalf W, Earl J, et al, European Registry of Hereditary Pancreatitis and Familial Pancreatic Cancer (EUROPAC), German National Case Collection for Familial Pancreatic Cancer (FaPaCa). Anticipation in familial pancreatic cancer. Gut 2006;55(2):252–8.

188. Eberle MA, Pfützer R, Pogue-Geile KL, et al. A new susceptibility locus for autosomal dominant pancreatic cancer maps to chromosome 4q32-34. Am J Hum Genet 2002;70(4):1044–8.

189. Pogue-Geile KL, Chen R, Bronner MP, et al. Palladin mutation causes familial pancreatic cancer and suggests a new cancer mechanism. PLoS Med 2006; 3(12):e516.

190. Earl J, Yan L, Vitone LJ, et al, European Registry of Hereditary Pancreatitis and Familial Pancreatic Cancer, German National Case Collection for Familial Pancreatic Cancer. Evaluation of the 4q32-34 locus in European familial pancreatic cancer. Cancer Epidemiol Biomarkers Prev 2006;15(10):1948–55.

191. Klein AP, Borges M, Griffith M, et al. Absence of deleterious palladin mutations in patients with familial pancreatic cancer. Cancer Epidemiol Biomarkers Prev 2009;18(4):1328–30.

192. Slater E, Amrillaeva V, Fendrich V, et al. Palladin mutation causes familial pancreatic cancer: absence in European families. PLoS Med 2007;4(4): e164.

193. Lieberman MD, Kilburn H, Lindsey M, et al. Relation of perioperative deaths to hospital volume among patients undergoing pancreatic resection for malignancy. Ann Surg 1995;222(5):638–45.

194. Raval MV, Bilimoria KY, Talamonti MS. Quality improvement for pancreatic cancer care: is regionalization a feasible and effective mechanism? Surg Oncol Clin N Am 2010;19(2):371–90.

195. Hampel H, Bennett RL, Buchanan A, et al, Guideline Development Group, American College of Medical Genetics and Genomics Professional Practice and Guidelines Committee and National Society of Genetic Counselors Practice Guidelines Committee. A practice guideline from the American College of Medical Genetics and Genomics and the National Society of Genetic Counselors: referral indications for cancer predisposition assessment. Genet Med 2015; 17(1):70–87.

196. Ozçelik H, Schmocker B, Di Nicola N, et al. Germline BRCA2 6174delT mutations in Ashkenazi Jewish pancreatic cancer patients. Nat Genet 1997;16(1):17–8.

197. Wang W, Chen S, Brune KA, et al. PancPRO: risk assessment for individuals with a family history of pancreatic cancer. J Clin Oncol 2007;25(11):1417–22.

198. LaDuca H, Stuenkel AJ, Dolinsky JS, et al. Utilization of multigene panels in hereditary cancer predisposition testing: analysis of more than 2,000 patients. Genet Med 2014;16(11):830–7.

199. Landrum MJ, Lee JM, Riley GR, et al. ClinVar: public archive of relationships among sequence variation and human phenotype. Nucleic Acids Res 2014; 42(Database issue):D980–5.

200. Thompson BA, Spurdle AB, Plazzer JP, et al, InSiGHT. Application of a 5-tiered scheme for standardized classification of 2,360 unique mismatch repair gene variants in the InSiGHT locus-specific database. Nat Genet 2014;46(2): 107–15.

201. Rulyak SJ, Brentnall TA. Inherited pancreatic cancer: surveillance and treatment strategies for affected families. Pancreatology 2001;1(5):477–85.

202. Canto MI, Goggins M, Yeo CJ, et al. Screening for pancreatic neoplasia in high-risk individuals: an EUS-based approach. Clin Gastroenterol Hepatol 2004;2(7): 606–21.

203. Poley JW, Kluijt I, Gouma DJ, et al. The yield of first-time endoscopic ultrasonography in screening individuals at a high risk of developing pancreatic cancer. Am J Gastroenterol 2009;104(9):2175–81.

204. Langer P, Kann PH, Fendrich V, et al. Five years of prospective screening of high-risk individuals from families with familial pancreatic cancer. Gut 2009; 58(10):1410–8.

205. Verna EC, Hwang C, Stevens PD, et al. Pancreatic cancer screening in a prospective cohort of high-risk patients: a comprehensive strategy of imaging and genetics. Clin Cancer Res 2010;16(20):5028–37.
206. Ludwig E, Olson SH, Bayuga S, et al. Feasibility and yield of screening in relatives from familial pancreatic cancer families. Am J Gastroenterol 2011;106(5): 946–54.
207. Canto MI, Hruban RH, Fishman EK, et al, American Cancer of the Pancreas Screening (CAPS) Consortium. Frequent detection of pancreatic lesions in asymptomatic high-risk individuals. Gastroenterology 2012;142(4):796–804 [quiz: e14–5].
208. Al-Sukhni W, Borgida A, Rothenmund H, et al. Screening for pancreatic cancer in a high-risk cohort: an eight-year experience. J Gastrointest Surg 2012;16(4): 771–83.
209. Canto MI, Harinck F, Hruban RH, et al, International Cancer of Pancreas Screening (CAPS) Consortium. International Cancer of the Pancreas Screening (CAPS) Consortium summit on the management of patients with increased risk for familial pancreatic cancer. Gut 2013;62(3):339–47 [Erratum appears in Gut 2014;63(12): 1978]. Hammell, Pascal [corrected to Hammel, Pascal]. Gut 2014;63(1):178. Hamell, Pascal [corrected to Hammell, Pascal].
210. Fong ZV, Winter JM. Biomarkers in pancreatic cancer: diagnostic, prognostic, and predictive. Cancer J 2012;18(6):530–8.
211. Ballehaninna UK, Chamberlain RS. The clinical utility of serum CA 19-9 in the diagnosis, prognosis and management of pancreatic adenocarcinoma: An evidence based appraisal. J Gastrointest Oncol 2012;3(2):105–19.
212. Brune K, Abe T, Canto M, et al. Multifocal neoplastic precursor lesions associated with lobular atrophy of the pancreas in patients having a strong family history of pancreatic cancer. Am J Surg Pathol 2006;30(9):1067–76.
213. Rulyak SJ, Kimmey MB, Veenstra DL, et al. Cost-effectiveness of pancreatic cancer screening in familial pancreatic cancer kindreds. Gastrointest Endosc 2003;57(1):23–9.
214. Rubenstein JH, Scheiman JM, Anderson MA. A clinical and economic evaluation of endoscopic ultrasound for patients at risk for familial pancreatic adenocarcinoma. Pancreatology 2007;7(5–6):514–25.
215. Rhim AD, Thege FI, Santana SM, et al. Detection of circulating pancreas epithelial cells in patients with pancreatic cystic lesions. Gastroenterology 2014; 146(3):647–51.
216. Bellin MD, Freeman ML, Gelrud A, et al, PancreasFest Recommendation Conference Participants. Total pancreatectomy and islet autotransplantation in chronic pancreatitis: recommendations from PancreasFest. Pancreatology 2014;14(1): 27–35.
217. Shapiro AM, Ricordi C, Hering BJ, et al. International trial of the Edmonton protocol for islet transplantation. N Engl J Med 2006;355(13):1318–30.
218. Mills PK, Beeson WL, Abbey DE, et al. Dietary habits and past medical history as related to fatal pancreas cancer risk among Adventists. Cancer 1988;61(12): 2578–85.
219. Skinner HG, Michaud DS, Giovannucci E, et al. Vitamin D intake and the risk for pancreatic cancer in two cohort studies. Cancer Epidemiol Biomarkers Prev 2006;15(9):1688–95.
220. Nöthlings U, Wilkens LR, Murphy SP, et al. Meat and fat intake as risk factors for pancreatic cancer: the multiethnic cohort study. J Natl Cancer Inst 2005;97(19): 1458–65 [Erratum appears in J Natl Cancer Inst 2006;98(11):796].

221. Waddell N, Pajic M, Patch AM, et al, Australian Pancreatic Cancer Genome Initiative. Whole genomes redefine the mutational landscape of pancreatic cancer. Nature 2015;518(7540):495–501.

222. Alexandrov LB, Nik-Zainal S, Wedge DC, et al, Australian Pancreatic Cancer Genome Initiative, ICGC Breast Cancer Consortium, ICGC MMML-Seq Consortium, ICGC PedBrain. Signatures of mutational processes in human cancer. Nature 2013;500(7463):415–21 [Erratum appears in Nature 2013;502(7470): 258]. Imielinsk, Marcin [corrected to Imielinski, Marcin].

223. Farmer H, McCabe N, Lord CJ, et al. Targeting the DNA repair defect in BRCA mutant cells as a therapeutic strategy. Nature 2005;434(7035):917–21.

224. Tutt AN, Lord CJ, McCabe N, et al. Exploiting the DNA repair defect in BRCA mutant cells in the design of new therapeutic strategies for cancer. Cold Spring Harb Symp Quant Biol 2005;70:139–48.

225. Pennington KP, Walsh T, Harrell MI, et al. Germline and somatic mutations in homologous recombination genes predict platinum response and survival in ovarian, fallopian tube, and peritoneal carcinomas. Clin Cancer Res 2014;20(3):764–75.

226. Ko AH, Dito E, Schillinger B, et al. Phase II study of fixed dose rate gemcitabine with cisplatin for metastatic adenocarcinoma of the pancreas. J Clin Oncol 2006;24(3):379–85.

227. Hess V, Pratsch S, Potthast S, et al. Combining gemcitabine, oxaliplatin and capecitabine (GEMOXEL) for patients with advanced pancreatic carcinoma (APC): a phase I/II trial. Ann Oncol 2010;21(12):2390–5.

228. Oettle H, Riess H, Stieler JM, et al. Second-line oxaliplatin, folinic acid, and fluorouracil versus folinic acid and fluorouracil alone for gemcitabine-refractory pancreatic cancer: outcomes from the CONKO-003 trial. J Clin Oncol 2014; 32(23):2423–9.

229. Sultana A, Smith CT, Cunningham D, et al. Meta-analyses of chemotherapy for locally advanced and metastatic pancreatic cancer. J Clin Oncol 2007;25(18): 2607–15.

230. Sultana A, Tudur Smith C, Cunningham D, et al. Meta-analyses of chemotherapy for locally advanced and metastatic pancreatic cancer: results of secondary end points analyses. Br J Cancer 2008;99(1):6–13.

231. Ciliberto D, Botta C, Correale P, et al. Role of gemcitabine-based combination therapy in the management of advanced pancreatic cancer: a meta-analysis of randomised trials. Eur J Cancer 2013;49(3):593–603.

232. Heinemann V, Boeck S, Hinke A, et al. Meta-analysis of randomized trials: evaluation of benefit from gemcitabine-based combination chemotherapy applied in advanced pancreatic cancer. BMC Cancer 2008;8:82.

233. Villarroel MC, Rajeshkumar NV, Garrido-Laguna I, et al. Personalizing cancer treatment in the age of global genomic analyses: PALB2 gene mutations and the response to DNA damaging agents in pancreatic cancer. Mol Cancer Ther 2011;10(1):3–8.

234. Sonnenblick A, Kadouri L, Appelbaum L, et al. Complete remission, in BRCA2 mutation carrier with metastatic pancreatic adenocarcinoma, treated with cisplatin based therapy. Cancer Biol Ther 2011;12(3):165–8.

235. Golan T, Kanji ZS, Epelbaum R, et al. Overall survival and clinical characteristics of pancreatic cancer in BRCA mutation carriers. Br J Cancer 2014;111(6): 1132–8.

236. US National Institutes of Health. Olaparib in gBRCA mutated pancreatic cancer who disease has not progressed on first line platinum-based chemotherapy (POLO). Available at: http://clinicaltrials.gov/show/NCT02184195.

237. Fogelman DR, Wolff RA, Kopetz S, et al. Evidence for the efficacy of Iniparib, a PARP-1 inhibitor, in BRCA2-associated pancreatic cancer. Anticancer Res 2011; 31(4):1417–20.

238. Guillotin D, Martin SA. Exploiting DNA mismatch repair deficiency as a therapeutic strategy. Exp Cell Res 2014;329(1):110–5.

Hereditary Gastric Cancer Syndromes

Hugh Colvin, MB, Bchir, MRCS[a],*, Ken Yamamoto, MD, PhD[b],
Noriko Wada, MD[a], Masaki Mori, MD, PhD[a]

KEYWORDS

- Hereditary gastric cancer syndromes • Diagnosis • Management
- Genetic counseling • Gastrectomy • Hereditary diffuse gastric cancer
- Familial intestinal gastric cancer
- Gastric adenocarcinoma and proximal polyposis of the stomach

KEY POINTS

- Hereditary gastric cancer syndromes are responsible for a small but distinct group of gastric cancers, which can be associated with a high penetrance of early-onset and aggressive gastric cancer.
- Endoscopy is used for disease surveillance, but clinicians must be wary that early cancers can be missed.
- For some individuals with hereditary gastric cancer syndromes, prophylactic total gastrectomy offers the only option for preventing the development of gastric cancer.
- Mutations of CDH1 is currently the only genetic marker of prognostic value, but is present in only a minority of families with hereditary diffuse gastric cancer.
- Significant opportunities for optimizing the management of individuals affected by hereditary gastric cancer syndromes exist, emphasizing the importance of continuing to manage affected families under research settings.

INTRODUCTION

Gastric cancer is one of the leading causes of global cancer mortality, causing more than 700,000 deaths per annum worldwide.[1–3] In most cases, environmental factors, including *Helicobacter pylori* infection,[4] smoking,[5,6] and diet,[7] account for much of the etiology of the disease. This article is dedicated to the small but distinct group of gastric cancers (1%–3%) that result from hereditary gastric cancer syndromes.[8]

There are 3 recognized syndromes that confer heritable predisposition to cancers primarily of the stomach. These syndromes are segregated according to their

The authors have nothing to disclose.
[a] Department of Gastroenterological Surgery, Osaka University Graduate School of Medicine, 2-2 Yamadaoka, Suita, Osaka 565-0871, Japan; [b] Department of Medical Chemistry, Kurume University School of Medicine, 67 Asahimachi, Kurume, Fukuoka 830-0011, Japan
* Corresponding author.
E-mail address: hcolvin@gesurg.med.osaka-u.ac.jp

histologic types or their macroscopic morphology and are (1) hereditary diffuse gastric cancer (HDGC), (2) familial intestinal gastric cancer (FIGC), and (3) gastric adenocarcinoma and proximal polyposis of the stomach (GAPPS). Of these syndromes, the genetic cause is known only in individuals with HDGC, and even then in a minority of this subgroup.[8]

Particularly in individuals affected by HDGC with pathologic mutations of cadherin-1 (CDH1), the seriousness of the condition is underlined by a high penetrance of early-onset and aggressive disease that is not always possible to detect by endoscopic surveillance; most individuals are therefore advised to undergo prophylactic total gastrectomy as a means of eliminating the risk of developing advanced-stage and incurable gastric cancer.[9,10] We discuss the nature of each of the hereditary gastric cancer syndromes and their management. These and other inherited syndromes associated with gastric cancers are summarized in **Table 1**.

IDENTIFICATION OF THOSE AT RISK

A thorough family history and the documentation of gastric and other relevant cancers occurring frequently and/or at young ages in a family is central to the identification of hereditary gastric cancer syndromes. The diagnosis of hereditary gastric cancer syndrome is based on the family history and information concerning the histologic subtype of gastric cancers that have occurred in the family. The positive diagnosis of hereditary gastric cancer syndrome in turn can allow other family members to be screened with the aim of identifying disease before progression to advanced and incurable stages. Given the potential for very early age of onset of hereditary gastric cancer, the importance of securing accurate cancer family history information as early as the pediatric age group is noted.

HEREDITARY DIFFUSE GASTRIC CANCER
Clinical Features

HDGC is an autosomal dominant syndrome, characterized by the development of highly aggressive diffuse type gastric cancer.[22–24] Fifteen percent to 50% of the families affected by HDGC have been identified to harbor germline mutations in the E-cadherin gene, CDH1.[11,12] In individual members of HDGC families who are carriers of pathogenic CDH1 mutations, the largest study to date has estimated the risk of developing gastric cancer to be 70% in men and 56% in women by the age of 80.[13] Individuals without previous knowledge of being at risk often present with advanced cancers that are associated with dismal prognosis.[22] The median age of invasive gastric cancer diagnosis for mutation carriers is 38, which is approximately 3 decades earlier than sporadic cases of gastric cancer[25]; however, diagnosis has been reported to occur over a wide range of ages from 14 to 82 years.[26,27]

Clinicians should be aware that women affected by HDGC associated with mutant CDH1 are also at significantly increased risk of developing lobular breast carcinoma,[28–32] with cases arising mostly after 40 years of age, and the lifetime cumulative risk being approximately 40% by the age of 80 years.[13,27] In some families affected by HDGC, there may also be an increased risk of developing colon cancers.[10]

Genetics

The earliest report of germline mutations of CDH1 in HDGC was made by Guilford and colleagues[22] in 1998 in Maori families in New Zealand. CDH1 is located on chromosome 16q22.1 and encodes E-cadherin, a cell adhesion protein that plays an important role in the maintenance of cellular polarity and epithelial tissue

Table 1
Hereditary gastric cancer syndromes and other cancer syndromes associated with gastric cancers

Syndromes	Main Characteristics	Associated Gene Mutations
Hereditary gastric cancer syndromes		
Hereditary diffuse gastric cancer	Autosomal dominant inheritance of diffuse-type gastric cancer, with high penetrance and early-onset of aggressive disease in cases arising from pathologic mutations of CDH1.	CDH1 in 15%–50%[11,12] of cases CTNNA1[13,14]
Familial intestinal gastric cancer	Autosomal dominant inheritance of intestinal-type gastric cancer in the absence of gastric polyposis.	Unknown
Gastric adenocarcinoma and proximal polyposis of the stomach	Autosomal dominant inheritance of fundic gland polyposis of the proximal stomach and the development of intestinal-type adenocarcinoma.	Unknown
Other cancer syndromes that can give rise to gastric cancers[a]		
Familial adenomatous polyposis	Autosomal dominant. Near complete penetration of early-onset colorectal cancer. Gastric cancer is uncommon (<2%).[15]	APC
Hereditary breast and ovarian cancer syndrome (when due to BRCA1/2 mutations)	Autosomal dominant. Breast and ovarian cancers. Gastric cancer is uncommon (1.7%).[16]	BRCA1 BRCA2
Juvenile-polyposis syndrome	Autosomal dominant. Polyps of the gastrointestinal tract and colorectal cancer. Gastric cancer is likely to be infrequent.[17]	SMAD4 BMPR1A
Li-Fraumeni syndrome	Autosomal dominant condition causing a variety of cancers: breast, brain, and adrenal glands and sarcomas. Gastric cancer is early onset and uncommon (4.9%).[18]	p53
Lynch syndrome	Autosomal dominant condition with high penetrance of early-onset colorectal cancer. Gastric cancers, predominantly of intestinal type, are uncommon (1.6%).[19]	Mismatch repair gene mutations[b]
Peutz-Jeghers syndrome	Autosomal dominant. Gastrointestinal hamartomatous polyps with mucocutaneous pigmentation. Gastric cancer is uncommon (2%–3%).[20,21]	STK11

[a] Only the most common cancers are listed alongside the estimated frequencies of gastric cancer arising in individuals affected by these syndromes.
[b] MLH1, MSH2, MSH6, PMS1, PMS2, and EPCAM, of which gastric cancers are most common in individuals affected by Lynch syndrome with MLH1 or MSH2 mutations.[19]
Adapted from Lynch HT, Silva E, Wirtzfeld D, et al. Hereditary diffuse gastric cancer: prophylactic surgical oncology implications. Surg Clin North Am 2008;88:759–78; with permission.

architecture.[33–35] It is a tumor suppressor gene and its inactivation follows the classic "2-hit hypothesis," with the "first-hit" being an inactivating germline (inherited) mutation in one allele of the CDH1 gene. The "second-hit" inactivation of the remaining E-cadherin allele is required for the complete loss of this protein's function and progression to neoplastic disease, and occurs later in life as a result of promoter methylation, mutation, or loss of heterozygosity.[36–40]

Clinically it is important to distinguish between CDH1 mutations that have been shown to be pathologic and lead to diffuse gastric cancers versus CDH1 DNA sequence alterations that are of uncertain significance. More than 100 known mutations of the CDH1 gene have been identified in HDGC and most of the mutations are clearly pathologic given they cause protein truncation; the presence of these mutations provide reliable prognostic information for affected families. However, the pathogenicity cannot be immediately established in approximately 20% of CDH1 sequence variations that are missense mutations.[41] These missense alterations can lead to the alteration of a single amino acid in the E-cadherin molecule, which may be inconsequential to the normal function of the protein. It has been proposed that the presence of the same missense mutations in 4 family members who develop gastric cancer (segregation analysis), together with assessment of the loss of E-cadherin function through in vitro[42,43] or in silico[44,45] methods are necessary to confirm the pathogenic nature of a particular missense mutation.[46]

The causative role of CDH1 mutations in HDGC is further supported by the observation that loss of CDH1 expression is also seen in sporadic cases of diffuse gastric cancer together with the existence of multiple mouse models, where knockout of the CDH1 gene demonstrates progression to diffuse-type gastric cancer.[38,47,48] It has been speculated that loss of E-cadherin expression may cause self-renewing cells to become inappropriately placed in the cell matrix of the lamina propria, resulting in the formation of signet ring cancer cells.[49]

When families affected by HDGC but without CDH1 mutations were screened for mutations in a preselected group of genes implicated in other gastrointestinal cancers, potentially causative mutations in genes other than CDH1 could be found in approximately 10% of families (**Fig. 1**).

Intriguingly, mutations in the α-E-catenin gene (cadherin-associated protein, alpha 1 [CTNNA1]), were found in a total of 3 families affected by HDGC. The protein product

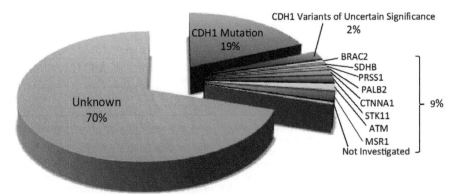

Fig. 1. The proportion of known and unknown mutations identified in 183 HDGC index families. (*Data from* Hansford S, Kaurah P, Li-Chang H, et al. Hereditary diffuse gastric cancer syndrome. JAMA Oncol 2015;1(1):23–32.)

of this gene also functions as an intercellular adhesion molecule similar to CDH1, adding support for α-E-catenin playing a role in HDGC.[13,14] Many other gene mutations were found in families affected by HDGC, but whether these really are pathogenic in HDGC will require further investigation before they can become a reliable and useful marker for counseling affected individuals as well as for deciding management strategies.[13]

Genetic Counseling and Testing of Hereditary Diffuse Gastric Cancer

The purpose of genetic testing is twofold: first, to identify the presence of pathologic CDH1 mutations in the index case, which in HDGC is associated with highly penetrant and aggressive disease and guides further management. Second, if a pathologic CDH1 mutation is identified, it allows for targeted mutational analysis of other family members to reliably distinguish between those who are or are not at risk of developing cancers.

There are 2 clinical criteria for selecting those who require genetic testing, one published by the British Columbia Cancer Agency Hereditary Diffuse Gastric Cancer Program[9] and the other by the International Gastric Cancer Linkage Consortium,[10] and are shown in **Boxes 1** and **2**, respectively.

It is also recommended that if carcinoma in situ or pagetoid spread of signet ring cells are detected adjacent to diffuse-type gastric cancer by an expert pathologist, these patients also should be referred for genetic testing regardless of family history, given these are histopathological features almost exclusively of HDGC.[50]

Before genetic testing, individuals should be counseled regarding the benefits of clarifying their CDH1 mutation status given the high penetrance of aggressive gastric cancers when the pathogenic mutations are present, and the effectiveness of prophylactic gastrectomy to prevent invasive gastric cancer. The significant short-term and long-term consequences associated with undergoing prophylactic gastrectomy also should also be discussed.

Box 1
Criteria for CDH1 mutation testing by British Columbia Cancer Agency Hereditary Diffuse Gastric Cancer Program

Modified testing criteria

- Family with 2 or more cases of gastric cancer, with at least 1 case of diffuse gastric cancer diagnosed before the age of 50 years

- Family with multiple cases of lobular carcinoma of the breast with or without diffuse gastric cancer in first-degree or second-degree relatives

- Isolated individuals from a low-incidence population diagnosed with diffuse gastric cancer at age younger than 35 years

Potential additional criteria

- Personal history but no family history of diffuse gastric cancer or lobular carcinoma of the breast

- Family with 3 or more cases of gastric cancer diagnosed at any age, one or more of which is a documented case of diffuse gastric cancer;

- Family with 1 or more cases of both diffuse gastric cancer and signet ring colon cancer

Adapted from Lynch HT, Silva E, Wirtzfeld D, et al. Hereditary diffuse gastric cancer: prophylactic surgical oncology implications. Surg Clin North Am 2008;88:761; with permission.

Box 2
Criteria for CDH1 mutation testing by International Gastric Cancer Linkage Consortium

- Two gastric cancer cases in family, 1 confirmed diffuse gastric cancer before the age of 50 years
- Three confirmed diffuse gastric cancer cases in first-degree or second-degree relatives independent of age
- Diffuse gastric cancer occurring before the age of 40
- Personal or family history of diffuse gastric cancer and lobular breast cancer, 1 diagnosed before the age of 50 years

Modified from Fitzgerald RC, Hardwick R, Huntsman D, et al. Hereditary diffuse gastric cancer: updated consensus guidelines for clinical management and directions for future research. J Med Genet 2010;47:436–44.

In most cases, it is sufficient for genetic testing to occur at the age of consent, given the probability of developing clinically significant lesions is fewer than 1% before the age of 20.[30] This is likely to be the best practice for most individuals, given there are many serious issues to come to terms with if diagnosed with HDGC. That said, some families with HDGC have an even earlier onset of gastric cancer, arising before 16 years of age, and so the timing of genetic testing requires careful and thoughtful adjustment on a case-by-case basis.[10]

DNA analysis is best conducted from blood samples in specialized centers. DNA sequencing is sufficient to detect most cases of CDH1 mutations, but large germline deletions occurring in 4% of affected families can be detected only by alternative techniques. If CDH1 mutations are not detected by DNA sequencing, additional tests should be conducted to look for the large germline mutations of CDH1 by techniques such as multiplex ligation-dependent probe amplification or comparative genomic hybridization.[11]

Since the publication of the most recent guidelines on genetic testing for individuals at risk of HDGC, new evidence has emerged that the presence of a CDH1 mutation in individuals with a family history of lobular breast cancer but without a family history of diffuse gastric cancer do not appear to be at significantly increased risk of gastric cancers. The necessity of intervention (including prophylactic total gastrectomy) in these individuals may have to be reconsidered.[51]

Endoscopic Surveillance

Endoscopy may not detect early lesions in HDGC, which are usually multifocal and lie hidden beneath the mucosal layer.[52] Therefore, there is no guarantee that endoscopy will detect lesions before progression onto more advanced and incurable stages. Endoscopy is thus reserved primarily for 2 groups of patients: (1) carriers of the HDGC mutation who either refuse or are unsuitable for prophylactic gastrectomy, or (2) members of HDGC families without mutations of CDH1 or where the mutations are of indeterminate clinical significance.[10,53]

Annual endoscopy for surveillance is recommended by the International Gastric Cancer Linkage Consortium for those fitting the criteria of HDGC but are not undergoing prophylactic gastrectomy.[10] The Cambridge protocol states endoscopy should be performed meticulously using white light and a high-definition visualization system. Careful inspection and targeted biopsies of any lesions, together with 6 random biopsies from the cardia, fundus, body, transitional zone, and antrum should be taken to secure at least 30 biopsies.[10] The effect of *H pylori* in HDGC is not understood, but given it is a World Heath Organization class 1 carcinogen, it is advised that *H pylori* status be checked and infected individuals undergo eradication.[10] The efficacy of chromoendoscopy in detecting lesions in the setting of HDGC has been inconsistent, and requires further evaluation.[54,55]

Surgical Management of Hereditary Diffuse Gastric Cancer

Preoperative considerations

In most individuals affected by HDGC associated with pathogenic mutations of CDH1, prophylactic gastrectomy is the only effective way of ensuring invasive gastric cancers are prevented, and therefore protecting the patient from the development of advanced-stage and incurable disease.[10,11,53] The high penetrance of pathologic CDH1 mutations in HDGC justifies prophylactic surgery, but at present, it is not possible to identify the large minority of mutation carriers who will not go on to develop gastric cancers and in whom gastrectomy would therefore have been unnecessary. Informed consent should be sought while discussing these points, as well as the short-term and long-term consequences of undergoing total gastrectomy. Prophylactic total gastrectomy should be performed in high-volume centers with an achievable postoperative mortality rate of less than 1%.[56]

The age at which prophylactic gastrectomy should be offered is not well understood. At present, most asymptomatic adults who are members of HDGC families are identified to be carriers of pathologic mutations of CDH1 will be offered gastrectomy soon after the diagnosis is made. This recommendation is made even in the setting of a negative endoscopy, because small foci of cancers are very often present when the resected specimens are examined carefully.[10] But the uniform presence of small foci of disease across most individuals also suggests that there exists a considerable length of time in which early lesions do not progress, laying the importance of continuing to study the natural history of CDH1 mutation–positive HDGC status.

Fertility after gastrectomy will be an important consideration for many women. Women are reported to have conceived and given birth to healthy infants after gastrectomy in the context of HDGC, as well as for nonmalignant disease,[57] but are susceptible to developing anemia, which can be treated by nutritional supplementation.[57–59]

Operative procedure

The operation itself consists of total gastrectomy with Roux-en-Y reconstruction, with intraoperative confirmation that the proximal resection is devoid of gastric mucosa by frozen section.[60] A radical lymph node dissection is deemed not necessary when gastrectomy is being performed for prophylaxis, given lymph node metastases are highly unlikely,[10,61] and this in turn allows for the sparing of the vagal nerve, which may be associated with improved quality of life in the long-term following the procedure.[62,63] Reports suggest laparoscopic total gastrectomy compared to open surgery is associated with improved postoperative recovery,[64–66] and the construction of a jejunal pouch is associated with improved quality of life,[67,68] although the benefits arising from these techniques are yet to be supported by robust evidence.

Management of Cancers at Other Sites

Given that women with HDGC associated with mutant CDH1 are at high risk of developing lobular breast cancer, they are advised from the age of 35 to perform self-examination on a monthly basis, have annual mammography and breast MRI, and have biannual clinical breast examination.[10] Evidence is insufficient regarding prophylactic mastectomy or chemoprevention with tamoxifen in these individuals.

Colonoscopic screening may be considered in HDGC families that report colorectal cancers.[10]

FAMILIAL INTESTINAL GASTRIC CANCER

FIGC is an autosomal dominant syndrome characterized by intestinal-type gastric cancer without gastric polyposis. The underlying genetic cause is unknown.[69] In the absence of any clear evidence for the best method of managing this syndrome, clinical surveillance and interventions ideally should be performed in a research environment to evaluate their efficacy with a view to improving the management of future generations of individuals affected by this syndrome.[60] The diagnostic criteria for FIGC, defined by the International Gastric Cancer Linkage Consortium, are listed in **Box 3**.

GASTRIC ADENOCARCINOMA AND PROXIMAL POLYPOSIS OF THE STOMACH

GAPPS is an autosomal dominant syndrome with incomplete penetrance of no known genetic cause. It is characterized by fundic gland polyposis that carpets the proximal stomach, while sparing the antrum, duodenum, and the colon. These polyps can be associated with dysplastic lesions and intestinal-type gastric cancer. Fundic gland polyposis with associated dysplasia has been described in affected individuals as young as 10, and the earliest reported case of adenocarcinoma occurred in a 33-year-old. All first-degree relatives should undergo gastroscopy and colonoscopy, the latter to exclude familial adenomatous polyposis and other gastrointestinal polyposis syndromes. Endoscopic surveillance can be difficult when there are a large number of polyps, and in these individuals gastrectomy may be considered. The diagnostic criteria for GAPPS, defined by Worthley and colleagues, are listed in **Box 4**.[70,71]

GASTRIC CANCER IN OTHER HEREDITARY CANCER SYNDROMES

Gastric cancers may arise in association with other hereditary cancer syndromes among mutation carriers (see **Table 1**), providing further evidence for the genetic etiology of this disease.[72] These syndromes should also be considered in the differential diagnosis when families are noted to have a predisposition to gastric and any other relevant cancers, alongside the hereditary gastric cancer syndromes. Even across

---

Box 3
Diagnostic criteria for familial intestinal gastric cancer by International Gastric Cancer Linkage Consortium

High-incidence countries (Portugal, Japan)

- At least 3 relatives should have intestinal gastric cancer and one of them should be a first-degree relative of the other two
- At least 2 successive generations should be affected
- In one of the relatives, gastric cancer should be diagnosed before the age of 50

Low-incidence countries (UK, USA)

- At least 2 first/second-degree relatives affected by intestinal gastric cancer, one diagnosed before the age of 50; or
- Three or more relatives with intestinal gastric cancer at any age

Modified from Caldas C, Carneiro F, Lynch HT, et al. Familial gastric cancer: overview and guidelines for management. J Med Genet 1999;36:873–80.

> **Box 4**
> **Diagnostic criteria for gastric adenocarcinoma and proximal polyposis of the stomach**
>
> - Gastric polyps restricted to the body and fundus with no evidence of colorectal or duodenal polyposis
> - More than 100 polyps carpeting the proximal stomach in the index case or more than 30 polyps in a first-degree relative of another case
> - Predominantly fundic gland polyps, some having regions of dysplasia (or a family member with either dysplastic fundic gland polyposis or gastric adenocarcinoma)
> - An autosomal dominant pattern of inheritance
> - Exclusions include other heritable gastric polyposis syndromes and use of proton pump inhibitors
>
> *Modified from* Worthley DL, Phillips KD, Wayte N, et al. Gastric adenocarcinoma and proximal polyposis of the stomach (GAPPS): a new autosomal dominant syndrome. Gut 2012;61:774–9.

the same syndrome, the incidence of gastric cancers can vary in different populations; from a practical viewpoint, this means surveillance protocol requires tailoring to suit different populations for identifying gastric cancers, the details of which are beyond the scope of this article.

FUTURE DIRECTIONS

The underlying genetic cause for many families affected by hereditary gastric cancer syndromes is yet to be identified. An unbiased approach using next-generation sequencing may uncover novel gene mutations that give rise to hereditary gastric cancer. Once validated for their role in hereditary gastric cancer syndromes, these identified gene mutations would be expected to provide valuable prognostic information as well to deepen our understanding of the mechanisms behind the disease process, which may also aid the development of novel treatments. Epigenetic factors also deserve serious consideration and thoughtful investigation.

Many of the current practices for managing individuals affected by inherited gastric cancer syndromes have much potential for refinement. For example, by improving our understanding of the natural course of each syndrome, as well as enhancing detection of early lesions through the use of modalities such as chromoendoscopy, it may be possible to delay the requirement of total gastrectomy or even better to avoid operating altogether on patients who will never go on to develop gastric cancers despite a strong family history of HDGC and harboring germline pathologic CDH1 mutations.

Optimal strategies for surveillance and prevention of breast and colorectal cancers among members of HDGC families have yet to be defined and will require further research.

SUMMARY

Hereditary gastric cancer syndromes are associated with an early age of onset of aggressive and invasive gastric cancer. In the setting of HDGC, endoscopic surveillance is unreliable at detecting cancers, leaving most patients with total gastrectomy as the only reliable method of avoiding the development of late-stage and incurable gastric cancer. To date, germline mutations of CDH1 have been reported in a significant proportion of HDGC families and have been used successfully as a genetic test for identifying those at risk of developing cancers and benefit from undergoing total gastrectomy. Many aspects of the syndromes described in this article, including the etiology, diagnosis, and possibility of nonoperative therapy, require further research to improve their management.

ONLINE SOURCES

National Institutes of Health Web site for general information on hereditary diffuse gastric cancer for clinicians: http://ghr.nlm.nih.gov/condition/hereditary-diffuse-gastric-cancer.

Familial gastric cancer study Web site, Cambridge, UK: http://www.cuh.org.uk/familial-gastric-cancer-study.

Support network for individuals and families affected by gastric cancer, including hereditary gastric cancer syndromes: http://www.nostomachforcancer.org.

REFERENCES

1. Jemal A, Bray F, Center MM, et al. Global cancer statistics: 2011. CA Cancer J Clin 2011;61:69–90.
2. Bakkelund KE, Nordrum IS, Fossmark R, et al. Gastric carcinomas localized to the cardia. Gastroenterol Res Pract 2012;2012:457831.
3. Mathers CD, Loncar D. Projections of global mortality and burden of disease from 2002 to 2030. PLoS Med 2006;3:2011–30.
4. IARC. Schistosomes, liver flukes and *Helicobacter pylori*. IARC Monogr Eval Carcinog Risks Hum 1994;61:121–62.
5. Ladeiras-Lopes R, Pereira AK, Nogueira A, et al. Smoking and gastric cancer: systematic review and meta-analysis of cohort studies. Cancer Causes Control 2008;19:689–701.
6. González CA, Pera G, Agudo A, et al. Smoking and the risk of gastric cancer in the European Prospective Investigation Into Cancer and Nutrition (EPIC). Int J Cancer 2003;107:629–34.
7. Kelley JR, Duggan JM. Gastric cancer epidemiology and risk factors. J Clin Epidemiol 2003;56:1–9.
8. Oliveira C, Pinheiro H, Figueiredo J, et al. Familial gastric cancer: genetic susceptibility, pathology, and implications for management. Lancet Oncol 2015;16:e60–70.
9. Lynch HT, Silva E, Wirtzfeld D, et al. Hereditary diffuse gastric cancer: prophylactic surgical oncology implications. Surg Clin North Am 2008;88:759–78.
10. Fitzgerald RC, Hardwick R, Huntsman D, et al. Hereditary diffuse gastric cancer: updated consensus guidelines for clinical management and directions for future research. J Med Genet 2010;47:436–44.
11. Oliveira C, Senz J, Kaurah P, et al. Germline CDH1 deletions in hereditary diffuse gastric cancer families. Hum Mol Genet 2009;18:1545–55.
12. Yamada H, Shinmura K, Ito H, et al. Germline alterations in the CDH1 gene in familial gastric cancer in the Japanese population. Cancer Sci 2011;102:1782–8.
13. Hansford S, Kaurah P, Li-Chang H, et al. Hereditary diffuse gastric cancer syndrome. JAMA Oncol 2015;1(1):23–32.
14. Majewski IJ, Kluijt I, Cats A, et al. An α-E-catenin (CTNNA1) mutation in hereditary diffuse gastric cancer. J Pathol 2013;229:621–9.
15. Wood LD, Salaria SN, Cruise MW, et al. Upper GI tract lesions in familial adenomatous polyposis (FAP): enrichment of pyloric gland adenomas and other gastric and duodenal neoplasms. Am J Surg Pathol 2014;38:389–93.
16. Friedenson B. BRCA1 and BRCA2 pathways and the risk of cancers other than breast or ovarian. MedGenMed 2005;7:60.

17. Brosens LA, Langeveld D, van Hattem WA, et al. Juvenile polyposis syndrome. World J Gastroenterol 2011;17:4839–44.
18. Masciari S, Dewanwala A, Stoffel EM, et al. Gastric cancer in individuals with Li-Fraumeni syndrome. Genet Med 2011;13:651–7.
19. Capelle L, Van Grieken NC, Lingsma HF, et al. Risk and epidemiological time trends of gastric cancer in Lynch syndrome carriers in the Netherlands. Gastroenterology 2010;138:487–92.
20. Van Lier MG, Wagner A, Mathus-Vliegen EM, et al. High cancer risk in Peutz-Jeghers syndrome: a systematic review and surveillance recommendations. Am J Gastroenterol 2010;105:1258–64 [author reply: 1265].
21. Van Lier MG, Westerman AM, Wagner A, et al. High cancer risk and increased mortality in patients with Peutz-Jeghers syndrome. Gut 2011;60:141–7.
22. Guilford P, Hopkins J, Harraway J, et al. E-cadherin germline mutations in familial gastric cancer. Nature 1998;392:402–5.
23. Gayther SA, Gorringe KL, Ramus SJ, et al. Identification of germ-line E-cadherin mutations in gastric cancer families of European origin. Cancer Res 1998;58:4086–9.
24. Grady WM, Willis J, Guilford PJ, et al. Methylation of the CDH1 promoter as the second genetic hit in hereditary diffuse gastric cancer. Nat Genet 2000;26:16–7.
25. Howlader N, Carneiro F, Lynch HT, et al. SEER cancer statistics review, 1975–2011. National Cancer Institute based on November 2013 SEER data submission. 2014. Available at: http://seer.cancer.gov/csr/1975_2011/. Accessed April 03, 2015.
26. Caldas C, Carneiro F, Lynch HT, et al. Familial gastric cancer: overview and guidelines for management. J Med Genet 1999;36:873–80.
27. Kaurah P, MacMillan A, Boyd N, et al. Founder and recurrent CDH1 mutations in families with hereditary diffuse gastric cancer. JAMA 2007;297:2360–72.
28. Keller G, Vogelsang H, Becker I, et al. Diffuse type gastric and lobular breast carcinoma in a familial gastric cancer patient with an E-cadherin germline mutation. Am J Pathol 1999;155:337–42.
29. Pharoah PD, Guilford P, Caldas C. Incidence of gastric cancer and breast cancer in CDH1 (E-cadherin) mutation carriers from hereditary diffuse gastric cancer families. Gastroenterology 2001;121:1348–53.
30. Blair V, Martin I, Shaw D, et al. Hereditary diffuse gastric cancer: diagnosis and management. Clin Gastroenterol Hepatol 2006;4:262–75.
31. Kriege M, Brekelmans CT, Boetes C, et al. Efficacy of MRI and mammography for breast-cancer screening in women with a familial or genetic predisposition. N Engl J Med 2004;351:427–37.
32. Guilford P, Blair V, More H, et al. A short guide to hereditary diffuse gastric cancer. Hered Cancer Clin Pract 2007;5:183–94.
33. Grunwald GB. The structural and functional analysis of cadherin calcium-dependent cell adhesion molecules. Curr Opin Cell Biol 1993;5:797–805.
34. Drubin DG, Nelson WJ. Origins of cell polarity. Cell 1996;84:335–44.
35. Nejsum LN, Nelson WJ. A molecular mechanism directly linking E-cadherin adhesion to initiation of epithelial cell surface polarity. J Cell Biol 2007;178:323–35.
36. Barber M, Murrell A, Ito Y, et al. Mechanisms and sequelae of E-cadherin silencing in hereditary diffuse gastric cancer. J Pathol 2008;216:295–306.
37. Corso G, Roviello F, Paredes J, et al. Characterization of the P373L E-cadherin germline missense mutation and implication for clinical management. Eur J Surg Oncol 2007;33:1061–7.
38. Humar B, Blair V, Charlton A, et al. E-cadherin deficiency initiates gastric signet-ring cell carcinoma in mice and man. Cancer Res 2009;69:2050–6.

39. Brooks-Wilson AR, Kaurah P, Suriano G, et al. Germline E-cadherin mutations in hereditary diffuse gastric cancer: assessment of 42 new families and review of genetic screening criteria. J Med Genet 2004;41:508–17.

40. Oliveira C, Sousa S, Pinheiro H, et al. Quantification of epigenetic and genetic 2nd hits in CDH1 during hereditary diffuse gastric cancer syndrome progression. Gastroenterology 2009;136:2137–48.

41. Carneiro F, Oliveira C, Suriano G, et al. Molecular pathology of familial gastric cancer, with an emphasis on hereditary diffuse gastric cancer. J Clin Pathol 2008;61:25–30.

42. Figueiredo J, Söderberg O, Simões-Correia J, et al. The importance of E-cadherin binding partners to evaluate the pathogenicity of E-cadherin missense mutations associated to HDGC. Eur J Hum Genet 2013;21(3):301–9.

43. Suriano G, Oliveira C, Ferreira P, et al. Identification of CDH1 germline missense mutations associated with functional inactivation of the E-cadherin protein in young gastric cancer probands. Hum Mol Genet 2003;12:575–82.

44. Suriano G, Seixas S, Rocha J, et al. A model to infer the pathogenic significance of CDH1 germline missense variants. J Mol Med 2006;84:1023–31.

45. Simões-Correia J, Figueiredo J, Lopes R, et al. E-cadherin destabilization accounts for the pathogenicity of missense mutations in hereditary diffuse gastric cancer. PLoS One 2012;7:e33783.

46. Fitzgerald RC, Caldas C. Clinical implications of E-cadherin associated hereditary diffuse gastric cancer. Gut 2004;53:775–8.

47. Mimata A, Fukamachi H, Eishi Y, et al. Loss of E-cadherin in mouse gastric epithelial cells induces signet ring-like cells, a possible precursor lesion of diffuse gastric cancer. Cancer Sci 2011;102:942–50.

48. Shimada S, Mimata A, Sekine M, et al. Synergistic tumour suppressor activity of E-cadherin and p53 in a conditional mouse model for metastatic diffuse-type gastric cancer. Gut 2012;61:344–53.

49. Humar B, Guilford P. Hereditary diffuse gastric cancer: a manifestation of lost cell polarity. Cancer Sci 2009;100:1151–7.

50. Oliveira C, Moreira H, Seruca R, et al. Role of pathology in the identification of hereditary diffuse gastric cancer: report of a Portuguese family. Virchows Arch 2005;446:181–4.

51. Xie ZM, Li LS, Laquet C, et al. Germline mutations of the E-cadherin gene in families with inherited invasive lobular breast carcinoma but no diffuse gastric cancer. Cancer 2011;117:3112–7.

52. Charlton A, Blair V, Shaw D, et al. Hereditary diffuse gastric cancer: predominance of multiple foci of signet ring cell carcinoma in distal stomach and transitional zone. Gut 2004;53:814–20.

53. Lim YC, di Pietro M, O'Donovan M, et al. Prospective cohort study assessing outcomes of patients from families fulfilling criteria for hereditary diffuse gastric cancer undergoing endoscopic surveillance. Gastrointest Endosc 2014;80:78–87.

54. Shaw D, Blair V, Framp A, et al. Chromoendoscopic surveillance in hereditary diffuse gastric cancer: an alternative to prophylactic gastrectomy? Gut 2005;54:461–8.

55. Chen Y, Kingham K, Ford JM, et al. A prospective study of total gastrectomy for CDH1-positive hereditary diffuse gastric cancer. Ann Surg Oncol 2011;18:2594–8.

56. Brennan M. Pre-emptive surgery and increasing demands for technical perfection. Br J Surg 2003;90:3–4.

57. Kaurah P, Fitzgerald R, Dwerryhouse S, et al. Pregnancy after prophylactic total gastrectomy. Fam Cancer 2010;9:331–4.

58. Peck D, Welch J, Waugh J, et al. Pregnancy following gastric resection. Am J Obstet Gynecol 1964;90:517–20.

59. Pisani B. Term gestation following total gastrectomy. J Am Geriatr Soc 1958;6: 99–102.

60. Kluijt I, Sijmons RH, Hoogerbrugge N, et al. Familial gastric cancer: guidelines for diagnosis, treatment and periodic surveillance. Fam Cancer 2012;11:363–9.

61. Sano T, Kobori O, Muto T. Lymph node metastasis from early gastric cancer: endoscopic resection of tumour. Br J Surg 1992;79:241–4.

62. Ukleja A. Dumping syndrome: pathophysiology and treatment. Nutr Clin Pract 2005;20:517–25.

63. Peyre CG, DeMeester SR, Rizzetto C, et al. Vagal-sparing esophagectomy: the ideal operation for intramucosal adenocarcinoma and Barrett with high-grade dysplasia. Ann Surg 2007;246:665–71 [discussion: 671–4].

64. Kim HS, Kim BS, Lee IS, et al. Comparison of totally laparoscopic total gastrectomy and open total gastrectomy for gastric cancer. J Laparoendosc Adv Surg Tech A 2013;23:323–31.

65. Shinohara T, Satoh S, Kanaya S, et al. Laparoscopic versus open D2 gastrectomy for advanced gastric cancer: a retrospective cohort study. Surg Endosc 2013;27: 286–94.

66. Lee M, Lee JH, Park do J, et al. Comparison of short- and long-term outcomes of laparoscopic-assisted total gastrectomy and open total gastrectomy in gastric cancer patients. Surg Endosc 2013;27:2598–605.

67. Fein M, Fuchs KH, Thalheimer A, et al. Long-term benefits of Roux-en-Y pouch reconstruction after total gastrectomy: a randomized trial. Ann Surg 2008;247: 759–65.

68. Gertler R, Rosenberg R, Feith M, et al. Pouch vs no pouch following total gastrectomy: meta-analysis and systematic review. Am J Gastroenterol 2009;104: 2838–51.

69. Corso G, Roncalli F, Marrelli D, et al. History, pathogenesis, and management of familial gastric cancer: original study of John XXIII's family. Biomed Res Int 2013; 2013:385132.

70. Worthley DL, Phillips KD, Wayte N, et al. Gastric adenocarcinoma and proximal polyposis of the stomach (GAPPS): a new autosomal dominant syndrome. Gut 2012;61:774–9.

71. Yanaru-Fujisawa R, Nakamura S, Moriyama T, et al. Familial fundic gland polyposis with gastric cancer. Gut 2012;61:1103–4.

72. McLean MH, El-Omar EM. Genetics of gastric cancer. Nat Rev Gastroenterol Hepatol 2014;11:664–74.

Genetic Testing in the Multidisciplinary Management of Melanoma

Omar M. Rashid, MD, JD[a,b], Jonathan S. Zager, MD[a],*

KEYWORDS

- Melanoma • Genetic targets • Genetic testing • Screening • Targeted therapy
- Somatic mutations • Mutations

KEY POINTS

- The genetic heterogeneity of melanoma has been a challenge to identifying genetic targets for prognosis and screening.
- BRAF mutation analysis has become a standard approach to the management of metastatic melanoma.
- The role of genetic screening in the management of melanoma is controversial.

INTRODUCTION
Clinical and Epidemiologic Overview

Skin cancer is one of the fastest growing cancer diagnoses in the United States. The lifetime risk for the general population of developing melanoma is 1 in 55 and that risk has increased approximately 2% annually since 1960.[1–3] Because of the association with sun exposure, efforts to reduce the incidence of melanoma have focused on educating the public on risk modification strategies to improve sun safety. However, despite these efforts, the incidence of skin cancer in general and melanoma specifically have continued to increase, especially in Western countries.[1–3] Although a personal history of sun exposure and sunburns is the most important risk factor, a family history of melanoma and previous personal history of skin cancers have also been used as criteria to help guide screening. There have been efforts to identify patients who have a genetic predisposition to be at increased risk for skin cancer. There has been an increased interest in understanding the genetic components of melanoma carcinogenesis and how that influences risk in patients with melanoma to better guide

The authors have nothing to disclose.

[a] Department of Cutaneous Oncology, Moffitt Cancer Center, 12902 Magnolia Drive, SRB 4.24012, Tampa, FL 33612, USA; [b] Bienes Comprehensive Cancer Center, Holy Cross Hospital, 4725 N Federal Highway, Fort Lauderdale, FL 33308, USA
* Corresponding author.
E-mail address: jonathan.zager@moffitt.org

screening, surveillance, and clinical management of this disease. This article reviews the hereditary factors associated with melanoma and the role of genetic testing in the multidisciplinary management of melanoma.

Risk Factors

Although genetic factors have been identified for melanoma, only 10% or less of all melanoma cases arise in families with clusters of melanoma.[4] Many of these families do not have specific genotypic risk factors identified for melanoma, and a significant fraction of these families harbor no detectable mutations in specific susceptibility genes. For example, although CDKN2A is a gene that may indicate an increased risk of melanoma, several studies have failed to demonstrate a population-wide correlation with actually developing melanoma.[4] The link between skin color and melanoma has been applied to study the prevalence of melanoma in ethnic groups. Although ethnic groups with a darker complexion have a lower melanoma risk, melanoma in such individuals more commonly presents in the palms, nail beds, and soles. In individuals with a lighter complexion, skin color is determined by a combination of behavior and genetics, including the MC1R pigment-controlling gene.[5,6]

A positive melanoma family history has been correlated with an increased individual risk of developing melanoma, and as such, population-based studies have been conducted to focus on families with clusters of melanoma cases. Studies have reported a nearly 3 times increased risk of melanoma in individuals with a family history of melanoma, a lifetime risk of nearly 3%, and even as high as 14% when 2 or more individuals were diagnosed by age 30 years in a single family.[7,8] In addition, the risk was even higher when the population had a high frequency of sun exposure.[9,10] Nearly 40% of families with at least 3 melanoma cases demonstrated mutations in the major hereditary melanoma susceptibility gene, CDKN2A; however, more than 50% of such high-risk families demonstrate no known genetic mutation.[11,12] Because of these findings, it is recommended that genetic counseling be sought for patients with (1) 3 or more primary melanomas, (2) melanoma and pancreatic cancer, (3) melanoma and astrocytoma, or (4) at least 3 cases of melanoma or pancreatic cancer in a first-degree relative or with 2 first-degree relatives with melanoma and astrocytoma.[13]

When assessing an individual's risk of developing additional melanoma primary lesions, factors such as skin type, family history, CDKN2A mutation, and sun exposure all play a role. For example, a family history has been shown to increase the risk of a subsequent primary melanoma from 5% to 30%.[14–17] Similarly, if a patient has a history of nonmelanoma skin cancer, the risk of developing melanoma is also increased, which is thought to be due to a combination of genetic and environment risk factors.[18,19] Although the exact genetic mechanisms remain under investigation, it is established that patients with a family history of melanoma should be actively screened for melanoma. The following sections review the genetic mechanisms under investigation in melanoma and provide an update on the status of genetic testing in the multidisciplinary management of melanoma (**Table 1**).

SOMATIC GENETIC ALTERATIONS ASSOCIATED WITH MELANOMA CARCINOGENESIS
Tyrosine Kinases

An important class of proteins to consider in understanding the carcinogenesis of melanoma includes the receptor tyrosine kinases (TKs), which have been implicated in the carcinogenesis of many tumor types. TKs, which are postulated to play a role in the development of melanoma, include the epidermal growth factor receptor (EGFR), Met receptor tyrosine kinase (c-MET), and Kit receptor TK (c-KIT). Although EGFR

Table 1
Germline and somatic mutations seen in melanoma

Gene	Location	Function	Application in Melanoma
N-RAS	1p13-p11 Somatic mutation	Encodes NRAS, cell cycle regulation	Under investigation
H-RAS	11p15.5 Somatic mutation	Encodes HRAS, transforming protein p21, cell cycle regulation	Under investigation
BRAF	7q34 Somatic mutation	Encodes BRAF, cell cycle regulation	Selection of patients for targeted therapy
CDKN2A	9p21.3 Germline mutation	Encodes CDKN2A, p16, p14ARF, cell cycle regulation	Selection of patients for closer screening and surveillance
TERT	10p15 Germline and somatic mutations	Encodes hTERT, regulation of telomerase and cellular senescence	Under investigation
POT1	7q31.33 Germline mutation	Encodes POT1, regulation of telomerase and cellular senescence	Under investigation
CDK4	12q14.1 Germline and somatic mutations	Encodes CDK4, cell cycle regulation	Under investigation
BAP1	3p12.31-p21.2 Germline and somatic mutations	Encodes BAP1, regulates DNA repair	Under investigation
PTEN	10q23.31 Germline mutation	Encodes PTEN, cell cycle regulation	Under investigation
MC1R	16q24.3 Somatic mutation	Encodes MC1R, encodes skin and hair pigment	Under investigation
MITF	3p14-p13 Germline and somatic mutations	Encodes MITF, regulates melanocyte development	Under investigation
BRCA2	13q12.3 Germline mutation	Encodes BRCA2, regulates DNA repair	Under investigation

Abbreviations: ARF, alternate reading frame; BRAF, v-Raf murine sarcoma viral oncogene homolog B; BAP1, BRCA-associated protein 1; CDK4, cyclin dependent kinase 4; hTERT, human telomerase reverse transcriptase; MC1R, melanocortin 1 receptor; MITF, microphthalmia-associated transcription factor; PTEN, phosphatase and tensin homologue.

activation can result in further activation of the mitogen-activated protein kinase and phosphoinositide 3-kinase (PI3K) signaling cascades, initial studies in melanoma have not demonstrated overexpression of EGFR.[20–23] However, there are data from melanoma cell lines that targeting the EGFR-RAS signaling pathway may have potential as a therapeutic target in melanoma.[24–26] c-MET has been shown to be overexpressed in metastatic melanoma and promote invasiveness in in vitro and in vivo animal models, and there are investigations underway to further assess its role as a targeted therapy.[27–36] c-KIT has been implicated in activating numerous signaling pathways, such as PI3K and RAS/ERK.[37–39] Similar to c-MET, there are in vitro and in vivo animal model data in melanoma to support the role of c-KIT in cancer progression, invasiveness, and survival.[40–49] In addition, the TK inhibitor imatinib may be an effective agent in treating melanoma, as case reports in rectal and anal mucosal melanoma demonstrated KIT overexpression and promising therapeutic responses to treatment, but further studies are still required.[50,51] Although these preliminary results are promising, the exact role of TKs in melanoma remains under investigation, and thus, the application to clinical management is not yet established.

RAS/RAF/MEK/ERK and Phosphoinositide 3-Kinase Pathways

Of the receptor TK-associated pathways in cancer, the most promising pathways for clinical application in melanoma have been the RAS/RAF/MEK/ERK and the PI3K pathways.[52] The most common TK mutation found in melanoma is N-RAS, which is seen in approximately one-third of primary melanomas and about one-fourth of metastatic lesions, yet these mutations are rarely present in benign skin lesions such as nevi.[53–56] Although H-RAS mutations have been identified in Spitz nevi, these lesions do not transform into melanoma, and the application to atypical Spitz nevi, including in cases where they may transform into melanoma, remains controversial.[57–59] The precise role of the different RAS mutations in melanoma carcinogenesis remains unclear and is a focus of research.[60,61] In contrast, the RAF family plays an important role in melanoma, and advances in research have already translated into a major impact on the management of melanoma with targeted therapy, as described in the following.

The RAF family consists of ARAF, BRAF, and CRAF; however, thus far BRAF mutations seem to be the most clinically relevant in melanoma. In fact, BRAF mutations have been identified in a variety of tumor cell lines, the highest occurrence in melanoma. Sixty-seven percent of sequenced melanoma tumor samples demonstrated a mutation in BRAF. An amino acid substitution (V600E) was, by far, the most common mutation both in cell lines and tumor samples.[62] Alterations in BRAF may be an early somatic event (see later), as germline mutations in BRAF are not commonly found in familial melanoma.[63–65] However, studies of benign cutaneous lesions and dysplastic nevi have identified the presence of this mutation, even though such lesions do not often progress to melanoma.[66–69] Although BRAF is thought to be a mechanism of inhibiting the progression of premalignant lesions to melanoma by inducing senescence, investigations are underway to clarify this mechanism.[70–74] In fact, the BRAF pathway has not been shown to promote melanoma carcinogenesis without failures in other pathways, such as p53 deficiency or changes in N-RAS expression.[74,75] Although BRAF V600E mutated melanoma is more likely to arise in less sun-exposed areas of the body, N-RAS mutated melanoma is more likely present in more sun-exposed areas, with significant differences between the two in genetic signatures of these 2 melanoma types.[75,76] The ERK pathway is another important factor under investigation, especially because in NRAS cells ERK activation is low in contrast to BRAF mutated melanoma.[76] The PI3K pathway has been implicated as an important factor in determining survival in melanoma because of its activation of AKT, which is inversely related to patient survival.[77] AKT3 activation has been identified in nearly two-thirds of sporadic melanoma samples; its role in cancer progression has been demonstrated in many in vitro and in vivo animal studies, whereas studies are underway to clarify its relevance to melanoma.[78]

Although the specific mechanisms of the role of BRAF in melanoma carcinogenesis and biology remain under investigation, BRAF regulation of melanoma cell survival has emerged as a target for therapy. The BRAF kinase inhibitor vemurafenib demonstrated improved overall and progression-free survival in stage IIIC and IV melanoma.[79] Accordingly, the US Food and Drug Administration (FDA) granted approval in 2011 for the use of vemurafenib in patients with BRAF V600E mutated unresectable metastatic melanoma. A second agent targeting BRAF has demonstrated promise. Dabrafenib, a selective BRAF kinase inhibitor, demonstrated improved progression-free survival in an international multi-institutional crossover study not designed to demonstrate an overall survival benefit.[80] The FDA in 2014 granted approval for the use of dabrafenib in the treatment of BRAF V600E mutated unresectable metastatic melanoma.

GERMLINE (HEREDITARY) GENETIC ALTERATIONS ASSOCIATED WITH MELANOMA PREDISPOSITION
CDKN2A (P16)

Of all the candidates for a genetic test to assess the risk of developing melanoma in the general population, CDKN2A has demonstrated the most promise (see **Table 1**). CDKN2A/p16 is a cyclin-dependent kinase inhibitor 2A located on chromosome 9p21.[11] It operates through the cyclin D1/cyclin-dependent kinase 4 complex to regulate the retinoblastoma gene pathway functioning as a tumor suppressor, controlling cell cycle progression, and blocking progression at G1/S for DNA damage repair.[11] It encodes p16INK4a and p14ARF, proteins that inhibit cellular senescence.[11] When the standard reading frame protein is not encoded, the exon 1 alternate reading frame (ARF) functions through the p53 pathway, which normally causes cell cycle arrest supporting blockade at G1/S and allows for DNA repair to thus prevent carcinogenesis. Taken together, the disruption of this pathway results in failure in tumor suppression and is actually accountable for 40% of all familial melanoma cases.[11]

Despite the prevalence of CDKN2A mutations in cases of familial melanoma, the penetrance of the melanoma phenotype in carriers of CDKN2A mutations has varied in the literature.[81] Although in Australia the penetrance has ranged from 30% to 91%, this contrasts to the United States (50%–76%) and Europe (13%–58%).[81] However, there was no difference in the cumulative risk of melanoma in CDKN2A mutation–positive families in Australia versus those in the United Kingdom.[82] Because of this variable penetrance, other genetic factors have been investigated as modifiers of the risk of developing melanoma in CDKN2A mutation carriers. For example, the melanocortin 1 receptor (MC1R), a somatic mutation, has been found to augment CDKN2A penetrance, and other genetic factors such as interleukin 9 (IL-9) and GSTT1, both somatic modifiers, have also been found to affect the risk of developing melanoma.[83] In addition to these identified genetic factors, it has been shown that CDKN2A mutation carriers who develop melanoma do so at a younger age than patients with CDKN2A wild-type melanoma, at a median age of 39 versus 54.3 years, respectively.[84]

Greater Breslow thickness was also found to correlate with the presence of a CDKN2A mutation; a 90% chance of the mutation was demonstrated in cases greater than 0.4 mm thick when investigating cases of melanoma in high cluster families (defined as at least 3 cases per family).[85] Patients with the CDKN2A mutation also had increased risks of pancreatic, breast, gastrointestinal, and lung cancers and Wilms tumor, suggesting additional genetic modifiers of the cancer phenotype in CDKN2A mutation carriers remain to be identified.[86] Although more specific CDKN2A variants have been identified, such as the CDKN2A exon 1β mutations (p14ARF), which demonstrated increased melanoma risk compared with individuals without the p16INK4a mutation, there is no commercially available genetic test for this mutation at this time.[87] Accordingly, studies have evaluated potential candidates for genetic testing in CDKN2A carriers to assess for the risk of other malignancies and hereditary syndromes. However, specific candidates have not yet been firmly established as appropriate for genetic testing.

Investigations of families with CDKN2A germline mutations indicate an increased incidence of pancreatic cancer and neural system tumors within certain subpopulations.[88] Specifically, in families with CDKN2A pathologic mutations that take the form of a so-called ankyrin repeat, there was a higher incidence of family clusters with both melanoma and pancreatic cancer cases rather than melanoma alone.[88] Families carrying a deletion CDKN2A exon 2 mutation (p16 Leiden) were also found to be at increased risk of melanoma and pancreatic cancer, in contrast to melanoma cluster families without that specific CDKN2A mutation that did not demonstrate an increased pancreatic cancer incidence.[88] However, other studies have not demonstrated an increased risk of pancreatic cancer in CDKN2A mutation families, and some CDKN2A mutation families demonstrated pancreatic cancer risk only.[88] Therefore, it is thought that other genetic factors may be contributing to the link between CDKN2A mutation and the phenotype of melanoma and pancreatic cancer.[88] Some CDKN2A mutation carriers also demonstrate the phenotype of the melanoma-astrocytoma syndrome.[88] The hallmark of this syndrome is the presence of melanoma in addition to tumors of the nervous system. This syndrome was only identified in the 1990s when individuals in high cluster melanoma case families were also found to have nervous system tumors, including neural cell tumors.[88] When these individuals were studied further, there was a loss of function in p14ARF, an ARF protein product of CDKN2A, strongly suggesting a link to CDKN2A.[88]

CDKN2A has been widely studied as a candidate gene for melanoma. Its mechanism through a cyclin-dependent kinase as a tumor suppressor has been established for oncogenesis in multiple studies. In addition, there have been some promising results that have demonstrated a link between CDKN2A mutations and a risk for developing cancer, including melanoma. However, these results have not been validated sufficiently to translate into a specific genetic test that assesses the risk of developing these phenotypes in the general population.

Telomeres

Telomeres are another important area of inquiry in the genetic understanding of melanoma carcinogenesis. Mutations in the telomerase reverse transcriptase (TERT) gene, on chromosome 5p, have been demonstrated in individuals with familial melanoma and other cancers such as bronchial, renal, ovarian, and bladder cancers, as well as in cases of sporadic melanoma.[89] The prevalence of TERT mutations in families with multiple melanoma cases is under investigation. Another telomere-associated gene has been implicated in melanoma; POT1 maintains telomere length by binding single-stranded repeats. Studies in multiple melanoma case families demonstrated correlations with POT1 missense mutations, including Ser270Asn, Tyr89Cys, Arg137His, and Gln623-His.[90] Supporting this mechanism is the finding of longer telomeres in POT1 mutated melanoma cases than in nonmutated cases.[90] Although these mutations were identified in 4% of non-CDKN2A melanoma families, the results have not been sufficiently validated to allow development of a genetic test that could be used to assess the risk of developing melanoma or to affect treatment.

Cyclin-Dependent Kinases

Another important candidate for melanoma genetic testing includes cyclin-dependent kinases, which regulate cell cycle progression and function in concert with CDK4 and 6. Although cyclin-dependent retinoblastoma protein phosphorylation results in changes in gene expression along the same pathway as CDKN2A, CDK4 mutations are not prevalent in sequenced melanoma samples.[91] Although families bearing CDK4 mutations demonstrated melanoma risk similar to that of CDKN2A families, CDK6 mutations have not been found in patients with melanoma.[92] It has also been demonstrated that patients with xeroderma pigmentosum, which results from defects in DNA repair, have a 1000 times increased likelihood of developing melanoma compared with the general population.[93] Another cyclin-dependent kinase–regulated tumor suppressor gene, BRCA-associated protein 1 (BAP1), was demonstrated as a factor in 84% of metastatic uveal melanoma somatic samples and has also been postulated to play a role in cutaneous melanoma.[94] Not only has BAP1 been implicated in sporadic and familial cases of melanoma but also there is evidence that BAP1 mutations are associated with paraganglioma, mesothelioma, and renal and lung cancer.[95] Although cyclin-dependent kinase–associated candidate genes remain under study, there is no established validated assay for genetic testing.

Phosphatase and Tensin Homologue, 9p21, and Additional Candidate Loci for Melanoma Predisposition

Phosphatase and tensin homologue (PTEN) is another important candidate for genetic testing in melanoma. PTEN is a phosphatase gene in which multiple mutations have been identified and have been implicated in the pathology of multiple organ systems.[96] PTEN mutations are associated with the PTEN hamartoma tumor syndromes, including Cowden and Bannayan-Riley-Ruvalcaba syndromes.[96] Diagnostic criteria for Cowden syndrome include mucocutaneous lesions and gangliocytoma.[96] Although the vast majority of patients with the PTEN mutation failed to demonstrate the phenotypic diagnostic criteria, they still had an 85% chance of developing cancer by age 70 years and a 6% chance of developing melanoma.[97] PTEN is located on chromosome 9p21. Loss of heterozygosity at 9p21 has been independently linked to melanoma carcinogenesis, and additional genes in this region are being sought.[98] In addition, the 1p22 locus has been correlated in melanoma cases that were CDKN2A and CDK4 mutation negative.[99] However, specific gene targets remain under investigation.[99] Recent studies have identified the 10q25.1 locus as a genetic association with melanoma, with single nucleotide polymorphisms significantly increasing the risk of melanoma, but specific genes have not been identified yet.[99] Other loci under investigation include 3p29, 17p11 to 12, and 18q22, but their link to melanoma have not been thoroughly validated.[100] Another candidate is the 20q11 locus, which encodes a signaling protein that controls hair color and is a MC1R antagonist, which has been correlated with an increased risk of melanoma.[101] However, no interaction between variants at this locus, MC1R variants, and melanoma risk have been proved to date (see later discussion).[101]

Melanocortin 1 Receptor

Mutations in MC1R have been correlated with red hair, fair skin, poor tanning, and increased skin cancer risk, and thus MC1R has been investigated as a candidate for genetic testing in melanoma.[102] Although some studies demonstrated a link between melanoma risk and MC1R mutation in patients with red hair, other studies demonstrated the link in MC1R mutants with dark hair, dark complexion, and good tanning ability.[102] In addition, an independent link between the R163Q DNA sequence variant of MC1R and melanoma was identified, as well as an increased risk of basal cell carcinoma in MC1R mutants whose other characteristics are traditionally considered low risk.[102] Similar findings have also been reported in cutaneous squamous cell carcinoma.[102] Patients with both CDKN2A and MC1R mutations had a significantly increased risk of melanoma; however, this increased risk only remained significant in individuals with dark hair.[103] Furthermore, patients with CDKN2A mutation had greater increased risk of melanoma when they expressed one or more MC1R variants, and this risk was seen among younger age groups.[103] For example, both Arg160Trp and Asp84Glu mutations of MC1R have been associated with increased melanoma risk in CDKN2A mutants.[104] There is some evidence that MC1R mutations may correlate with improved survival and may thus provide prognostic information.[104]

Microphthalmia-Associated Transcription Factor

The microphthalmia-associated transcription factor (MITF) regulates melanocyte function; the E318K mutation has been implicated in melanoma, and thus MITF is another candidate for melanoma genetic testing.[105] Not only has this mutation been found to be in higher prevalence in melanoma cases but it has also been identified in CDKN2A and CDK4-negative melanoma cases.[105] That correlation was found in patients who had a light complexion, nevi, freckles, more than 1 primary melanoma, and amelanotic melanoma.[105] Although population-based studies in the United Kingdom and Australia demonstrated an increased risk of melanoma correlated with the E318K MTIF mutation, a similar correlation was not demonstrated in a population-based Polish study.[105] It remains under investigation and has not yet been established for genetic testing in clinical practice.

BRCA

Although BRCA2 mutations have been established as an important genetic factor in carcinogenesis in other cancers, their role in melanoma remains uncertain and under investigation. Despite initial reports of an increased risk of melanoma in BRCA2 carriers as high as 2.6 times that of the general population, further studies have not demonstrated the same significantly increased risk of melanoma.[106] A Dutch study reported a lower risk of developing melanoma in BRCA2 carriers.[106] Studies of melanoma cases in the Ashkenazi Jewish population have failed to demonstrate any increased rate of either BRCA2 or BRCA1 positivity.[106]

The Current Role of Genetic Testing in the Clinical Management of Melanoma

Although genetic testing is available for CDKN2A, the most established genetic risk factor for melanoma, its role in clinical practice remains controversial. Advocates for genetic testing cite the importance of accurate diagnosis, improving patient compliance with screening for early detection, and the value of a negative test result for individuals in a mutation-bearing family.[107] However, as discussed earlier, many patients who have a genetic predisposition still test negative for CDKN2A mutations. Furthermore, individuals in a family with CDKN2A mutation who test negative for CDKN2A are still at an increased risk of developing melanoma compared with the general population. In contrast, somatic genetic testing of melanoma tumors to identify which patients may benefit from targeted therapy has made significant progress. The dramatic advances made with the success of BRAF-targeted therapy has changed significantly the landscape of the multidisciplinary management of metastatic melanoma with routine testing for the BRAFV600E mutation. The clinical applications of genetic testing for assessing the risk of developing melanoma remain unclear, and instead, the clinical assessment of risk remains based primarily on personal and family history.

Clinical Assessment of Melanoma Risk

Personal and family history are important risk factors for melanoma.[107] Furthermore, environmental factors such as sun exposure also increase the risk of developing melanoma. Therefore, education about sun safety and early signs of melanoma is critical, including regular skin examinations by the appropriately skilled providers.[107] Patients with a personal history of melanoma and/or a strong family history of melanoma whereby multiple first- or second-degree relatives have been diagnosed with melanoma should undergo semiannual examinations starting at age 10 years until nevi are considered stable, then annually thereafter.[107] These patients should also be taught skin self-examination techniques (parents for the pediatric population), to be performed on a monthly basis. Observation of lesions may be aided by techniques such as full-body photography and dermoscopy.[107] A cost-utility analysis has demonstrated the benefits of screening in the high-risk population.[107] The same criteria for biopsy of suspicious lesions should be applied to this population, and prophylactic removal of nevi without suspicious features should not be advocated.[107] Furthermore, it is important to consider that these patients are more likely to develop melanoma spontaneously rather than from a premalignant lesion.[107] For individuals at normal risk, monthly self skin examinations and yearly whole-body skin examinations from a qualified physician are recommended for early detection of melanoma.

SUMMARY

The genetics of melanoma is complex as is the literature that attempts to describe it. A critical first step for researchers and readers alike is to distinguish clearly between somatic (tumor) DNA changes and germline (heritable) genetic alterations. Germline genetic testing to clarify heritable increased predisposition to melanoma is an important component of this book. As described earlier, germline mutations in the CDKN2A gene have been associated with increased risk of developing melanoma. Clinical testing is available to identify germline CDKN2A mutations. Expert opinion regarding the use of CDKN2A is somewhat divided. Current evidence does not support population-based testing of CDKN2A to identify individuals at increased risk. However, there is literature support for testing members of high risk melanoma families. A negative test result (no CDKN2A germline mutation found) is not associated with melanoma risk equal to the general population. That patient, a member of a high risk melanoma family, remains at increased risk, and increased clinical vigilance is still required (**Table 2**). Based on this complexity, the National Cancer Institute recommends that consideration for germline genetic testing be undertaken after thorough evaluation by a certified genetic counselor. Specific groups for which genetic counseling evaluation is recommended include patients with (1) 3 or more primary melanomas, (2) melanoma and pancreatic cancer, (3) melanoma and astrocytoma, and (4) at least 3 cases of melanoma or pancreatic cancer in a first-degree relative or with 2 first-degree relatives with melanoma and astrocytoma.[13] The importance of a thorough cancer family history when caring for patients with melanoma, and indeed all patients, cannot be overstated (see **Table 2**). Completion of a diligent family history can be lifesaving, as it may direct

Table 2
Relative indications for genetic counseling and increased frequency of clinical surveillance in patients with melanoma

Indications for Genetic Counseling	Indications for Close Skin Surveillance
A patient diagnosed with 3 or more primary melanomas	Personal history of melanoma
A patient diagnosed with melanoma and pancreatic cancer	More than 1 first-degree relative diagnosed with melanoma
A patient diagnosed with melanoma and astrocytoma	More than 1 second-degree relative diagnosed with melanoma
More than 2 first-degree relatives with melanoma or pancreatic cancer	Personal history of environmental factors such as sun exposure and skin damage
More than 1 first-degree relative with melanoma and astrocytoma	

increased screening and surveillance to those at greatest risk and most in need. Please see the article by Drs Venne and Scheuner for a review of state-of-the-art family history documentation techniques.

Somatic genetic testing of melanoma tumors plays an important role in optimizing care for patients with melanoma. However, a major challenge in understanding the genetics of melanoma carcinogenesis and the development of genetic targets for therapy has been the considerable genomic heterogeneity of melanoma tumors. Although technological limitations have historically slowed the progression of therapeutic somatic genetics, advances have recently been made. Perhaps the most dramatic example of this progress is the emerging role of BRAF mutations in the clinical management of melanoma described earlier. The potential of somatic genetic testing for melanoma is illustrated by advances in ocular melanoma and the availability of commercial tests, although their precise role and clinical application remains controversial.[108] A concise expanded review of advances in melanoma somatic genetics and associated targeted molecular therapies can be found at http://www.cancer.gov/types/skin/hp/skin-genetics-pdq#section/all.[109]

In conclusion, dramatic gains have been made in understanding the germline and somatic genetics of melanoma. However, the clinical applications of these gains remain limited and in need of continued investigation. That said, there is clearly enormous potential for advancing the understanding of melanoma genetics. Progress in this field will improve our ability to discern who is at risk of the disease and produce additional targeted molecular therapies with improved clinical efficacy.

REFERENCES

1. Siegel R, Ma J, Zou Z, et al. Cancer statistics, 2014. CA Cancer J Clin 2014; 64(1):9–29.
2. Ries L, Melbert D, Krapcho M, et al, National Cancer Institute. SEER cancer statistics review, 1975–2005. Bethesda (MD): National Cancer Institute; 2008.
3. Rigel DS. Cutaneous ultraviolet exposure and its relationship to the development of skin cancer. J Am Acad Dermatol 2008;58(5 Suppl 2):S129–32.
4. Berwick M, Orlow I, Hummer AJ, et al. The prevalence of CDKN2A germ-line mutations and relative risk for cutaneous malignant melanoma: an international population-based study. Cancer Epidemiol Biomarkers Prev 2006;15(8):1520–5.
5. Scherer D, Kumar R. Genetics of pigmentation in skin cancer–a review. Mutat Res 2010;705(2):141–53.
6. Fitzpatrick TB. The validity and practicality of sun-reactive skin types I through VI. Arch Dermatol 1988;124(6):869–71.
7. Brandt A, Sundquist J, Hemminki K. Risk of incident and fatal melanoma in individuals with a family history of incident or fatal melanoma or any cancer. Br J Dermatol 2011;165(2):342–8.
8. Fallah M, Pukkala E, Sundquist K, et al. Familial melanoma by histology and age: joint data from five Nordic countries. Eur J Cancer 2014;50(6):1176–83.
9. Olsen CM, Carroll HJ, Whiteman DC. Familial melanoma: a meta-analysis and estimates of attributable fraction. Cancer Epidemiol Biomarkers Prev 2010;19(1):65–73.
10. Hemminki K, Zhang H, Czene K. Incidence trends and familial risks in invasive and in situ cutaneous melanoma by sun-exposed body sites. Int J Cancer 2003; 104(6):764–71.
11. Goldstein AM, Chan M, Harland M, et al. High-risk melanoma susceptibility genes and pancreatic cancer, neural system tumors, and uveal melanoma across GenoMEL. Cancer Res 2006;66(20):9818–28.

12. Bishop JN, Harland M, Bishop DT. The genetics of melanoma. Br J Hosp Med 2006;67(6):299–304.
13. Hampel H, Bennett RL, Buchanan A, et al. A practice guideline from the American College of Medical Genetics and Genomics and the National Society of Genetic Counselors: referral indications for cancer predisposition assessment. Genet Med 2015;17(1):70–87.
14. Goggins WB, Tsao H. A population-based analysis of risk factors for a second primary cutaneous melanoma among melanoma survivors. Cancer 2003; 97(3):639–43.
15. Slingluff CL Jr, Vollmer RT, Seigler HF. Multiple primary melanoma: incidence and risk factors in 283 patients. Surgery 1993;113(3):330–9.
16. Giles G, Staples M, McCredie M, et al. Multiple primary melanomas: an analysis of cancer registry data from Victoria and New South Wales. Melanoma Res 1995;5(6):433–8.
17. Begg CB, Orlow I, Hummer AJ, et al. Lifetime risk of melanoma in CDKN2A mutation carriers in a population-based sample. J Natl Cancer Inst 2005;97(20):1507–15.
18. Karagas MR, Greenberg ER, Mott LA, et al. Occurrence of other cancers among patients with prior basal cell and squamous cell skin cancer. Cancer Epidemiol Biomarkers Prev 1998;7(2):157–61.
19. Chen J, Ruczinski I, Jorgensen TJ, et al. Nonmelanoma skin cancer and risk for subsequent malignancy. J Natl Cancer Inst 2008;100(17):1215–22.
20. Bastian BC, LeBoit PE, Hamm H, et al. Chromosomal gains and losses in primary cutaneous melanomas detected by comparative genomic hybridization. Cancer Res 1998;58(10):2170–5.
21. Koprowski H, Herlyn M, Balaban G, et al. Expression of the receptor for epidermal growth factor correlates with increased dosage of chromosome 7 in malignant melanoma. Somat Cell Mol Genet 1985;11(3):297–302.
22. Udart M, Utikal J, Krahn GM, et al. Chromosome 7 aneusomy. A marker for metastatic melanoma? Expression of the epidermal growth factor receptor gene and chromosome 7 aneusomy in nevi, primary malignant melanomas and metastases. Neoplasia 2001;3(3):245–54.
23. Bardeesy N, Kim M, Xu J, et al. Role of epidermal growth factor receptor signaling in RAS-driven melanoma. Mol Cell Biol 2005;25(10):4176–88.
24. Dlugosz AA, Hansen L, Cheng C, et al. Targeted disruption of the epidermal growth factor receptor impairs growth of squamous papillomas expressing the v-ras(Ha) oncogene but does not block in vitro keratinocyte responses to oncogenic ras. Cancer Res 1997;57(15):3180–8.
25. Gangarosa LM, Sizemore N, Graves-Deal R, et al. A raf-independent epidermal growth factor receptor autocrine loop is necessary for Ras transformation of rat intestinal epithelial cells. J Biol Chem 1997;272(30):18926–31.
26. Sibilia M, Fleischmann A, Behrens A, et al. The EGF receptor provides an essential survival signal for SOS-dependent skin tumor development. Cell 2000; 102(2):211–20.
27. Bottaro DP, Rubin JS, Faletto DL. Identification of the hepatocyte growth factor receptor as the c-met proto-oncogene product. Science 1991;251:802–4.
28. Wiltshire RN, Duray P, Bittner ML, et al. Direct visualization of the clonal progression of primary cutaneous melanoma: application of tissue microdissection and comparative genomic hybridization. Cancer Res 1995;55:3954–7.
29. Natali PG, Nicotra MR, Di Renzo MF, et al. Expression of the c-Met/HGF receptor in human melanocytic neoplasms: demonstration of the relationship to malignant melanoma tumour progression. Br J Cancer 1993;68(4):746–50.

30. Vande Woude GF, Jeffers M, Cortner J, et al. Met-HGF/SF: tumorigenesis, invasion and metastasis. Ciba Found Symp 1997;212:119–30.

31. Rusciano D, Lorenzoni P, Burger MM. Expression of constitutively activated hepatocyte growth factor/scatter factor receptor (c-met) in B16 melanoma cells selected for enhanced liver colonization. Oncogene 1995;11(10):1979–87.

32. Otsuka T, Takayama H, Sharp R, et al. c-Met autocrine activation induces development of malignant melanoma and acquisition of the metastatic phenotype. Cancer Res 1998;58(22):5157–67.

33. Noonan FP, Recio JA, Takayama H, et al. Neonatal sunburn and melanoma in mice. Nature 2001;413(6853):271–2.

34. Recio JA, Noonan FP, Takayama H, et al. Ink4a/arf deficiency promotes ultraviolet radiation-induced melanomagenesis. Cancer Res 2002;62(22):6724–30.

35. McGill GG, Haq R, Nishimura EK, et al. c-Met expression is regulated by MITF in the melanocyte lineage. J Biol Chem 2006;281(15):10365–73.

36. Garraway LA, Widlund HR, Rubin MA, et al. Integrative genomic analyses identify MITF as a lineage survival oncogene amplified in malignant melanoma. Nature 2005;436(7047):117–22.

37. Montone KT, van Belle P, Elenitsas R, et al. Proto-oncogene c-kit expression in malignant melanoma: protein loss with tumor progression. Mod Pathol 1997; 10(9):939–44.

38. Shen SS, Zhang PS, Eton O, et al. Analysis of protein tyrosine kinase expression in melanocytic lesions by tissue array. J Cutan Pathol 2003;30(9):539–47.

39. Isabel Zhu Y, Fitzpatrick JE. Expression of c-kit (CD117) in Spitz nevus and malignant melanoma. J Cutan Pathol 2006;33(1):33–7.

40. Huang S, Luca M, Gutman M, et al. Enforced c-KIT expression renders highly metastatic human melanoma cells susceptible to stem cell factor-induced apoptosis and inhibits their tumorigenic and metastatic potential. Oncogene 1996;13:2339–47.

41. Yoshida H, Kunisada T, Kusakabe M, et al. Distinct stages of melanocyte differentiation revealed by anlaysis of nonuniform pigmentation patterns. Development 1996;122(4):1207–14.

42. Grichnik JM, Burch JA, Burchette J, et al. The SCF/KIT pathway plays a critical role in the control of normal human melanocyte homeostasis. J Invest Dermatol 1998;111(2):233–8.

43. Sviderskaya EV, Wakeling WF, Bennett DC. A cloned, immortal line of murine melanoblasts inducible to differentiate to melanocytes. Development 1995; 121(5):1547–57.

44. Willmore-Payne C, Holden JA, Tripp S, et al. Human malignant melanoma: detection of BRAF- and c-kit-activating mutations by high-resolution amplicon melting analysis. Hum Pathol 2005;36(5):486–93.

45. Willmore-Payne C, Holden JA, Hirschowitz S, et al. BRAF and c-kit gene copy number in mutation-positive malignant melanoma. Hum Pathol 2006;37(5): 520–7.

46. Nakahara M, Isozaki K, Hirota S, et al. A novel gain-of-function mutation of c-kit gene in gastrointestinal stromal tumors. Gastroenterology 1998;115(5):1090–5.

47. Fukuda R, Hamamoto N, Uchida Y, et al. Gastrointestinal stromal tumor with a novel mutation of KIT proto-oncogene. Intern Med 2001;40(4):301–3.

48. Curtin JA, Busam K, Pinkel D, et al. Somatic activation of KIT in distinct subtypes of melanoma. J Clin Oncol 2006;24(26):4340–6.

49. Beadling C, Jacobson-Dunlop E, Hodi FS, et al. KIT gene mutations and copy number in melanoma subtypes. Clin Cancer Res 2008;14(21):6821–8.

50. Hodi FS, Friedlander P, Corless CL, et al. Major response to imatinib mesylate in KIT-mutated melanoma. J Clin Oncol 2008;26(12):2046–51.

51. Lutzky J, Bauer J, Bastian BC. Dose-dependent, complete response to imatinib of a metastatic mucosal melanoma with a K642E KIT mutation. Pigment Cell Melanoma Res 2008;21(4):492–3.

52. Hanahan D, Weinberg RA. The hallmarks of cancer. Cell 2000;100(1):57–70.

53. Jafari M, Papp T, Kirchner S, et al. Analysis of ras mutations in human melanocytic lesions: activation of the ras gene seems to be associated with the nodular type of human malignant melanoma. J Cancer Res Clin Oncol 1995;121(1):23–30.

54. van Elsas A, Zerp SF, van der Flier S, et al. Relevance of ultraviolet-induced N-ras oncogene point mutations in development of primary human cutaneous melanoma. Am J Pathol 1996;149(3):883–93.

55. Papp T, Pemsel H, Zimmermann R, et al. Mutational analysis of the N-ras, p53, p16INK4a, CDK4, and MC1R genes in human congenital melanocytic naevi. J Med Genet 1999;36:610–4.

56. Albino AP, Nanus DM, Mentle IR, et al. Analysis of ras oncogenes in malignant melanoma and precursor lesions: correlation of point mutations with differentiation phenotype. Oncogene 1989;4:1363–74.

57. Bastian BC, LeBoit PE, Pinkel D. Mutations and copy number increase of HRAS in Spitz nevi with distinctive histopathological features. Am J Pathol 2000;157:967–72.

58. Barnhill RL. The Spitzoid lesion: rethinking Spitz tumors, atypical variants, 'Spitzoid melanoma' and risk assessment. Mod Pathol 2006;19:S21–33.

59. Smith KJ, Barrett TL, Skelton HG 3rd, et al. Spindle cell and epithelioid cell nevi with atypia and metastasis (malignant Spitz nevus). Am J Surg Pathol 1989;13(11):931–9.

60. Sharpless NE, Kannan K, Xu J, et al. Both products of the mouse Ink4a/Arf locus suppress melanoma formation in vivo. Oncogene 2003;22(32):5055–9.

61. Ackermann J, Frutschi M, Kaloulis K, et al. Metastasizing melanoma formation caused by expression of activated N-RasQ61Kon an INK4a-deficient background. Cancer Res 2005;65(10):4005–11.

62. Davies H, Bignell GR, Cox C, et al. Mutations of the BRAF gene in human cancer. Nature 2002;417(6892):949–54.

63. Lang J, Boxer M, MacKie R. Absence of exon 15 BRAF germline mutations in familial melanoma. Hum Mutat 2003;21(3):327–30.

64. Casula M, Colombino M, Satta MP, et al. BRAF gene is somatically mutated but does not make a major contribution to malignant melanoma susceptibility: the Italian Melanoma Intergroup Study. J Clin Oncol 2004;22(2):286–92.

65. Laud K, Kannengiesser C, Avril MF, et al. BRAF as a melanoma susceptibility candidate gene? Cancer Res 2003;63(12):3061–5.

66. Pollock PM, Harper UL, Hansen KS, et al. High frequency of BRAF mutations in nevi. Nat Genet 2003;33(1):19–20.

67. Kumar R, Angelini S, Snellman E, et al. BRAF mutations are common somatic events in melanocytic nevi. J Invest Dermatol 2004;122(2):342–8.

68. Saldanha G, Purnell D, Fletcher A, et al. High BRAF mutation frequency does not characterize all melanocytic tumor types. Int J Cancer 2004;111(5):705–10.

69. Yazdi AS, Palmedo G, Flaig MJ, et al. Mutations of the BRAF gene in benign and malignant melanocytic lesions. J Invest Dermatol 2003;121(5):1160–2.

70. Michaloglou C, Vredeveld LC, Soengas MS, et al. BRAFE600-associated senescence-like cell cycle arrest of human naevi. Nature 2005;436(7051):720–4.

71. Wellbrock C, Ogilvie L, Hedley D, et al. V599EB-RAF is an oncogene in melanocytes. Cancer Res 2004;64(7):2338–42.

72. Sharpless NE, DePinho RA. Cancer: crime and punishment. Nature 2005; 436(7051):636–7.

73. Wajapeyee N, Serra RW, Zhu X, et al. Oncogenic BRAF induces senescence and apoptosis through pathways mediated by the secreted protein IGFBP7. Cell 2008;132(3):363–74.

74. Chudnovsky Y, Adams AE, Robbins PB, et al. Use of human tissue to assess the oncogenic activity of melanoma-associated mutations. Nat Genet 2005;37(7): 745–9.

75. Bhatt KV, Hu R, Spofford LS, et al. Mutant B-RAF signaling and cyclin D1 regulate Cks1/S-phase kinase-associated protein 2-mediated degradation of p27Kip1 in human melanoma cells. Oncogene 2007;26(7):1056–66.

76. Shields JM, Thomas NE, Cregger M, et al. Lack of extracellular signal-regulated kinase mitogen-activated protein kinase signaling shows a new type of melanoma. Cancer Res 2007;67(4):1502–12.

77. Dai DL, Martinka M, Li G. Prognostic significance of activated Akt expression in melanoma: a clinicopathologic study of 292 cases. J Clin Oncol 2005;23(7): 1473–82.

78. Stahl JM, Sharma A, Cheung M, et al. Deregulated Akt3 activity promotes development of malignant melanoma. Cancer Res 2004;64(19):7002–10.

79. Chapman PB, Hauschild A, Robert C, et al. Improved survival with vemurafenib in melanoma with BRAF V600E mutation. N Engl J Med 2011;364(26):2507–16.

80. Hauschild A, Grob JJ, Demidov LV, et al. Dabrafenib in BRAF-mutated metastatic melanoma: a multicentre, open-label, phase 3 randomised controlled trial. Lancet 2012;380(9839):358–65.

81. Bishop DT, Demenais F, Goldstein AM, et al. Geographical variation in the penetrance of CDKN2A mutations for melanoma. J Natl Cancer Inst 2002;94(12): 894–903.

82. Cust AE, Harland M, Makalic E, et al. Melanoma risk for CDKN2A mutation carriers who are relatives of population-based case carriers in Australia and the UK. J Med Genet 2011;48(4):266–72.

83. Santillan AA, Cherpelis BS, Glass LF, et al. Management of familial melanoma and nonmelanoma skin cancer syndromes. Surg Oncol Clin N Am 2009;18(1): 73–98.

84. van der Rhee JI, Krijnen P, Gruis NA, et al. Clinical and histologic characteristics of malignant melanoma in families with a germline mutation in CDKN2A. J Am Acad Dermatol 2011;65(2):281–8.

85. Pedace L, De Simone P, Castori M, et al. Clinical features predicting identification of CDKN2A mutations in Italian patients with familial cutaneous melanoma. Cancer Epidemiol 2011;35(6):e116–20.

86. Mukherjee B, Delancey JO, Raskin L, et al. Risk of non-melanoma cancers in first-degree relatives of CDKN2A mutation carriers. J Natl Cancer Inst 2012; 104(12):953–6.

87. Binni F, Antigoni I, De Simone P, et al. Novel and recurrent p14 mutations in Italian familial melanoma. Clin Genet 2010;77(6):581–6.

88. Goldstein AM, Fraser MC, Struewing JP, et al. Increased risk of pancreatic cancer in melanoma-prone kindreds with p16INK4 mutations. N Engl J Med 1995; 333(15):970–4.

89. Horn S, Figl A, Rachakonda PS, et al. TERT promoter mutations in familial and sporadic melanoma. Science 2013;339(6122):959–61.

90. Shi J, Yang XR, Ballew B, et al. Rare missense variants in POT1 predispose to familial cutaneous malignant melanoma. Nat Genet 2014;46(5):482–6.
91. Zuo L, Weger J, Yang Q, et al. Germline mutations in the p16INK4a binding domain of CDK4 in familial melanoma. Nat Genet 1996;12(1):97–9.
92. Veinalde R, Ozola A, Azarjana K, et al. Analysis of Latvian familial melanoma patients shows novel variants in the noncoding regions of CDKN2A and that the CDK4 mutation R24H is a founder mutation. Melanoma Res 2013;23(3):221–6.
93. Bradford PT, Goldstein AM, Tamura D, et al. Cancer and neurologic degeneration in xeroderma pigmentosum: long term follow-up characterises the role of DNA repair. J Med Genet 2011;48(3):168–76.
94. Harbour JW, Onken MD, Roberson ED, et al. Frequent mutation of BAP1 in metastasizing uveal melanomas. Science 2010;330(6009):1410–3.
95. Wiesner T, Obenauf AC, Murali R, et al. Germline mutations in BAP1 predispose to melanocytic tumors. Nat Genet 2011;43(10):1018–21.
96. Zhou XP, Waite KA, Pilarski R, et al. Germline PTEN promoter mutations and deletions in Cowden/Bannayan-Riley-Ruvalcaba syndrome result in aberrant PTEN protein and dysregulation of the phosphoinositol-3-kinase/Akt pathway. Am J Hum Genet 2003;73(2):404–11.
97. Tan MH, Mester JL, Ngeow J, et al. Lifetime cancer risks in individuals with germline PTEN mutations. Clin Cancer Res 2012;18(2):400–7.
98. Ohta M, Berd D, Shimizu M, et al. Deletion mapping of chromosome region 9p21-p22 surrounding the CDKN2 locus in melanoma. Int J Cancer 1996; 65(6):762–7.
99. Gillanders E, Juo SH, Holland EA, et al. Localization of a novel melanoma susceptibility locus to 1p22. Am J Hum Genet 2003;73(2):301–13.
100. Höiom V, Tuominen R, Hansson J. Genome-wide linkage analysis of Swedish families to identify putative susceptibility loci for cutaneous malignant melanoma. Genes Chromosomes Cancer 2011;50(12):1076–84.
101. Maccioni L, Rachakonda PS, Scherer D, et al. Variants at chromosome 20 (ASIP locus) and melanoma risk. Int J Cancer 2013;132(1):42–54.
102. Kanetsky PA, Panossian S, Elder DE, et al. Does MC1R genotype convey information about melanoma risk beyond risk phenotypes? Cancer 2010;116(10): 2416–28.
103. Fargnoli MC, Gandini S, Peris K, et al. MC1R variants increase melanoma risk in families with CDKN2A mutations: a meta-analysis. Eur J Cancer 2010;46(8): 1413–20.
104. Helsing P, Nymoen DA, Rootwelt H, et al. MC1R, ASIP, TYR, and TYRP1 gene variants in a population-based series of multiple primary melanomas. Genes Chromosomes Cancer 2012;51(7):654–61.
105. Sturm RA, Fox C, McClenahan P, et al. Phenotypic characterization of nevus and tumor patterns in MITF E318K mutation carrier melanoma patients. J Invest Dermatol 2014;134(1):141–9.
106. Gromowski T, Masojć B, Scott RJ, et al. Prevalence of the E318K and V320I MITF germline mutations in Polish cancer patients and multiorgan cancer risk – a population-based study. Cancer Genet 2014;207(4):128–32.
107. Hansson J. Familial melanoma. Surg Clin North Am 2008;88(4):897–916.
108. Harbour JW, Roberson ED, Anbunathan H, et al. Recurrent mutations at codon 625 of the splicing factor SF3B1 in uveal melanoma. Nat Genet 2014;45(2): 133–5.
109. Available at: http://www.cancer.gov/types/skin/hp/skin-genetics-pdq#section/all. Accessed January 5, 2015.

Multiple Endocrine Neoplasia

Genetics and Clinical Management

Jeffrey A. Norton, MD[a],*, Geoffrey Krampitz, MD[a],
Robert T. Jensen, MD[b]

KEYWORDS

- Endocrine neoplasia • Genetics • Clinical management
- Multiple endocrine neoplasia

KEY POINTS

- Early diagnosis of the multiple endocrine neoplasia (MEN) syndromes is critical for optimal clinical outcomes; before the MEN syndromes can be diagnosed, they must be suspected.
- Genetic testing for germline alterations in both the MEN type 1 (MEN1) gene and RET proto-oncogene is crucial to identifying those at risk in affected kindreds and directing timely surveillance and surgical therapy to those at greatest risk of potentially life-threatening neoplasia.
- Pancreatic, thymic, and bronchial neuroendocrine tumors are the leading cause of death in patients with MEN1 and should be aggressively considered by at least biannual computed tomography imaging.
- Patients with MEN-2a or 2b who are from a kindred and have a RET gene mutation identified should undergo total thyroidectomy after a pheochromocytoma is excluded.

MULTIPLE ENDOCRINE NEOPLASIA TYPE 1

Multiple endocrine neoplasia type 1 (MEN1) is inherited as an autosomal dominant disorder.[1,2] It has a prevalence of 2 to 3 per 100,000[3] and is reported to be present in 0.22% to 0.25% of autopsies.[4] The gene causing MEN1 is located on the long arm of chromosome 11 (11q13)[5,6] and is composed of 10 exons (9 coding).[2,4] The MEN1 gene is a tumor suppressor gene. It encodes a 610 amino acid nuclear protein

The authors have nothing to disclose.
[a] Department of Surgery, Stanford University School of Medicine, 300 Pasteur Drive, Stanford, CA 94305, USA; [b] Cell Biology Section, Digestive Diseases Branch, National Institute of Arthritis, Diabetes, Digestive and Kidney Disease, National Institutes of Health, Bethesda, MD 20892-2560, USA
* Corresponding author. Department of Surgery, Stanford University School of Medicine, 300 Pasteur Drive, H3591, Stanford, CA 94305.
E-mail address: janorton@stanford.edu

called menin. Abnormalities of this gene result in mutations, deletions, and/or truncations of the menin protein.[4,7,8] The exact mechanism by which alterations of menin result in endocrine tumors is still unclear. Menin interacts with several proteins, many of which have important roles in transcriptional regulation, genomic stability, cell division, and cell cycle control.[2,4,7,8] The crystal structure of menin supports its role as a key scaffolding protein that regulates gene transcription.[9,10]

Patients with MEN1 usually develop primary hyperparathyroidism (HPT) as the initial disorder of the syndrome (90%–100%),[1,11–13] followed by pancreatic neuroendocrine tumors (pNETs) that can either be functional (20%–70%), of which gastrinoma is the most common, or nonfunctional (80%–100%) (pituitary adenomas [20%–65%], adrenal tumors [10%–73%], and thyroid adenomas [0%–10%]).[2,12,14,15] Patients with MEN1 also have a high occurrence of other endocrine and nonendocrine tumors, including carcinoid tumors (thymic 0%–8%, gastric 7%–35%, bronchial 0%–8%, and rarely intestinal), skin and subcutaneous tumors (angiofibromas 88%, collagenomas 72%, lipomas 34%, and melanoma), central nervous system tumors (meningiomas, ependymomas, and schwannomas 0%–8%), and smooth muscle tumors (leiomyomas and leiomyosarcomas 1%–7%).[2,15–26] In early studies, thyroid disease was also reported in patients with MEN1; but in a recent cross-sectional study of 95 patients with MEN1,[27] the rate of co-occurrence of a thyroid incidentaloma was the same as matched non-MEN1 patients (45% vs 51%), respectively. In addition, other nonendocrine malignant tumors are also being reported to occur in MEN1.[11] These tumors include lymphomas, renal cell cancer, melanoma, leiomyosarcoma, thrombotic thrombocytopenia purpura, myeloma, ovarian tumors, gastrointestinal stromal tumor,[28] seminoma, chondrosarcoma, mesothelioma, and thymomas.[11,29–37] However, whether the incidence of these nonendocrine tumors is truly increased or not is unclear.

EARLY DIAGNOSIS OF MULTIPLE ENDOCRINE NEOPLASIA TYPE 1

Before MEN1 can be diagnosed, it must be suspected. Suspicion should be raised in any patient with a family history of endocrine tumors of the pancreas, family members with pituitary or parathyroid disease, or a family history of endocrinopathy; in patients with renal colic with NETs; in any patient with Zollinger-Ellison syndrome (ZES) (20%–25% have it as part of the MEN1 syndrome); with a young age onset of a functional pNET; with multiple pNETs; with HPT with multiple gland involvement or with hyperplasia or with a pNET associated with hypercalcemia or another endocrinopathy.[1,2] In most patients (83%), MEN1 clinically presents after 21 years of age.[38] In the 17% of patients with MEN1 presenting at less than 21 years of age, which should lead to suspicion of the diagnosis, the most frequent abnormalities were HPT (75%), pituitary adenoma (34%), insulinoma (12%), nonfunctional pNET (9%), and gastrinoma (2%).[38] Genetic screening for MEN1 is recommended when an individual has 2 or more MEN1–related tumors, multiple abnormal parathyroid glands before 30 years of age, recurrent HPT at a young age, gastrinoma and HPT or multiple pNETs at any age, plus a family history of kidney stones or endocrine tumors that are part of the syndrome.[39,40] Genetic testing includes sequencing of the entire coding region of the MEN1 gene (exons 2–10) and identifies mutations in about 80% of patients with familial MEN1[1,41,42] (Table 1).

PARATHYROID DISEASE IN MULTIPLE ENDOCRINE NEOPLASIA TYPE 1

Primary HPT is the most common endocrine abnormality in MEN1. It reaches nearly 100% penetrance by 50 years of age. HPT is usually the first manifestation of MEN1

Table 1
Basic facts about the different endocrine neoplasia familial syndromes

Familial Endocrine Syndrome	Chromosome	Gene	Pattern of Inheritance	Glands Involved	Extraglandular Manifestations	Cause of Death
MEN1	11	Menin	Autosomal dominant	Parathyroid, pancreas, pituitary, thyroid, adrenal	Bronchus, thymus, stomach, lipomas, skin tumors	pNET, bronchial or thymic NET
MEN-2a	10	RET	Autosomal dominant	Thyroid, adrenal, parathyroid	None	MTC
MEN-2b (MEN-3)	10	RET	Autosomal dominant	Thyroid, adrenal	Marfanoid habitus, mucosal neuromas, corneal nerve hypertrophy, intestinal ganglioneuromatosis	MTC
FMTC	10	RET	Autosomal dominant	Thyroid	None	Natural causes
MEN-4	12	CDKN1B/p27Kip1	Autosomal dominant	Parathyroid, GEP, pituitary	None	Unclear

Abbreviations: FMTC, familial medullary thyroid carcinoma; GEP, gastroenteropancreatic neuroendocrine tumors; MTC, medullary thyroid carcinoma.

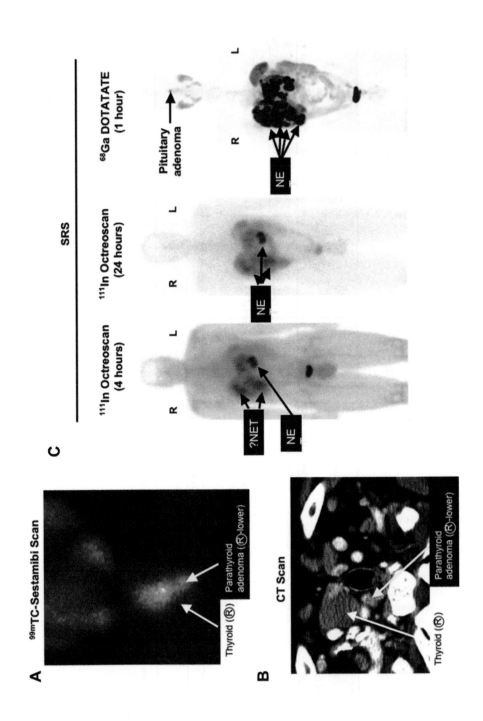

with a typical age of onset of 20 to 25 years. Decreased bone density and kidney stones are common. HPT often occurs at the same time as ZES and surgery to correct the HPT greatly ameliorates the clinical findings of ZES.[43,44] As in sporadic cases, biochemical testing for HPT is critical to the diagnosis.[45,46] Total or ionized serum level of calcium and intact serum parathyroid hormone levels are measured and both should be elevated. 24 hour urinary calcium should also be measured and will be elevated. Opinions differ as to the timing of parathyroid surgery in MEN1 as well as to the type of operation that should be performed. Early surgery may delay the lifetime exposure to the biochemical manifestations of HPT, whereas waiting until the parathyroid glands enlarge may make the operation easier. Patients with MEN1 and HPT typically have multiple abnormal glands. The tumors are asymmetric in size and should be considered as independent clonal adenomas.[47] Imaging studies are not useful for initial operations because all 4 parathyroid glands must be identified but are necessary and very useful in reoperations (**Fig. 1**). Some have recommended in patients with MEN1 a minimally invasive parathyroidectomy should be considered with selective removal of only the enlarged glands, whereas others recommend subtotal parathyroidectomy (3.5 glands removed) or a total parathyroidectomy with inplant.[13,40–48] The current operation that is recommended by most experts is a subtotal parathyroidectomy (3.5 gland resection) with removal of the cervical thymus. Intraoperative parathyroid hormone level monitoring is recommended to be certain that sufficient abnormal parathyroid tissue has been removed.[45,48] A viable 50-mg amount of normal parathyroid tissue should be left in the neck and marked with a hemoclip. Total parathyroid resection and transplantation of parathyroid tissue to the nondominant forearm used to be recommended, but it has been shown to have too high an incidence of hypoparathyroidism caused by graft failure.[49] Because of the multiple abnormal parathyroid gland nature of this disease, there is a high probability of recurrent HPT years after surgery if less than 3.5 parathyroid gland resections are performed.[50] Patients should be followed for this possibility. Calcium-sensing receptor agonists (calcimimetics) are a new class of drugs that can act directly on the parathyroid gland, decrease parathyroid hormone release, and may even decrease parathyroid tissue growth. A small number of patients with MEN1 and HPT have been treated with the calcium-sensing receptor agonist cinacalcet, and it has been effective in the control of the HPT.[51,52] These agents may play an important role in the management of these patients in the future.[53] Parathyroid carcinoma has been reported in patients with MEN1[54,55]; however, it is uncommon, occurring in only 0.28% of all patients with MEN1. The clinical presentation is similar to that seen in patients without MEN1 with parathyroid carcinoma.[55] Patients with MEN1 commonly develop bone disease with osteoporosis thought secondary to the HPT.[56,57] However, recent studies show that menin has important effects in bone particularly in regulating osteoblast activity, which plays a key role in bone development, remodeling, and maintenance.[58] Some patients with

◄─────────────────────────────────

Fig. 1. Sestamibi scan (A), neck computed tomography (CT) scan (B), and somatostatin receptor scintigraphy (SRS) (C) in a patient with MEN1 with recurrent primary HPT and metastatic pNET. Patient is a 45-year-old man with recurrent primary HPT after an operation in which they removed 2 abnormal parathyroid glands, and now he has recurrent disease. Sestamibi scan (A) shows an abnormal right inferior parathyroid gland (*yellow arrow*), and the same abnormal gland is demonstrated on a 4-dimensional neck CT scan with intravenous contrast (*yellow arrow*) (B). Octreoscan shows an abnormal pNET in the tail of the pancreas with possible liver metastases (C) left at 4 hours and middle panel 24 hours after labeled octreotide, whereas gallium-68 (^{68}Ga)-DOTATATE (C, *right panel*) clearly shows more tumor and also a pituitary adenoma. ^{99m}TC, technetium.

MEN1 require multiple reoperations to control the recurrent or persistent HPT, and reoperation can be difficult and associated with increased morbidity. Recently ethanol ablation of abnormal parathyroids[59] has been described to be able to successfully control the HPT in such patients with MEN1 with a low rate of hypocalcemia and no permanent complications.

PITUITARY TUMORS IN MULTIPLE ENDOCRINE NEOPLASIA TYPE 1

Anterior pituitary adenomas are the initial clinical manifestation of MEN1 in 25% of cases.[2,8] Its prevalence in MEN1 is between 20% and 60%; in a recent study of all patients (N = 144) with pituitary adenomas seen in one institution over a 6-year period, 7.7% had MEN1.[60] Most of these anterior pituitary tumors are microadenomas (<1 cm in diameter). Every type of anterior pituitary tumor has been reported to occur in MEN1, with the most common being a prolactinoma. Screening for anterior pituitary tumors requires measuring serum levels of prolactin and insulinlike growth factor 1 and MRI of the pituitary. Patients should be questioned for loss of peripheral vision. Visual fields are assessed formally if any suspicion of change or there is evidence of a pituitary tumor. Because these tumors occur in patients of childbearing age, undiagnosed pregnancy may cause a confusingly elevated prolactin level. Treatment of pituitary tumors in MEN1 is the same as sporadic pituitary tumors. Bromocriptine and cabergoline are used to treat prolactinomas. Octreotide and lanreotide are used to treat growth hormone–secreting tumors. Transsphenoidal surgery is the treatment of choice for discrete pituitary microadenomas or macroadenomas and may be curative. The major surgical morbidity of transsphenoidal hypophysectomy is permanent diabetes insipidus. Even in patients who are successfully treated, long-term follow-up is indicated because tumors may recur.

PANCREATIC NEUROENDOCRINE TUMORS IN MULTIPLE ENDOCRINE NEOPLASIA TYPE 1

The prevalence of pNETs in MEN1 is between 30% and 75% clinically and between 80% and 100% in postmortem studies.[2,11,61] The pathologic findings of pNETs in MEN1 is typically multicentric and multifocal with multiple endocrine tumors throughout the pancreas and the duodenum in patients with MEN1/ZES (**Fig. 2**). Unfortunately the only reliable method of establishing the presence of pNETs in patients with MEN1 not associated with a clinical syndrome (nonfunctional pNETS [NF-pNETs]) is to perform detailed imaging studies. Although NF-pNETs can secrete several peptides, including chromogranin A, neuron-specific enolase, pancreatic polypeptide, neurotensin, or ghrelin, these do not result in a distinct clinical syndrome; a recent study demonstrates their assessment in plasma in patients with MEN1 have low diagnostic accuracy for NF-pNETs.[62] The frequency with which pNETs are detected by imaging depends to a large extent on the imaging modality. Cross-sectional imaging studies (computed tomography [CT], MRI, transabdominal ultrasound) frequently (35%) miss tumors less than 2 cm; indium In 111 pentetreotide (Octreoscan) misses 25% to 30% less than 1 cm; gallium-68 (^{68}Ga)–DOTATOC/PET misses 20% to 30% less than 0.5 cm; and endoscopic ultrasound (EUS) can detect pNETs down to 0.1 to 0.2 cm.[63] ^{68}Ga-DOTATE is less available than Octreoscan but is more sensitive and frequently images more tumors than Octreoscan (see **Fig. 1**). Studies in patients with MEN1 show that EUS is the most sensitive single modality to detect pNETs.[64] In one recent comparative study,[65] EUS was markedly superior to Carbon[11] 5-Hydroxytryptophan scanning, somatostatin receptor scintigraphy (SRS), and CT/MRI for the detection of pNET. However, in another recent prospective study, the findings of MRI and

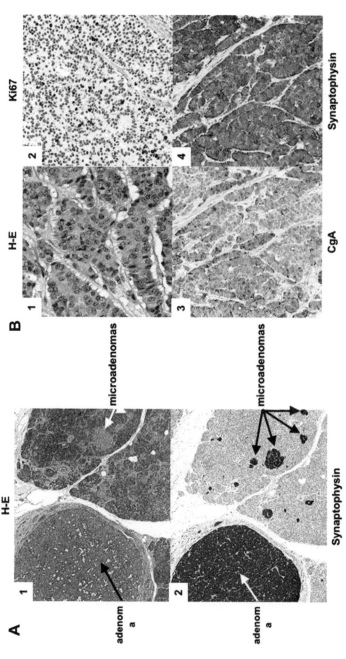

Fig. 2. Histologic appearance of the pancreas in 2 separate patients with MEN1. (*A*) Histologic sections of a pancreas in a patient with multiple neuroendocrine microadenomas in a background of islet cell hyperplasia. (*Panel 1*) The stain demonstrates clusters of enlarged microadenomas, the largest of which is 0.35 cm (hematoxylin-eosin [H-E], original magnification ×40). (*Panel 2*) Staining for synaptophysin highlights the multiple (>4) neuroendocrine microadenomas (immunohistochemical stain, original magnification ×40). (*B*) Histologic sections of a pNET (World Health Organization grade 2) from another patient with MEN1. (*Panel 1*) Stain shows tumor cells in a trabecular pattern with stippled chromatin and prominent nucleoli (H-E, original magnification ×400). (*Panel 2*) The Ki67 proliferation index is 13% (Immunohistochemistry for chromogranin A and synaptophysin, original magnification ×200). (*Panels 3 and 4*) Staining for chromogranin A (CgA) (*panel 3*) and synaptophysin (*panel 4*) are positive (immunohistochemical stain, original magnification ×200). (*Courtesy of* Drs Allison Zemek and Teri Longacre, Department of Pathology, Stanford University School of Medicine, Stanford, CA.)

EUS were complementary in patients with MEN1 for the detection of pNETs.[66] Tumors vary from microadenomas to adenomas to carcinomas (see **Fig. 2**) with lymph node and liver metastases. The most characteristic MEN1 pancreatic lesion on pathology studies is the presence of diffuse microadenomatosis (<0.5 mm).[67–69] Molecular studies in multiple pNETs or gastrinomas from patients with MEN1 assessing loss of heterozygosity at various loci and X-chromosome inactivation studies demonstrate that the multiple pNETs arise as independent events.[70] Although microadenomatosis of the pancreas is almost invariably seen, in various studies, only 0% to 13% of patients with MEN1 are reported to develop large (>2 cm) and/or symptomatic NF-pNETs,[2] with many patients not developing larger pNETs even over long periods of time. At present the molecular events that lead to this variability in growth of pancreatic microadenomas in different patients with MEN1 are unknown, and there are well-established predictive factors requiring sequential imaging as the only means to evaluate the growth over time.[2,71] Most studies in patients with MEN1 show no genotype-phenotype correlations[72,73]; however, a few recent studies have reported various MEN1 gene mutations more frequently in patients with aggressive tumors or with decreased survival; but they are not widely used or generally established for clinical use. These mutations include inactivating mutations of the MEN1 gene; the presence of exon 2 or nonsense/frameshift mutation in exon 2, 9, and 10; the presence of mutations affecting the June D interacting domain; and the presence of mutations affecting the checkpoint kinase 1 interacting domain.[74–76] Islet cell hyperplasia is rare. Duodenal gastrinomas in MEN1 are usually small (<1 cm), submucosal, multifocal,[77–80] and, as seen in sporadic ZES, occur primarily in the proximal duodenum.[81,82] Lymph node metastases occur in 45% to 95% of both duodenal and pancreatic gastrinomas, demonstrating that they are equally malignant; however, liver metastases occur less frequently in patients with duodenal NETs than pNETs, demonstrating that they are not equally aggressive.[2,83] pNETs contain, in decreasing frequency, chromogranin A, pancreatic polypeptide, glucagon, insulin, proinsulin, somatostatin, gastrin, vasoactive intestinal polypeptide, serotonin, calcitonin, growth-hormone releasing factor, and neurotensin.[2,84] Just because tumors may stain positive for these hormones by immunohistochemistry does not mean that they are associated with a clinical syndrome.[2,84,85] A functional pNET, by definition, demonstrates excessive secretion of hormones associated with symptoms of hormonal excess.[86,87] Malignant pNETs are rare before 30 years of age; however, 50% of middle-aged patients with MEN1 have evidence for a malignant pNET. A prospective study in patients with MEN1/ZES demonstrated that 14% of all patients had pNETs/gastrinomas demonstrating aggressive growth that was associated with decreased survival,[88] which is a lower rate than seen in patients with sporadic ZES, wherein 25% are reported to show an aggressive growth pattern.[89]

One of the most significant controversies concerning patients with MEN1 is the role of surgery in the management of various aspects of pNETs.[1,2,80,83,90–94] Almost all agree that surgical resection should be undertaken for MEN1 patients who develop insulinomas (18%), or other rare functional pNETs, such as VIPomas, glucagonomas, Growth Hormone Releasing Factor (<5%), or very rarely functional somatostatinomas (<1%). However, there is no agreement on surgery's role in patients with the most frequent functional pNET, gastrinomas causing the Zollinger-Ellison syndrome, that occur in 54% of patients or NF-pNETs that develop in 80% to 100% of patients.[1,2,85,95–100] There are several reasons for this controversy. In contrast to patients with insulinoma or the other rarer functional pNETs, in which surgery is frequently curative,[1,2,99,100] surgery for patients with MEN1 with ZES or with NF-pNETs is seldom curative. Therefore, surgical interventions must be carefully considered in a true risk-benefit analysis. This risk-benefit ratio is difficult to calculate for several reasons. A primary factor is that the natural history of patients with ZES, pNET, and MEN1 is changing and largely unknown[1,11] **(Fig. 3)**. In early series, before effective medical control of gastric acid hypersecretion caused by ZES existed, most patients with MEN1 died of the complications of the uncontrolled acid hypersecretion[23,101,102] **(Fig. 4)**. With the development of effective medical therapies (histamine H2-receptor antagonists [1970–80s] and proton pump inhibitors [PPIs] [1985-present]), the gastric acid secretion became an uncommon cause of death (<20%)[2,11,103] (see **Fig. 4**). In contrast, death from the malignant behavior of an NET has increased in frequency to greater than 60% in recent series[11,86,104–106] (see **Fig. 4**). Patients with MEN1 are now living longer (mean age at death: 55–60 years) (see **Fig. 3**),[11,104] and the death rate from other malignant tumors is increasing.[11] This finding is particularly true of thymic NETs (carcinoids). Currently, thymic carcinoids are the cause of death in approximately 10% to 25% of patients with MEN1.[11,105] These carcinoids are the most lethal NETs in MEN1.[11,18,23,107] Further, a wide range of other tumors are increasingly reported in patients with MEN1. Even though malignant NETs are reported as a cause of death of patients with MEN1 in various series, the exact source of the metastatic NET is usually not clearly established. This point is illustrated by the fact that a given patient may have a pNET and a carcinoid tumor (gastric, thymic, or pulmonary), so the source of the metastatic disease is unclear. This consideration is further complicated by the fact that small NF-pNETs have an excellent long-term survival[2,11,83,90,92]; in fact, their survival is not different from patients without pNETs.[90,98] An additional factor affecting the role of surgery is the fact that patients with MEN1 and pNETs may have life-threatening symptoms secondary to unregulated hormonal overproduction of the tumor. Examples include peptic ulcer disease and diarrhea secondary to gastrinoma, hypercortisolism secondary to ectopic ACTH secretion, and hypoglycemia secondary to an insulinoma. In the past, surgery was frequently the only hope to ameliorate and control these symptoms. However, effective drugs can control these symptoms, making surgery less necessary. Specifically, PPIs can control acid hypersecretion in all patients with MEN1/ZES[103]; long-acting somatostatin analogues can control severe diarrhea in VIPoma and necrolytic migratory pruritic rash in glucagonoma[108]; diazoxide can control hypoglycemia in insulinoma.[2,86,87,109] Lastly, surgery may be associated with both short-term and long-term complications that may result in morbidity and mortality. For example, some studies suggest that patients with MEN1 have an increased incidence of diabetes mellitus[11,110,111] and that pancreatic resections exacerbate this condition.[112] Furthermore, because microscopic pNETs are almost invariably left in the pancreas, curative surgery may require a total pancreatectomy, which can result in a greatly impaired quality of life and a difficult management course. Each of these factors (unknown natural history, low cure rate without aggressive surgery, excellent prognosis for small pNETs in MEN1/ZES-NF-pNETs, good medical control of functional pNETs, short-term/long-term surgical side-effects) has made it difficult to calculate the true risk/benefit ratio of surgery for pNETs in patients with MEN1. There are currently no clear markers that identify the cases that are at greatest risk for progression and death caused by a malignant pNET. In recent studies, several clinical/laboratory/tumoral features are reported to have prognostic value in patients with MEN1.[11,32,88,90] These features include the presence of thymic carcinoids, the presence of more than one functional hormonal pNET syndrome, the need for greater than 3 parathyroid surgical procedures, the presence of either liver metastases or distant metastases from the pNET, aggressive primary tumor growth (invasion into superior mesenteric vein, bile duct obstruction), large pNETs (>4 cm), pNETs with areas of poor vascular enhancement on CT,[113]

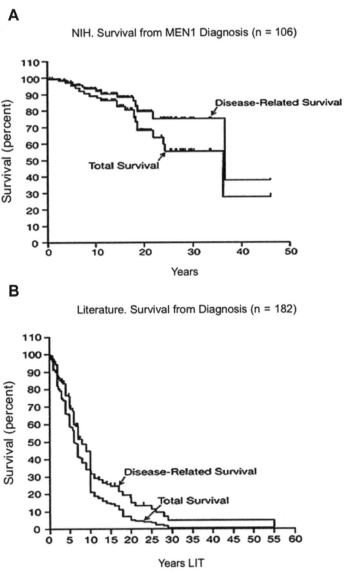

Fig. 3. Survival of patients with MEN1 with pNETs. Shown are total survival and disease-related survival from 2 groups of patients with MEN1 and pNETs. Data in the upper panel (*A*) are the survival from the time of diagnosis of MEN1 for 106 patients with MEN1/ZES followed at the National Institutes of Health (NIH). The bottom panel (*B*) shows survival data from the time of MEN1 diagnosis for 182 patients with MEN1 with pNETs from pooled literature (LIT) data from case reports and small series. The survival curves are plotted as Kaplan/Meier plots. (*Adapted from* Ito T, Igarashi H, Uehara H, et al. Causes of death and prognostic factors in multiple endocrine neoplasia type 1: a prospective study: comparison of 106 MEN1/Zollinger-Ellison syndrome patients with 1613 literature MEN1 patients with or without pancreatic endocrine tumors. Medicine (Baltimore) 2013;92(3):63; with permission.)

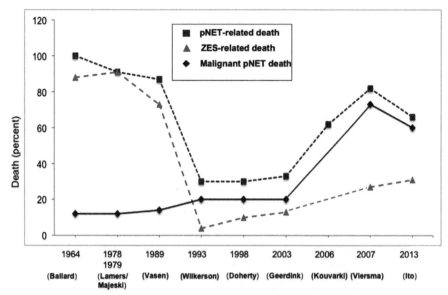

Fig. 4. Death rates and causes of death in patients with MEN1 from different series over time. The percentage of patients in various studies of patients with MEN1 reported to have a pNET-related death (death from any pNET cause including hormonal syndrome or malignant tumor), death caused by ZES (acid, tumor), or death caused by a malignant pNET are shown. As a percentage of all deaths, there was marked decrease with time in deaths caused by ZES, primarily because of the increased ability to control gastric acid hypersecretion, which is also reflected in the decrease with time in the percentage of all deaths that were pNET related; then with control of the hormone excess state there was an increase in the percentages of all deaths caused by malignant pNETs or pNET related. (*Data from Refs.*[11,23,39,74,101,104,232–234])

calcifications on CT,[114] and serial imaging with evidence for progression by increasing tumor size or new lesions.[11,23]

Gastrinomas (ZES) are the most common functional pNET in MEN1.[1,95] Recent studies show the duodenal but not pancreatic gastrinomas develop by hyperplasia of duodenal G cells.[115] With increasing hyperplasia and subsequent loss of heterozygosity (LOH) at the 11q13 MEN1 locus, duodenal microgastrinomas arise.[115] ZES is diagnosed by demonstrating an elevated fasting serum level of gastrin (off PPIs) with a concomitant increased gastric acid output (>10 mEq/h). Correlates for a poor prognosis with MEN1/ZES are pancreatic tail primary tumors, hepatic metastases, tumors that make both gastrin and adrenocorticotropic hormone (ACTH), distant metastases, and severe hypergastrinemia (defined as a level >3000).[11,88] Various surgical approaches have been performed in an attempt to cure patients with MEN1/ZES. However, patients with MEN1 typically have multiple, small duodenal gastrinomas associated with lymph node metastases in greater than 50% of cases,[116,117] in addition to multiple pNETs, which are uncommonly the cause of the ZES (<15%)[79,81,118] (see **Fig. 2**). Almost all studies show that local removal of duodenal gastrinomas is associated with persistent ZES.[1,5,118–122] However, Whipple pancreaticoduodenectomy has been reportedly associated with biochemical cure.[2,80,117,123–125] This latter approach is controversial because the symptoms of ZES are well controlled with PPIs; studies show patients with MEN1/ZES have an outstanding long-term survival on PPIs (up to 100% at 15 years); and the immediate and long-term morbidity/mortality of the Whipple procedure may be too great.[2,83,87,98] An argument for the more aggressive surgical procedure is that with even longer follow-up a higher percentage of these patients with MEN1/ZES develop malignant gastric carcinoid tumors that may also affect survival (**Fig. 5**B).[106] Therefore, the surgical approach to these patients will likely remain controversial until more data on the natural history becomes available. The authors' approach, because of its excellent quality of life and outlook, is to currently recommend only local resection (excision of duodenal tumors and/or enucleation of pancreatic head tumors with lymph node sampling and distal pancreatectomy for body/tail tumors that are >2 cm). Lymph node sampling is recommended because it has prognostic value[126–128] and perhaps can increase the cure rate. Although uncommonly curative, it is associated with acceptable morbidity and mortality and long-term tumor control and survival with a high quality of life. If patients have larger (>2.0–2.5 cm) pancreatic head tumors with positive lymph nodes, then the authors agree that more radical resection (proximal pancreaticoduodenectomy) may be considered in selected cases,

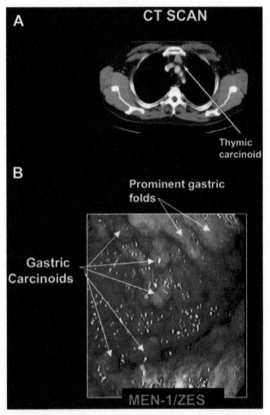

Fig. 5. (*A*) Thymic carcinoid on CT, (*B*) type 2 gastric carcinoids on endoscopy. (*A*) CT scan of a small resectable thymic carcinoid in the anterior mediastinum of a patient with MEN1. Unfortunately this is an uncommon finding in patients with MEN1 with these tumors that are usually first discovered when advanced disease is present. (*B*) Upper endoscopy of the stomach of a patient with ZES and MEN1 who had been treated with PPIs to reduce gastric acid secretion for many years. Image shows prominent gastric folds (*arrows top right*) consistent with ZES and multiple gastric carcinoids (*lower right arrows*) each of which is labeled. This patient illustrates the difficulty of removing all NETs endoscopically in many of these patients with MEN1 with type 2 gastric carcinoids.

although the authors' usual operation is to locally resect these tumors and not to perform a pancreaticoduodenectomy.[129] The authors' recommendations are consistent with those of both large neuroendocrine tumor societies' guidelines recently published (ie, the North American Neuroendocrine Tumor Society [NANET][125,130] and the European Neuroendocrine Tumor Society [ENET][87]) as well as the clinical practice guidelines for MEN1 published by the Endocrine Society.[1]

Insulinoma is the second most common functional pNET in MEN1.[2,129,131,132] Approximately 10% to 18% of patients with MEN1 will develop insulinoma, and 5% to 10% of insulinomas occur in the setting of MEN1. Insulinoma is the first manifestation of MEN1 in up to 10% of patients.[2,133] Patients have hypoglycemia and neuroglycopenic symptoms (altered mental status and seizures). This manifestation characteristically occurs at a young age (<35 years). Fasting hypoglycemia (glucose <45 mg/dL) and concomitant hyperinsulinemia (levels >5 uU/mL) are diagnostic.[86] Insulinomas are generally small (<2 cm) and distributed uniformly throughout the pancreas.[1,133] Because patients with MEN1 have multiple pNETS, it may not be clear which tumor is secreting the excessive insulin. However, studies have reported that the insulinoma in MEN1 is most commonly a dominant (>2 cm) pNET that is frequently identified by conventional imaging studies like CT or MRI, usually in the body and tail of the pancreas.[99,134–136] Medical control of the hypoglycemia is not as effective as that with other functional tumors making surgery more important for symptom relief. Insulinomas in the pancreatic body and tail are removed by a distal pancreatectomy. Tumors in the head are enucleated. Preoperative endoscopic and intraoperative ultrasound can provide precise localization of the tumor and may facilitate excision by imaging the relationship to the pancreatic duct. Patients with MEN1 with an insulinoma and no imaging evidence of a dominant tumor should undergo calcium angiogram.[137,138] This angiogram will localize the section of the pancreas containing the insulinoma. Surgical resection can usually be done laparoscopically if the lesion is well localized preoperatively. Patients need to be followed for subsequent development of recurrent tumor and hypoglycemia.[133] In a recent study[139] of 73 patients with MEN1 with insulinoma after distal pancreatectomy (63%), total/cephalic pancreatectomy (12%), or enucleations (25%), at a median follow-up of 9 years, 82% remained hypoglycemia free. The recurrence rate was higher with enucleation, but the long-term complication rate was much greater (43%–55%) with resections than with enucleation (0%) ($P = .002$).[139] This finding led to the conclusion that, although resection is associated with a lower recurrence rate, enucleation alone may be an alternative because of its lower long-term morbidity.[139]

NF-pNETs are a frequent problem in patients with MEN1, occurring as microadenomas in 80% to 100% on pathology examination (see **Fig. 2**), in 25% to 60% by imaging studies, and causing symptoms in up to 12% in different studies.[2,90,98,140] For NF-pNETs in asymptomatic patients with MEN1, there is controversy over the role of surgery, the timing of surgery, and the type of surgery performed. Studies have demonstrated that patients with small NF-pNETs (<2 cm) have an excellent long-term survival; in fact, it is the same as patients with MEN1 without any pNET.[83,90,98] Several groups recommend avoiding surgery if the NF-pNET is less than 2 cm or slowly growing.[83,89,90,98] Others recommend surgery for tumors that are 1 cm.[141,142] Still others recommend routine surgery for all patients in whom a pNET is identified by any method, even if it is identified biochemically and not imaged.[93] Another approach [64,143] is to perform serial EUS on patients with small pNETs (<1–2 cm) and operate if growth occurs. At present there is no consensus as to what size or change in size should be used for intervention. This lack of consensus is caused in large part by a lack of information on the natural history of NF-pNETs, especially those less than 1.5 to 2.0 cm in size that are asymptomatic. Recently several studies have attempted to address this question by following patients with MEN1 with serial EUSs that have been shown to be reliable for assessing changes in pNET size[144] and to be able to detect additional small (<0.5 cm), new NF-pNETs as well as changes in existing NF-pNETs.[64,71,145,146] These studies show that most NF-pNETs less than 1.5 to 2.0 cm remain stable or even decrease in size, with most of the rest only increasing in size slowly. At present too few patients have been studied in this manner to allow specific criteria about what rate of change or other alteration in the NF-pNET should lead to surgical intervention. It has been suggested that if change occurs, biopsy may help identify which patients should undergo surgery. The goal of surgery in MEN1 with NF-pNETs is to control tumor growth and prevent progression. Recent studies[11,132] identify the following factors as suggestive of poor prognosis: higher fasting serum levels of gastrin, presence of more than one functional hormonal syndrome, need for greater than 3 parathyroid surgical procedures, presence of distant metastases from pNET, aggressive primary tumor growth (invasion into the SMV, bile duct obstruction), large pNETs (>4 cm), pNETs with areas of poor vascular enhancement on CT,[113] calcifications,[114] and imaging evidence of progression.[11] EUS and fine-needle or core-needle biopsy can be especially useful for determining the malignant potential by measuring the Ki67 rate (see **Fig. 2**).[66,125,143,147] Further, ^{68}Ga-DOTATOC PET/CT can be used to better stage the true extent of tumor in patients with MEN1.[41] It is very useful because it is a sensitive whole-body study; it may identify other primary NETs like pituitary, bronchus, thymus, stomach, and ileum.[148–150] It is more sensitive than Octreoscan, which uses ^{111}In-labeled pentetreotide with single-photon emission computed tomography imaging (see **Fig. 1**). ^{68}Ga-DOTATOC PET/CT was originally available only in Europe, and now it is becoming available in the United States. The standard operation for NF-pNETs is distal or subtotal pancreatic resection with intraoperative ultrasound and enucleation of tumors from the pancreatic head and duodenum. For bulky (>2.0–2.5 cm) tumors in the head of the pancreas, proximal pancreaticoduodenectomy or the Whipple procedure may be necessary. Dissection of lymph nodes along the celiac axis and hepatoduodenal ligament is also indicated. Extensive pancreaticoduodenal resection is associated with an increased risk and is primarily indicated for clearly malignant tumors, as these tumors must be controlled. At present, because these patients have excellent long-term survival (see **Fig. 3**), the authors recommend surgical exploration only in patients with MEN1 with NF-pNETs greater than 2 cm or symptomatic. This recommendation is consistent with the guidelines by both large neuroendocrine tumor societies (ie, NANETs[125,130] and ENETs[87]) as well as the clinical practice guidelines for MEN1 published by the Endocrine Society.[1]

MANAGEMENT OF RARE FUNCTIONAL PANCREATIC NEUROENDOCRINE TUMORS IN MULTIPLE ENDOCRINE NEOPLASIA TYPE 1

Glucagonomas occur in 3% (range 1%–6%) of patients with MEN1, VIPomas in 3% (range 1%–12%), and GRFomas and somatostatinomas in less than 1%.[2,151] All guidelines agree that if unresectable disease is not present and patients have no medical contraindication to surgery,[112] these patients should undergo surgical exploration for potential cure and control of the malignant nature of the pNET.[1,2,125,130,151]

STOMACH, THYMIC, AND BRONCHIAL NEUROENDOCRINE TUMORS AND ADRENAL CORTICAL TUMORS

Patients with MEN1 develop type II gastric carcinoid tumors (7%–35%) (see **Fig. 5**), bronchial carcinoid tumors (0%–8%) (**Fig. 6**), thymic carcinoid tumors (0%–8%),

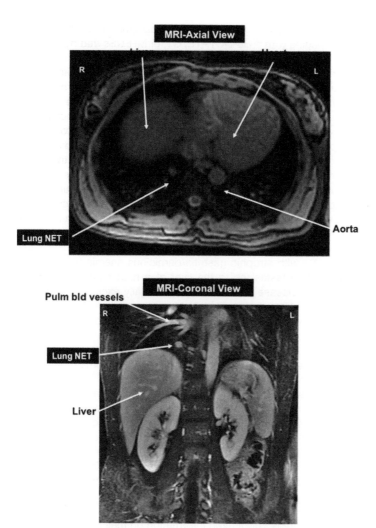

Fig. 6. MRI axial view (*top*) and coronal view (*bottom*) of right lower lobe bronchial NET in a patient with MEN1. Axial and coronal MRI images, respectively, of a small bronchial carcinoid tumor (Lung NET) in the right lower lobe of the lung in a patient with MEN1 who presented for routine follow-up. She underwent a right lower lobectomy and had positive lymph node metastases at surgery.

and adrenal cortical tumors (27%–36%, <2% symptomatic).[2,11,17,26,152,153] In a recent study of patients with MEN1[2] who died, 45% had adrenal cortical tumors, 19% gastric carcinoid tumors, 10% lung carcinoid tumor, and 6% thymic carcinoid tumor. Of these less common tumors listed, the tumor that seems to cause death most frequently was the thymic carcinoid tumor (see **Fig. 5**). It was second only to pNETs as the cause of death in patients with MEN1.[11] Unfortunately, thymic NETs in patients with MEN1 are rarely discovered when completely resectable; most present with advanced disease encasing great vessels, invading surrounding tissues, and frequently with bone and/or liver metastases.[2,11,18,154] In contrast to thymic carcinoids occurring in a non-MEN1 setting, thymic carcinoids occurring in patients with MEN1 are rarely associated with ectopic hormone production, such as Cushing syndrome.[2,17] Early diagnosis by awareness and imaging with ^{68}Ga-DOTATE, CT, or MRI followed by complete surgical resection are the mainstays of treatment.

Type 2 gastric carcinoid tumors occur almost entirely in patients with MEN1 with ZES[2,155] and are thought to be secondary to the trophic action of chronic hypergastrinemia on the gastric enterochromaffin-like (ECL) cells combined with the presence of LOH at the MEN1 locus on 11q13[156] (see **Fig. 5**). Studies show that almost all patients with MEN1/ZES have gastric ECL cell proliferative changes, which are currently thought to be precursor changes leading to the development of gastric carcinoids in these patients.[25] A large prospective study[25] found gastric ECL proliferative changes were present in all patients with MEN1/ZES studied; the changes were advanced in greater than 50% of the patients and more severe than that seen in patients with sporadic ZES without MEN1. The natural history is unclear because before the mid 1980s most patients with ZES underwent a total gastrectomy and, thus, did not develop these tumors. More recent studies show these type 2 gastric carcinoids (5%–6% all gastric carcinoids) are more aggressive than the more common type 1 found in patients without MEN1 with atrophic gastritis/pernicious anemia (70%–80% all gastric carcinoids). Type 2 metastasizes to the liver at a higher rate (10%–30%).[26,106,155] Those with localized disease (>70%–90%) are usually excised endoscopically after assessing the extent of invasion by EUS; but in some patients, the tumors are present in excessive numbers and a larger size. In these latter patients, the gastric NETs can be invasive so that additional treatments may be needed. In some cases, aggressive surgical resection (subtotal or total gastrectomy and D-2 lymph node dissection) is recommended and additional treatment with long-acting somatostatin analogues or cholecystokinin B receptor antagonists is administered.[1,155,157,158] Because most gastric carcinoids develop asymptomatically and because they can be more aggressive than type 1 gastric carcinoids that occur in atrophic gastritis, it is recommended that all patients with ZES/MEN1 undergo regular endoscopic evaluation (annually).

Curative resection (lobectomy with lymph node dissection) is recommended for bronchopulmonary NETs (see **Fig. 6**) and radical median sternotomy with thymectomy for thymic carcinoid tumors[1,11] (see **Fig. 5**). Although most bronchopulmonary NETs can be completely resected,[153] unfortunately this is not the case for most thymic carcinoids, which are very aggressive tumors and metastasize early, especially to bone.[2,11,18,154] Thymic carcinoids were not recognized as part of the MEN1 syndrome until the 1980s, so there is only limited information on their natural history.[11,154] Controversy exists as to the best method for their early detection, whether surgical resection should be performed even if distant metastatic disease is present, whether the recommendation of routine thymic resection during parathyroid surgery for HPT reduces the risk of the subsequent development of thymic carcinoids, and whether radiation or some other ant-tumor treatment should be given after surgical resection.[2,11,18,154] Current guidelines recommend screening CT or MRI screening of the chest every 1 to 2 years[1] and continued cervical thymectomy when parathyroid glands are removed; many recommend aggressive resection even with metastatic disease to prevent local complications.[1,18]

Adrenal tumors in patients with MEN1 are frequent (27%–36%); however, they are usually small (<3–4 cm) (>80%), nonfunctional (85%), benign (>86%), and asymptomatic (>98%).[2,11,129] These tumors may cause primary hyperaldosteronism and primary hypercortisolism and may become malignant.[129] At present adrenal tumors in patients with MEN1 are generally treated as that for non-MEN1 adrenal tumors.[1] Some studies suggest important differences in adrenal tumors in patients with MEN1 and non-MEN1 patients.[129] At present the exact screening time, tumor size that should be appropriated for surgical intervention, and frequency of assessment of functionality have not been systematically studied and defined to detect early malignant change or functionality in patients with MEN1.

MANAGEMENT OF METASTATIC DISEASE IN MULTIPLE ENDOCRINE NEOPLASIA TYPE 1

Of the MEN1–associated tumors, metastatic disease most commonly occurs with pancreatic, thymic, and bronchial NETs and occasionally in gastric carcinoid tumors. For example, approximately 60% of patients with duodenal gastrinomas or pNETs have metastatic disease at the time of diagnosis.[11,159] The presence of liver metastases initially or their development subsequently is associated with a poor prognosis and decreasing survival.[2,11,18,83,154] One of the unique problems confounding the treatment of patients with MEN1 is often the fact that the exact primary source of the liver metastases is unclear. It may be a pNET, a duodenal gastrinoma, thymic carcinoid, or another carcinoid like the stomach or bronchial. For example, there are several reports of patients with MEN1/ZES with liver metastases from a NET that is not the gastrinoma.[160,161] Liver metastases in patients with MEN1 and a pNET and without apparent carcinoid tumors like thymic, pulmonary, or stomach are almost always attributed to the pNET. This ambiguity may be resolved because recently pathologists are using different immunohistochemical studies to try to determine the true primary source of the metastasis (ie, PAX8, TTF-1, CDX-2, and so forth).[162] This distinction of the true source of the metastases is becoming more important because recent studies with several therapies used in patients with advanced metastatic NET disease (somatostatin analogues, everolimus, sunitinib, chemotherapeutic agents) demonstrate that pNETs and gastrointestinal (GI)-NETs (carcinoids) respond differently.[130,161,163,164] Management of metastatic disease in patients with MEN1 is generally comparable with the management of patients without MEN1.[130,161,163,164] However, for patients with multiple primary endocrine tumors, vigilance must be taken when evaluating new findings on cross-sectional imaging to be certain which tumor is metastatic and/or progressing. The oncologic management of metastatic NETs has improved with new drugs showing response rates primarily in pNETs. The Food and Drug Administration (FDA) has recently approved 2 agents for the treatment of metastatic pNETs, the mammalian target of rapamycin inhibitor everolimus[165] and the tyrosine kinase inhibitor sunitinib.[166] Both have shown promising antitumor effects in recent studies. For advanced GI-NETs, 2 double-blind, randomized, placebo-controlled somatostatin analogue studies (PROMID,[167] CLARINET[168]) as well as other studies[163] show both the somatostatin–long-acting analogue octreotide-LAR and lanreotide autogel have antiproliferative effects, respectively. In addition, other novel therapies are being evaluated for the treatment of advanced pNETs and GI-carcinoids, including the use of radiolabeled somatostatin analogues ([90]yttrium, [177]lutetium-labeled analogues) using the finding that almost all well-differentiated GI-NETs overexpress at least one subtype of somatostatin receptor, which can be used to image as well as target these cytotoxic agents; this approach is currently undergoing phase III trials.[169]

In summary, the importance of the authors' initial comments regarding the timely diagnosis of MEN1 cannot be overstated. *Again, before MEN1 can be diagnosed it must be suspected.* Suspicion should be raised in any patient with a family history of endocrine tumors of the pancreas, family members with pituitary or parathyroid disease, or a family history of endocrinopathy; in patients with renal colic with NETs; in any patient with ZES (20%–25% have it as part of the MEN1 syndrome); with a young age onset of a functional pNET; with multiple pNETs; with HPT with multiple gland involvement or with hyperplasia or with a pNET associated with hypercalcemia or another endocrinopathy.[1,2] Genetic screening for MEN1 is recommended when an individual has 2 or more MEN1–related tumors, multiple abnormal parathyroid glands before 30 years of age, recurrent HPT at a young age, gastrinoma and HPT or multiple pNETs at any age, plus a family history of kidney stones or endocrine tumors that are part of the syndrome.[39,40]

Patients with MEN1 are living longer and less frequently dying from the hormonal effects of tumors. However, the potentially malignant nature of some tumors, like pNETs, bronchial NETs, and thymic NETs, are accounting for an increasingly high proportion of deaths. Additionally, there is a possibility that these patients may have a higher incidence of other malignant nonendocrine tumors.[10] Awareness of these possibilities and the use of improved imaging modalities, like CT, MRI, EUS, SRS, and ^{68}Ga-DOTATOC PET/CT, should diagnose these tumors earlier and in a more treatable state.

Multiple Endocrine Neoplasia Type 4

Recently a new MEN1–related syndrome has been defined and recognized entitled MEN-4.[170,171] It has long been known that in patients with the MEN1 syndrome clinically 70% to 85% were found to have mutations in the MEN1 gene with familial disease and 30% of patients with sporadic MEN1.[1,7,10] In studies that also assess large deletions, the percentage with MEN1 mutations in patients with familial MEN1 can increase to 90%.[1,10,172] Thus, a percentage of patients with MEN1 features seem to have the disease based on some other genetic alteration.[172] Recently it has been established that germline mutations in the cyclin-dependent kinase (CDK) inhibitor gene CDKN1B is responsible for causing MEN-X, a syndrome in rats with features of both the human MEN1 and MEN-2 syndromes.[173] Subsequently, several patients with MEN1 features without a MEN1 gene mutation have been described who have mutations in the CDKN1B gene.[170,171,174] The CCDKN1B gene encodes for a member of the CDK inhibitor family, p27 (also called KIP1), a nuclear protein that is important in regulating the cell cycle, particularly the transition from the G1 to S phase.[170,171,175] The CDKN1B gene, similar to the MEN1 gene, functions as a tumor suppressor gene.[170,171] Alterations in other cyclin-dependent kinase genes have also been reported in patients with clinical MEN1 features but no MEN1 gene mutations.[176] In a study of 196 patients with clear MEN1 or suspected MEN1 but no MEN1 gene mutation,[176] the relative frequency of the various CDK mutations were p15 (1.0%), p18 (0.5%), p21 (0.5%), and p27 (1.5%).[176] In other studies, it is estimated that 3% of patients with MEN1 features have CDK1B mutations.[171]

Multiple Endocrine Neoplasia Type 2

Multiple endocrine neoplasia type 2 is composed of 3 distinct clinical subtypes: MEN-2a, MEN-2b, and familial medullary thyroid carcinoma (FMTC). MEN-2 is a rare syndrome with an incidence of 1 in 200,000 live births.[177] Each subtype is an autosomal dominant familial cancer syndrome associated with a germline mutation of variable penetrance in the RET proto-oncogene.[178] Because 50% of children of an affected parent will manifest MEN-2, the syndrome occurs in every generation of a family. The principle feature of all MEN-2 subtypes is medullary thyroid carcinoma (MTC), a cancer of the parafollicular calcitonin secreting C cells. Calcitonin and carcinoembryonic antigen (CEA) are sensitive and, in the case of calcitonin, specific blood markers for MTC. Patients with MEN-2 have a 100% risk of developing MTC by 70 years of age, and MTC is the most important determinant of mortality in these patients. If MTC has spread beyond the thyroid, the prognosis is poor. Further, patient survival is greatly improved when MTC is treated surgically early in the course of the disease. Therefore, the emphasis on treating patients with MEN-2 is screening and early detection of MTC.[178] MEN-2 is subgrouped into 2 variants called MEN-2a and MEN-2b (sometimes called MEN-3).[179] Common features of the 2 groups are multicentric, bilateral MTC, occurring in all patients and bilateral pheochromocytomas occurring in 50% of patients.[180] MEN-2a is the most common manifestation of MEN-2, accounting for 55% of cases. MTC is often the first manifestation of MEN-2a, usually occurring between 20 and 30 years of age. MEN-2a is characterized by MTC and pheochromocytomas plus primary HPT apparent in 20% to 30% of patients and a normal physical appearance and body habitus.[178]

MEN-2b is a more rare form, accounting for approximately 5% to 10% of all cases. MEN-2b is marked by an early onset of a more aggressive form of MTC. MTC develops within the first year of life, and patients die before the 30 years of age.[181] Patients with MEN-2b do not have parathyroid disease but do have a characteristic appearance, including Marfanoid habitus, pectus abnormalities, mesodermal abnormalities, corneal nerve hypertrophy, labial and mucosal neuromas, and intestinal ganglioneuromatosis.[178–180,182] FMTC is another hereditary endocrine syndrome. It is the second most common variant. It accounts for 35% of cases. FMTC is the mildest subtype of MTC, and patients usually do not die of MTC. Patients only have MTC without any of the other features seen in MEN-2a or 2b.[183] The diagnosis of FMTC should be considered when at least 4 family members develop MTC without other endocrine findings.

DISCOVERY OF THE MEDULLARY THYROID CARCINOMA SYNDROMES

In 1961, Sipple[184] first described an association among malignant tumors of the thyroid, bilateral adrenal pheochromocytomas, and parathyroid hyperplasia. Later Steiner and colleagues[185] further characterized a kindred with pheochromocytomas, MTC, and parathyroid hyperplasia. They noted that the syndrome was transmitted in an autosomal dominant fashion with high penetrance similar to MEN1. However, because MTC and pheochromocytomas were defining features, they reasoned that MEN-2 is genetically different from MEN1.[185] Early diagnosis of MTC is based on a radioimmunoassay for calcitonin, which was an excellent blood marker for MTC. Further, studies demonstrated that both calcium and pentagastrin stimulated C cells to rapidly secrete calcitonin; this could be used for the early diagnosis of MTC. Curative thyroidectomy was based on stimulated plasma calcitonin levels in patients from families with MEN-2a.

In 1966, Williams and Pollock[159] described 2 patients with neuromatosis, pheochromocytomas, and MTC who died at a young age. Both had pheochromocytomas, multiple mucosal and ocular neuromas, ganglioneuromatosis of the intestine, and metastatic medullary carcinoma of the thyroid. In 1968, Schimke and colleagues noted that marfanoid body habitus, coarse facial features, and characteristic skeletal abnormalities (pectus carinatum, saber shin) were part of this syndrome. They postulated that the entire syndrome was explained by an inheritable defect in neural crest–derived tissues.[186] This syndrome is now called MEN-2b; importantly, primary HPT is not part of this disease.

FMTC is the least malignant form of MEN-2, and patients seldom die of this form of MTC. These patients do not have other clinical manifestations of MEN-2.[155] It was first described by Farndon and colleagues.[183] The clinical diagnosis and onset of MTC in FMTC usually occurs later in life in the fifth or sixth decade.[187]

RET PROTO-ONCOGENE

RET is a proto-oncogene composed of 21 exons located on chromosome 10 (10q11.2) encoding a transmembrane receptor tyrosine kinase for members of the glial cell line–derived neurotrophic factor family (GDNF) and associated ligands (artemin, neurturin, persephin).[188–191] The RET protein is composed of 3 functional domains: an extracellular ligand-binding domain, a transmembrane domain, and a cytoplasmic tyrosine kinase domain. The extracellular domain contains 4 cadherinlike repeats and a cysteine-rich region. The cysteine-rich region is important for disulfide bond formation needed for maintaining the native tertiary structure allowing for receptor dimerization. The intracellular domain contains 2 tyrosine kinase subdomains that are involved in several intracellular signal transduction pathways.[192] Coupling RET, its coreceptors, GNDF-family receptor alpha (GFRα 1–4),[193] and GNDF-family ligands leads to RET dimerization to form a heterohexamer complex that results in transcellular kinase activation and signaling. RET is involved in several cellular signaling pathways during development regulating the enteric nervous system progenitor cells and neural crest and kidney progenitor cells.[194–201] Basic studies suggest that RET is a component of the signaling pathway required for renal organogenesis and enteric neurogenesis.[202,203] Inactivating mutations in RET associated with Hirschsprung disease[204–209] and renal agenesis have been identified.[202,203,210–214]

Genetic linkage analysis has mapped the MEN-2a locus to chromosome 10.[215,216] The RET gene has been found to be expressed in both familial and sporadic human pheochromocytomas and MTC.[190] RET mutations have been identified in exons 7 and 8 in patients with MEN-2a and FMTC.[217] Mulligan and colleagues[218] identified specific missense mutations in the RET gene at codons encoding for cysteine residues within the transition point between the extracellular and transmembrane domains. Subsequently, MEN-2b was shown to be associated with a T644M mutation affecting the intracellular tyrosine kinase domain of the RET proto-oncogene.[219] In MEN-2a and 2b, RET mutations act by constitutively activating the kinase. MEN-2a mutations alter the disulfide bond between receptor monomers creating an activating homodimer. On the other hand, the MEN-2b mutation altered the substrate specificity for the receptor.[220]

GENETIC TESTING AND RISK STRATIFICATION

Since the identification of mutations in the RET gene as the causative agents in MEN-2, genetic tests have been developed and refined to clinically detect these defects.[221–224] Mutations vary among kindreds but are consistently inherited within kindreds. In addition, investigators determined that new direct genetic analysis supplanted established linkage-based tests, because the latter was precluded by recombination events and required the selection of informative genetic markers. There was an invariable correlation between mutation and disease. Importantly, 2 affected individuals that were presymptomatic were identified by genetic testing. Thus, this new direct genetic analysis offered an important early diagnostic tool for the disorder. Today, genetic testing can detect nearly 100% of mutation carriers. It is the standard of care for all first-degree relatives of patients with newly diagnosed MTC. However, because of the varying clinical effects of RET mutations, strategies based on clinical phenotype, age of onset, and aggressiveness of MTC are still needed to guide therapy. Guidelines for the age of genetic testing and prophylactic thyroidectomy based on the inherited syndrome have been identified[225] and revised. Recommendations on the diagnostic workup and timing of prophylactic thyroidectomy and the extent of surgery are based on a classification into 4 risk levels using the genotype-phenotype correlation.[187] The American Thyroid Association classified mutations according to the risk of developing early, more aggressive MTC from A to D in increasing levels.[226]

GENOTYPE AND PHENOTYPE

Since the initial discovery of RET mutations responsible for MEN-2, as many as 50 different point mutations across 7 exons (exons 8, 10, 11, 13–16) have been identified.[227] Different mutations in the RET gene produce varying phenotypes for the disease, including age of onset and aggressiveness of MTC and the presence or absence of other endocrine neoplasms, such as pheochromocytoma or HPT. Approximately 85% of patients with MEN-2 have a mutation at exon 11 codon 634, whereas mutations in codons 609, 611, 618, and 620 account for 10% to 15% of cases.[187] Particularly early aggressive behavior and metastases in MEN-2a and MEN-2b are associated with C634 and M918T mutations, respectively, requiring early intervention.[199] On the other hand, an A883F mutation displays a more indolent form of MTC compared with an M918T mutation for MEN-2b.[228] In addition, polymorphism at codon 836 is associated with early metastases in patients with hereditary or sporadic MTC.[229]

PROPHYLACTIC THYROIDECTOMY

Untreated patients with MEN-2 ultimately develop MTC and succumb to their disease. Thus, diagnostic tools for detecting MTC in patients at risk for MEN-2 were developed even before the genetic origins were known. Parafollicular cells secrete calcitonin, and blood levels of this hormone serve as a sensitive tumor marker as well as an indicator of the cancer. Intravenously administered calcium and pentagastrin are potent calcitonin secretagogues that markedly enhance the sensitivity of the calcitonin assay. Although the pentagastrin-stimulated calcitonin test provided a sensitive diagnostic test for C-cell hyperplasia or carcinoma, it lacked the capacity to predict which patients would develop particularly aggressive forms of MTC and require early intervention and which patients would have a more indolent course and could be followed with biochemical surveillance. Because early detection and intervention are paramount to patient survival, genetic tests were needed to prospectively identify patients with MEN-2 at risk for accelerated MTC and requiring immediate treatment.

In 1995, shortly after mutations in RET were found to cause MEN-2, thyroidectomies were performed solely on the identification of these gene mutations in patients. Using polymerase chain reaction–based testing (confirmed by haplotype analysis) for 19 known RET mutations, Wells and colleagues[230] studied 132 members of 7 kindreds with MEN-2a. Twenty-one of the 58 subjects at risk for the disease had germline mutations in the RET oncogene associated with MEN-2a. Plasma calcitonin levels were elevated in 9 of the 21 subjects. However, 12 subjects had normal levels of calcitonin. After undergoing genetic counseling, 13 of the 21 subjects with detected germline mutations in RET, including 6 with normal serum calcitonin levels, underwent total thyroidectomies with central lymph node dissections. All of the surgically resected thyroid glands demonstrated medullary hyperplasia, many with evidence of MTC. Further, there was no evidence of lymph node metastasis in any subject at the time of surgery. In addition, postoperative plasma calcitonin levels normalized in subjects who had elevated levels preoperatively. The study showed that for family members who have germline mutations in the RET proto-oncogene, total thyroidectomy is indicated irrespective of plasma calcitonin levels.[230] Genetic screening and timely thyroidectomy in kindred members who have germline-mutated RET alleles characteristic of MEN-2 can prevent MTC, the most common cause of death in these syndromes.[192]

A major issue is the age to perform screening and prophylactic thyroidectomy. In patients from a family with MEN-2 and a RET mutation, most clinicians recommend that the individual should be screened at 5 years of age and the thyroid gland be removed, if affected. In this setting, central compartment lymph node dissection is unnecessary as it can increase the occurrence of postoperative hypoparathyroidism. In patients with MEN-2b, the surgery should be done at an early age as soon as the diagnosis is established. Because these patients commonly have a more aggressive tumor, central lymph node dissection should always be done. In patients with FMTC, screening should be done at 21 years of age; thyroidectomy without central lymph node dissection should be done in patients with inherited mutations. Postoperatively at 6 months, physical examination and serum levels of calcitonin and CEA are measured. If calcitonin and CEA levels are undetectable or normal for 5 years, no additional studies are necessary.

Multiple Endocrine Neoplasia Type 2

MEN-2 (also termed MEN-2a) accounts for 80% of the familial MTC syndromes (**Fig. 7**). In MEN-2, besides MTC, 50% of patients develop pheochromocytomas and 30% develop primary HPT depending on the RET codon mutation.[231] Patients with MEN-2 may also develop cutaneous lichen amyloidosis, Hirschsprung disease, and prominent corneal nerves. C cells secrete calcitonin and CEA. Either calcitonin or CEA levels in the blood serve as an excellent marker for MTC. Pentagastrin or calcium-stimulated serum calcitonin levels may serve as a more sensitive marker for

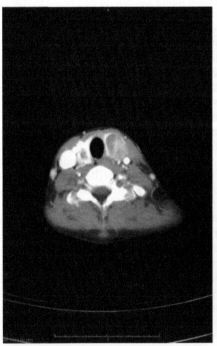 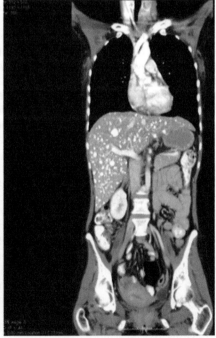

Fig. 7. Metastatic MTC in a patient with MEN-2a. Patient with MEN-2a who presented with bilateral neck nodules that were found to be primary MTC (*left panel*). Mass in left lobe was 4 cm, and the right was 2 cm. Coronal CT of the abdomen shows multiple diffuse bilateral liver metastases (*right panel*).

MTC and have been used for early diagnosis and to document surgical cure. Unlike sporadic MTC that is usually unilateral, familial forms of MTC are always bilateral. The tumor is multicentric and occupies the superior and central portion of each lobe. MTC initially remains confined to the thyroid gland, but subsequently it spreads to the central portion followed by other regional lymph nodes. Then it spreads to distant sites, including the liver, lung, bone, and brain. The tumor is very firm and has a fibrous acellular stroma that has staining properties similar to amyloid. On immunohistochemistry, it stains positive for calcitonin.

Pheochromocytomas develop in 50% of patients with MEN-2a and 2b[231] (**Fig. 8**). The clinical findings and behavior is the same in both syndromes. The mean age at presentation is 36 years, and the diagnosis is made after MTC in 40% of cases and before MTC in 10%. In this setting, the pheochromocytomas are benign and confined to the adrenal gland. Sixty-five percent of the time, these tumors are bilateral; with a 10-year follow-up, patients with a surgically excised unilateral pheochromocytoma will develop a contralateral tumor. It is critical to exclude the diagnosis of pheochromocytoma in patients with MEN-2 before doing any invasive procedures because sudden death may occur if a pheochromocytoma is not detected and patients are not appropriately prepared with an alpha-adrenergic blocking drug. Deaths have been reported during surgical procedures and childbirth. Patients suspected of having a pheochromocytoma should have measurement of plasma-free metanephrine and normetanephrine levels or a 24-hour urine for vanillylmandelic acid, metanephrines and total catecholamines. CT and MRI are used to image pheochromocytomas. The sensitivity and specificity are similar for the two procedures: 90% to 100% and 70% to 80%, respectively.

The pheochromocytoma has priority and should be removed before the thyroid surgery. Preoperative preparation with an alpha-adrenergic blocking drug like phenoxybenzamine is done; when patients are well blocked, a beta-adrenergic drug is added

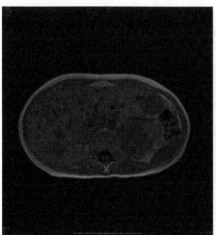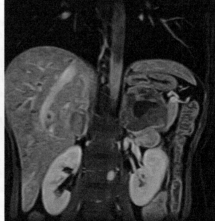

Fig. 8. MRI of bilateral pheochromocytomas in same patient with MEN-2a with metastatic MTC to the liver. Axial MRI (*left panel*) shows bilateral pheochromocytomas. Left adrenal tumor is larger than the right and measures 6 cm compared with 3 cm on right. Patient's liver also shows multiple bilateral metastases that were proven to be from MTC. Coronal image (*right panel*) also demonstrates both adrenal pheochromocytomas as axial. Left adrenal has some cystic areas.

to keep the heart rate less than 100 beats per minute. Despite the fact that the pheochromocytomas are usually bilateral, if only one adrenal seems to contain a tumor, unilateral adrenalectomy is recommended.[231] This procedure is recommended because there has been a very high risk of addisonian crisis in these patients following bilateral adrenalectomy. Some other surgeons have recommended bilateral subtotal adrenalectomy for these patients in an attempt to preserve cortical function. Although this approach may have merit, there has been limited follow-up and documentation of long-term adrenal function or recurrent pheochromocytomas with this procedure. Adrenalectomy can usually be accomplished laparoscopically, and this approach greatly reduces morbidity. In patients who undergo bilateral adrenalectomy, corticosteroid and mineralocorticoid replacement is necessary.

Primary HPT develops in 20% to 30% of patients with MEN-2a. The mean age of onset is 36 years. It may occur before any other manifestation of MTC in 5% of patients. The hypercalcemia is minimal, and most patients are without symptoms. The parathyroid glands are asymmetrically enlarged and contain hyperplastic nodules. Pathologically it is labeled pseudonodular hyperplasia. The operation of choice is subtotal parathyroidectomy or 3.5 gland parathyroidectomy.

MULTIPLE ENDOCRINE NEOPLASIA TYPE 2B

MEN-2b accounts for 5% of hereditary MTC. These patients all have MTC and bilateral pheochromocytomas, a characteristic phenotype; but they do not develop primary HPT. Patients with MEN-2b have this characteristic appearance that includes marfanoid habitus, prolonged facies, muscular skeletal abnormalities (pectus, saber shins, bowing of the extremities), ocular abnormalities (inability to cry tears and corneal nerve hypertrophy), mucosal neuromas usually on the tip of the tongue, and intestinal ganglioneuromatosis. Most have GI symptoms characterized by pain, diarrhea, constipation, bloating, and even megacolon. These symptoms may occur in children and young adults with this syndrome.

The MTC is uniformly aggressive and spreads to distant sites early in these patients. It occurs during infancy, and early diagnosis is critical. In approximately 50% of MEN-2b cases, de novo germline RET mutations give rise to the disease. In patients with de novo MEN-2b, the mutated allele generally comes from the father. Babies are at a high risk in this setting because the parents are asymptomatic and the disease is not expected. This is unfortunate because there is only a narrow window during which thyroidectomy may be curative. Even in the most advantageous setting whereby thyroidectomy was performed during the neonatal period, most babies are not cured.

FAMILIAL MEDULLARY THYROID CARCINOMA

FMTC accounts for 15% of hereditary MTC. These patients only have MTC that occurs at a late age and is less aggressive than the other familial forms. The diagnosis is made when an individual can identify 10 affected individuals occurring in a kindred older than 50 years with an adequate history and biochemical data to exclude pheochromocytoma and primary HPT in affected individuals.

The strongest predictor of survival for patients with MTC is the stage of disease at the time of thyroidectomy. The 10-year disease-specific survival of MTC is 90% with localized disease, 78% with lymph node metastases, and 40% with distant metastases. Only 10% of patients with metastases to cervical lymph nodes are cured with extensive lymph node dissection. The prognosis is excellent for patients with FMTC who have a preoperative calcitonin level less than 150 pg/mL, an MTC smaller than 1 cm, and no lymph node metastases. The 10-year survival approaches 100% if basal and stimulated calcitonin levels are undetectable after thyroidectomy. In patients with MTC confined to the thyroid gland, the standard operation is total thyroidectomy and resection of all lymph nodes in the central zone of the neck. The neck dissection is more extensive in patients with advanced nodal disease.

A reliable indicator of progression of MTC is the calcitonin or CEA doubling time. A calcitonin doubling time between 6 months and 2 years is associated with a 5-year survival of 92% and a 10-year survival of 37%, whereas a doubling rate of less than 6 months is associated with a 25% and 8% survival, respectively. In patients with MTC, the calcitonin level is most predictive of prognosis; but in some patients, the CEA level is more correlative, so both should be measured. If the postoperative serum calcitonin level increases to more than 150 to 200 pg/mL, a total-body CT scan should be performed. In the absence of distant metastases and the presence of cervical lymph node disease, a neck dissection should be performed. Prior studies suggested that this strategy may cure approximately 30% of patients, but a more recent long-term follow-up indicates that these patients will eventually recur. Some studies suggest that external beam radiation should be administered after neck dissection; however, this treatment has not improved outcomes.

SUMMARY OF MULTIPLE ENDOCRINE NEOPLASIA TYPE 2

MEN-2 is caused by a mutation in the RET proto-oncogene. It is inherited as an autosomal dominant trait. It is broken down into 3 clinical syndromes: MEN-2a, MEN-2b, and FMTC. Each of the 3 syndromes has MTC with complete penetrance. The MTC is the most lethal in MEN-2b, intermediate in 2a, and least virulent in FMTC. Patients with MEN-2a and 2b also have a 50% chance of developing pheochromocytomas that may be bilateral, and patients with MEN-2a may also get primary HPT caused by parathyroid hyperplasia. In children from kindreds with MEN-2a or 2b, total thyroidectomy is indicated once the RET gene mutation is detected and pheochromocytoma is excluded.

MANAGEMENT OF METASTATIC DISEASE IN MULTIPLE ENDOCRINE NEOPLASIA TYPE 2, MULTIPLE ENDOCRINE NEOPLASIA TYPE 3, AND FAMILIAL MEDULLARY THYROID CARCINOMA

Development of distant metastatic disease in individuals who were not diagnosed by screening is common in MTC. The survival of patients with distant metastases from MTC is 51% at 1 year, 26% at 5 years, and 10% at 10 years. When patients develop distant metastases from MTC and calcitonin levels increase, they may also develop secretory diarrhea that is especially difficult to control. Management of metastatic disease in patients with inherited forms of MTC is similar to management in sporadic MTC. Loperamide, codeine, or octreotide acetate (Sandostatin) may help control the diarrhea in some cases. Tumor debulking or selective arterial embolization may provide symptomatic improvement in others. Two new compounds have recently been approved by the FDA for the treatment of metastatic MTC and include Vandetanib and Cabozantinib, and were shown to prolong progression-free survival in phase III clinical trials.

REFERENCES

1. Thakker RV, Newey PJ, Walls GV, et al. Clinical practice guidelines for multiple endocrine neoplasia type 1 (MEN1). J Clin Endocrinol Metab 2012;97(9): 2990–3011.

2. Jensen RT, Berna MJ, Bingham MD, et al. Inherited pancreatic endocrine tumor syndromes: advances in molecular pathogenesis, diagnosis, management and controversies. Cancer 2008;113(7 suppl):1807–43.

3. Giusti F, Cavalli L, Cavalli T, et al. Hereditary hyperparathyroidism syndromes. J Clin Densitom 2013;16(1):69–74.

4. Thakker RV. Multiple endocrine neoplasia type 1 (MEN1). Best Pract Res Clin Endocrinol Metab 2010;24(3):355–70.

5. Brandi ML, Marx SJ, Aurbach GD, et al. Familial multiple endocrine neoplasia type I: a new look at pathophysiology. Endocr Rev 1987;8(4):391–405.

6. Marx SJ, Agarwal SK, Kester MB, et al. Germline and somatic mutation of the gene for multiple endocrine neoplasia type 1 (MEN1). J Intern Med 1998; 243(6):447–53.

7. Lemos MC, Thakker RV. Multiple endocrine neoplasia type 1 (MEN1): analysis of 1336 mutations reported in the first decade following identification of the gene. Hum Mutat 2008;29:22–32.

8. Agarwal SK. Exploring the tumors of multiple endocrine neoplasia type 1 in mouse models for basic and preclinical studies. Int J Endocr Oncol 2014;1: 153–61.

9. Huang J, Gurung B, Wan B, et al. The same pocket in menin binds both MLL and JUND but has opposite effects on transcription. Nature 2012;482(7386): 542–6.

10. Matkar S, Thiel A, Hua X. Menin: a scaffold protein that controls gene expression and cell signaling. Trends Biochem Sci 2013;38(8):394–402.

11. Ito T, Igarashi H, Uehara H, et al. Causes of death and prognostic factors in multiple endocrine neoplasia type 1: a prospective study: comparison of 106 MEN1/Zollinger-Ellison syndrome patients with 1613 literature MEN1 patients with or without pancreatic endocrine tumors. Medicine (Baltimore) 2013;92(3): 135–81.

12. Gibril F, Schumann M, Pace A, et al. Multiple endocrine neoplasia type 1 and Zollinger-Ellison syndrome: a prospective study of 107 cases and comparison with 1009 cases from the literature. Medicine (Baltimore) 2004;83(1):43–83.

13. Benya RV, Metz DC, Venzon DJ, et al. Zollinger-Ellison syndrome can be the initial endocrine manifestation in patients with multiple endocrine neoplasia-type I. Am J Med 1994;97(5):436–44.

14. Burgess JR, David R, Parameswaran V, et al. The outcome of subtotal parathyroidectomy for the treatment of hyperparathyroidism in multiple endocrine neoplasia type 1. Arch Surg 1998;133(2):126–9.

15. Skogseid B, Rastad J, Gobl A, et al. Adrenal lesion in multiple endocrine neoplasia type 1. Surgery 1995;118(6):1077–82.

16. Burgess JR, Harle RA, Tucker P, et al. Adrenal lesions in a large kindred with multiple endocrine neoplasia type 1. Arch Surg 1996;131(7):699–702.

17. Darling TN, Skarulis MC, Steinberg SM, et al. Multiple facial angiofibromas and collagenomas in patients with multiple endocrine neoplasia type 1. Arch Dermatol 1997;133(7):853–7.

18. Gibril F, Chen YJ, Schrump DS, et al. Prospective study of thymic carcinoids in patients with multiple endocrine neoplasia type 1. J Clin Endocrinol Metab 2003; 88(3):1066–81.

19. Hofmann M, Schilling T, Heilmann P, et al. Multiple endocrine neoplasia associated with multiple lipomas. Med Klin (Munich) 1998;93(9):546–9.

20. Marx S, Spiegel AM, Skarulis MC, et al. Multiple endocrine neoplasia type 1: clinical and genetic topics. Ann Intern Med 1998;129(6):484–94.

21. Raef H, Zou M, Baitei EY, et al. A novel deletion of the MEN1 gene in a large family of multiple endocrine neoplasia type 1 (MEN1) with aggressive phenotype. Clin Endocrinol (Oxf) 2011;75(6):791–800.
22. Teh BT, Zedenius J, Kytola S, et al. Thymic carcinoids in multiple endocrine neoplasia type 1. Ann Surg 1998;228(1):99–105.
23. Wilkinson S, Teh BT, Davey KR, et al. Cause of death in multiple endocrine neoplasia type 1. Arch Surg 1993;128(6):683–90.
24. Asgharian B, Chen YJ, Patronas NJ, et al. Meningiomas may be a component tumor of multiple endocrine neoplasia type 1. Clin Cancer Res 2004;10(3): 869–80.
25. Asgharian B, Turner ML, Gibril F, et al. Cutaneous tumors in patients with multiple endocrine neoplasm type 1 (MEN1) and gastrinomas: prospective study of frequency and development of criteria with high sensitivity and specificity for MEM-1. J Clin Endocrinol Metab 2004;89:5328–36.
26. Berna MJ, Annibale B, Marignani M, et al. A prospective study of gastric carcinoids and enterochromaffin-like cell changes in multiple endocrine neoplasia type 1 and Zollinger-Ellison syndrome: identification of risk factors. J Clin Endocrinol Metab 2008;93(5):1582–91.
27. Lodewijk L, Bongers PJ, Kist JW, et al. Thyroid incidentalomas in patients with multiple endocrine neoplasia type 1. Eur J Endocrinol 2015;172:337–42.
28. Papillon ERA, Calender A, Chabre O, et al. A malignant gastrointestinal stromal tumour in a patient with multiple endocrine neoplasia type 1. Eur J Gastroenterol Hepatol 2001;13:207–11.
29. De Toma G, Plocco M, Nicolanti V, et al. Type B1 thymoma in multiple endocrine neoplasia type 1 (MEN-1) syndrome. Tumori 2001;87(4):266–8.
30. Denker PS, Wright D, Hilscher JR, et al. Hypernephroma associated with multiple endocrine neoplasia type I: a case report. J Urol 1986;136(4):896–8.
31. Dong Q, Debelenko LV, Chandrasekharappa SC, et al. Loss of heterozygosity at 11q13: analysis of pituitary tumors, lung carcinoids, lipomas, and other uncommon tumors in subjects with familial multiple endocrine neoplasia type 1. J Clin Endocrinol Metab 1997;82(5):1416–20.
32. Goudet P, Murat A, Cardot-Bauters C, et al. Thymic neuroendocrine tumors in multiple endocrine neoplasia type 1: a comparative study on 21 cases among a series of 761 MEN1 from the GTE (Groupe des Tumeurs Endocrines). World J Surg 2009;33(6):1197–207.
33. Kojima Y, Ito H, Hasegawa S, et al. Resected invasive thymoma with multiple endocrine neoplasia type 1. Jpn J Thorac Cardiovasc Surg 2006;54(4):171–3.
34. Mallek R, Mostbeck G, Walter RM, et al. Contrast MRI in multiple endocrine neoplasia type 1 (MEN) associated with renal cell carcinoma. Eur J Radiol 1990;10(2):105–8.
35. Nishimura Y, Yamashita K, Yumita W, et al. Multiple endocrine neoplasia type 1 with unusual concomitance of various neoplastic disorders. Endocr J 2004; 51(1):75–81.
36. Tanabe T, Yasuo M, Tsushima K, et al. Mediastinal seminoma in a patient with multiple endocrine neoplasia type 1. Intern Med 2008;47(18):1615–9.
37. Toshimori H, Okamoto M, Nakatsuru K, et al. Multiple endocrine neoplasia type 1 associated with malignant lymphoma and other complications. Intern Med 1996; 35(11):849–54.
38. Goudet P, Dalac A, Le Bras A, et al. MEN1 disease occurring before 21 years old. A 160-patient cohort study from the GTE (Groupe d'étude des Tumeurs Endocrines). J Clin Endocrinol Metab 2015;100(4):1568–77.

39. Vasen HF, Lamers CB, Lips CJ. Screening for the multiple endocrine neoplasia syndrome type I. A study of 11 kindreds in The Netherlands. Arch Intern Med 1989;149(12):2717–22.

40. Marx SJ, Vinik AI, Santen RJ, et al. Multiple endocrine neoplasia type I: assessment of laboratory tests to screen for the gene in a large kindred. Medicine (Baltimore) 1986;65(4):226–41.

41. Skogseid B, Oberg K. Experience with multiple endocrine neoplasia type 1 screening. J Intern Med 1995;238(3):255–61.

42. Waldmann J, Fendrich V, Habbe N, et al. Screening of patients with multiple endocrine neoplasia type 1 (MEN-1): a critical analysis of its value. World J Surg 2009;33(6):1208–18.

43. Macleod AF, Ayers B, Young AE, et al. Resolution of hypergastrinaemia after parathyroidectomy in multiple endocrine neoplasia syndrome type I (MEN type I). Clin Endocrinol (Oxf) 1987;26(6):693–8.

44. Norton JA, Cornelius MJ, Doppman JL, et al. Effect of parathyroidectomy in patients with hyperparathyroidism in patients with hyperparathyroidism, Zollinger-Ellison syndrome and multiple endocrine neoplasia type 1: a prospective study. Surgery 1987;102:958–66.

45. Norton JA, Venzon DJ, Berna MJ, et al. Prospective study of surgery for primary hyperparathyroidism (HPT) in multiple endocrine neoplasia-type 1 and Zollinger-Ellison syndrome: long-term outcome of a more virulent form of HPT. Ann Surg 2008;247(3):501–10.

46. Marx SJ. Multiplicity of hormone-secreting tumors: common themes about cause, expression, and management. J Clin Endocrinol Metab 2013;98(8):3139–48.

47. Marx SJ, Menczel J, Campbell G, et al. Heterogeneous size of the parathyroid glands in familial multiple endocrine neoplasia type 1. Clin Endocrinol (Oxf) 1991;35(6):521–6.

48. Nilubol N, Weisbrod AB, Weinstein LS, et al. Utility of intraoperative parathyroid hormone monitoring in patients with multiple endocrine neoplasia type 1-associated primary hyperparathyroidism undergoing initial parathyroidectomy. World J Surg 2013;37:1966–72.

49. Lairmore TC, Govednik CM, Quinn CE, et al. A randomized, prospective trial of operative treatments for hyperparathyroidism in patients with multiple endocrine neoplasia type 1. Surgery 2014;156(6):1326–34.

50. Versnick M, Popadich A, Sidhu S, et al. Minimally invasive parathyroidectomy provides a conservative surgical option for multiple endocrine neoplasia type 1-primary hyperparathyroidism. Surgery 2013;154(1):101–5.

51. Filopanti M, Verga U, Ermetici F, et al. MEN1-related hyperparathyroidism: response to cinacalcet and its relationship with the calcium-sensing receptor gene variant Arg990Gly. Eur J Endocrinol 2012;167:157–64.

52. Del Prete M, Marotta V, Ramundo V, et al. Impact of cinacalcet hydrochloride in clinical management of primary hyperparathyroidism in multiple endocrine neoplasia type 1. Minerva Endocrinol 2013;38:389–94.

53. Giusti F, Tonelli F, Brandi ML. Primary hyperparathyroidism in multiple endocrine neoplasia type 1: when to perform surgery? Clinics (Sao Paulo) 2012;67(Suppl 1):141–4.

54. del Pozo C, García-Pascual L, Balsells M, et al. Parathyroid carcinoma in multiple endocrine neoplasia type 1. Case report and review of the literature. Hormones (Athens) 2011;4:326–31.

55. Singh Ospina N, Sebo TJ, Thompson GB, et al. Prevalence of parathyroid carcinoma in 348 patients with multiple endocrine neoplasia type 1-case report and

review of the literature. Clin Endocrinol (Oxf) 2014. http://dx.doi.org/10.1111/cen.12714.

56. Burgess JR, David R, Greenaway TM, et al. Osteoporosis in multiple endocrine neoplasia type 1: severity, clinical significance, relationship to primary hyperparathyroidism, and response to parathyroidectomy. Arch Surg 1999;134:1119–23.

57. Kann PH, Bartsch D, Langer P, et al. Peripheral bone mineral density in correlation to disease-related predisposing conditions in patients with multiple endocrine neoplasia type 1. J Endocrinol Invest 2012;35:573–9.

58. Kanazawa I, Canaff L, Abi Rafeh J, et al. Osteoblast menin regulates bone mass in vivo. J Biol Chem 2015;290:3910–24.

59. Singh Ospina N, Thompson GB, Lee RA, et al. Safety and efficacy of percutaneous parathyroid ethanol ablation in patients with recurrent primary hyperparathyroidism and multiple endocrine neoplasia type 1. J Clin Endocrinol Metab 2015;100:E87–90.

60. Nunes VS, Souza GL, Perone D, et al. Frequency of multiple endocrine neoplasia type 1 in a group of patients with pituitary adenoma: genetic study and familial screening. Pituitary 2014;17:30–7.

61. Thakker RV. Multiple endocrine neoplasia type 1. Indian J Endocrinol Metab 2012;16(Suppl 2):S272–4.

62. de Laat JM, Pieterman CR, Weijmans M, et al. Low accuracy of tumor markers for diagnosing pancreatic neuroendocrine tumors in multiple endocrine neoplasia type 1 patients. J Clin Endocrinol Metab 2013;98:4143–51.

63. Alexander HR, Norton JA, Bartlett DL, et al. Prospective study of somatostatin receptor scintigraphy and its effect on operative outcome in patients with Zollinger-Ellison syndrome. Ann Surg 1998;228:228–2238.

64. Langer P, Kann PH, Fendrich V, et al. Prospective evaluation of imaging procedures for the detection of pancreaticoduodenal endocrine tumors in patients with multiple endocrine neoplasia type 1. World J Surg 2004;28(12):1317–22.

65. van Asselt SJ, Brouwers AH, van Dullemen HM, et al. EUS is superior for detection of pancreatic lesions compared with standard imaging in patients with multiple endocrine neoplasia type 1. Gastrointest Endosc 2015;81:159–67.

66. Barbe C, Murat A, Dupas B, et al. Magnetic resonance imaging versus endoscopic ultrasonography for the detection of pancreatic tumours in multiple endocrine neoplasia type 1. Dig Liver Dis 2012;44(3):228–34.

67. Thompson NW, Lloyd RV, Nishiyama RH, et al. MEN I pancreas: a histological and immunohistochemical study. World J Surg 1984;8:561–74.

68. Anlauf M, Schlenger R, Perren A, et al. Microadenomatosis of the endocrine pancreas in patients with and without the multiple endocrine neoplasia type 1 syndrome. Am J Surg Pathol 2006;30(5):560–74.

69. Kloppel G, Willemer S, Stamm B, et al. Pancreatic lesions and hormonal profile of pancreatic tumors in multiple endocrine neoplasia type I. An immunocytochemical study of nine patients. Cancer 1986;57(9):1824–32.

70. Debelenko LV, Zhuang Z, Emmert-Buck MR, et al. Allelic deletions on chromosome 11q13 in multiple endocrine neoplasia type 1-associated and sporadic gastrinomas and pancreatic endocrine tumors. Cancer Res 1997;57(11):2238–43.

71. Thomas-Marques L, Murat A, Delemer B, et al. Prospective endoscopic ultrasonographic evaluation of the frequency of nonfunctioning pancreaticoduodenal endocrine tumors in patients with multiple endocrine neoplasia type 1. Am J Gastroenterol 2006;101(2):266–73.

72. Wautot V, Vercherat C, Lespinasse J, et al. Germline mutation profile of MEN1 in multiple endocrine neoplasia type 1: search for correlation between phenotype and the functional domains of the MEN1 protein. Hum Mutat 2002;20(1): 35–47.

73. Giraud S, Zhang CX, Serova-Sinilnikova O, et al. Germ-line mutation analysis in patients with multiple endocrine neoplasia type 1 and related disorders. Am J Hum Genet 1998;63(2):455–67.

74. Kouvaraki MA, Shapiro SE, Cote GJ, et al. Management of pancreatic endocrine tumors in multiple endocrine neoplasia type 1. World J Surg 2006;30(5):643–53.

75. Thevenon J, Bourredjem A, Faivre L, et al. Higher risk of death among MEN1 patients with mutations in the JunD interacting domain: a Groupe d'etude des Tumeurs Endocrines (GTE) cohort study. Hum Mol Genet 2013;22:1940–8.

76. Bartsch DK, Slater EP, Albers M, et al. Higher risk of aggressive pancreatic neuroendocrine tumors in MEN1 patients with MEN1 mutations affecting the CHES1 interacting MENIN domain. J Clin Endocrinol Metab 2014;99:E2387–91.

77. Tonelli F, Fratini G, Falchetti A, et al. Surgery for gastroenteropancreatic tumours in multiple endocrine neoplasia type 1: review and personal experience. J Intern Med 2005;257(1):38–49.

78. MacFarlane MP, Fraker DL, Alexander HR, et al. Prospective study of surgical resection of duodenal and pancreatic gastrinomas in multiple endocrine neoplasia type 1. Surgery 1995;118(6):973–9 [discussion: 979–80].

79. Anlauf M, Garbrecht N, Henopp T, et al. Sporadic versus hereditary gastrinomas of the duodenum and pancreas: distinct clinicopathological and epidemiological features. World J Surg 2006;12(34):5440–6.

80. Lopez CL, Falconi M, Waldmann J, et al. Partial pancreaticoduodenectomy can provide cure for duodenal gastrinoma associated with multiple endocrine neoplasia type 1. Ann Surg 2013;257(2):308–14.

81. Pipeleers-Marichal M, Somers G, Willems G, et al. Gastrinomas in the duodenums of patients with multiple endocrine neoplasia type 1 and the Zollinger-Ellison syndrome. N Engl J Med 1990;322(11):723–7.

82. Thom AK, Norton JA, Axiotis CA, et al. Location, incidence and malignant potential of duodenal gastrinomas. Surgery 1991;110:1086–93.

83. Norton JA, Alexander HR, Fraker DL, et al. Comparison of surgical results in patients with advanced and limited disease with multiple endocrine neoplasia type 1 and Zollinger-Ellison syndrome. Ann Surg 2001;234(4):495–506.

84. LeBodic MF, Heymann MF, Lecomte M, et al. Immunohistochemical study of 100 pancreatic tumors in 28 patients with multiple endocrine neoplasia, type 1. Am J Surg Pathol 1996;20(11):1378–84.

85. Tonelli F, Giudici F, Fratini G, et al. Pancreatic endocrine tumors in multiple endocrine neoplasia type 1 syndrome: review of literature. Endocr Pract 2011; 17(Suppl 3):33–40.

86. Ito T, Igarashi H, Jensen RT. Pancreatic neuroendocrine tumors: clinical features, diagnosis and medical treatment: advances. Best Pract Res Clin Gastroenterol 2012;26:737–53.

87. Jensen RT, Cadiot G, Brandi ML, et al. ENETS consensus guidelines for the management of patients with digestive neuroendocrine neoplasms: functional pancreatic endocrine tumor syndromes. Neuroendocrinology 2012;95(2): 98–119.

88. Gibril F, Venzon DJ, Ojeaburu JV, et al. Prospective study of the natural history of gastrinoma in patients with MEN1: definition of an aggressive and a nonaggressive form. J Clin Endocrinol Metab 2001;86(11):5282–93.

89. Weber HC, Venzon DJ, Lin JT, et al. Determinants of metastatic rate and survival in patients with Zollinger-Ellison syndrome: a prospective long-term study. Gastroenterology 1995;108:1637–49.

90. Triponez F, Dosseh D, Goudet P, et al. Epidemiology data on 108 MEN 1 patients from the GTE with isolated nonfunctioning tumors of the pancreas. Ann Surg 2006;243(2):265–72.

91. You YN, Thompson GB, Young WF Jr, et al. Pancreatoduodenal surgery in patients with multiple endocrine neoplasia type 1: operative outcomes, long-term function, and quality of life. Surgery 2007;142(6):829–36 [discussion: 836.e1].

92. Norton JA, Fraker DL, Alexander HR, et al. Surgery to cure the Zollinger-Ellison syndrome. N Engl J Med 1999;341(9):635–44.

93. Akerstrom G, Hessman O, Skogseid B. Timing and extent of surgery in symptomatic and asymptomatic neuroendocrine tumors of the pancreas in MEN1. Langenbecks Arch Surg 2002;386:558–69.

94. Singh MH, Fraker DL, Metz DC. Importance of surveillance for multiple endocrine neoplasia-1 and surgery in patients with sporadic Zollinger-Ellison syndrome. Clin Gastroenterol Hepatol 2012;10(11):1262–9.

95. Adkisson CD, Stauffer JA, Bowers SP, et al. What extent of pancreatic resection do patients with MEN-1 require? JOP 2012;13(4):402–8.

96. Lopez CL, Waldmann J, Fendrich V, et al. Long-term results of surgery for pancreatic neuroendocrine neoplasms in patients with MEN1. Langenbecks Arch Surg 2011;396(8):1187–97.

97. Jensen RT. Management of the Zollinger-Ellison syndrome in patients with multiple endocrine neoplasia type 1. J Intern Med 1998;243(6):477–88.

98. Triponez F, Goudet P, Dosseh D, et al. Is surgery beneficial for MEN1 patients with small (< or = 2 cm), nonfunctioning pancreaticoduodenal endocrine tumor? An analysis of 65 patients from the GTE. World J Surg 2006;30(5): 654–62.

99. Giudici F, Nesi G, Brandi ML, et al. Surgical management of insulinomas in multiple endocrine neoplasia type 1. Pancreas 2012;41(4):547–53.

100. Norton JA, Fang TD, Jensen RT. Surgery for gastrinoma and insulinoma in multiple endocrine neoplasia type 1. J Natl Compr Canc Netw 2006;4(2):148–53.

101. Ballard HS, Frame B, Harstock RT. Familial endocrine adenoma-peptic ulcer disease. Medicine (Baltimore) 1964;43:481–515.

102. Majewski JT, Wilson SD. The MEN-I syndrome: an all or none phenomenon? Surgery 1979;86(3):475–84.

103. Ito T, Igarashi H, Uehara H, et al. Pharmacotherapy of Zollinger-Ellison syndrome. Expert Opin Pharmacother 2013;14(3):307–21.

104. Vierimaa O, Ebeling TM, Kytola S, et al. Multiple endocrine neoplasia type 1 in Northern Finland: clinical features and genotype phenotype correlation. Eur J Endocrinol 2007;157(3):285–94.

105. Machens A, Schaaf L, Karges W, et al. Age-related penetrance of endocrine tumours in multiple endocrine neoplasia type 1 (MEN1): a multicentre study of 258 gene carriers. Clin Endocrinol (Oxf) 2007;67(4):613–22.

106. Norton JA, Melcher ML, Gibril F, et al. Gastric carcinoid tumors in multiple endocrine neoplasia-1 patients with Zollinger-Ellison syndrome can be symptomatic, demonstrate aggressive growth, and require surgical treatment. Surgery 2004; 136(6):1267–74.

107. Teh BT, Hayward NK, Walters MK, et al. Genetic studies of thymic carcinoids in multiple endocrine neoplasia type 1. J Med Genet 1994;31:261–2.

108. Wickenhauser C, Aichelmann E, Neuhaus H, et al. Glucagon-secreting malignant neuroendocrine tumor of the pancreas. Med Klin (Munich) 2000;95(8): 466–9 [in German].

109. Jadoul M, Koppeschaar HP, Bax MA, et al. Insulinomas in MEN-I patients: early detection and treatment of insulinomas in patients with the multiple endocrine neoplasia syndrome type-I. Neth J Med 1990;37(3–4):95–102.

110. McCallum RW, Parameswaran V, Burgess JR. Multiple endocrine neoplasia type 1 (MEN 1) is associated with an increased prevalence of diabetes mellitus and impaired fasting glucose. Clin Endocrinol (Oxf) 2006;65(2):163–8.

111. van Wijk JP, Dreijerink KM, Pieterman CR, et al. Increased prevalence of impaired fasting glucose in MEN1 gene mutation carriers. Clin Endocrinol (Oxf) 2012;76(1):67–71.

112. King J, Kazanjian K, Matsumoto J, et al. Distal pancreatectomy: incidence of postoperative diabetes. J Gastrointest Surg 2008;12(9):1548–53.

113. Worhunsky DJ, Krampitz GW, Poullos PD, et al. Pancreatic neuroendocrine tumours: hypoenhancement on arterial phase computed tomography predicts biological aggressiveness. HPB (Oxford) 2013;16(4):304–11.

114. Poultsides GA, Huang LC, Chen Y, et al. Pancreatic neuroendocrine tumors: radiographic calcifications correlate with grade and metastasis. Ann Surg Oncol 2012;19(7):2295–303.

115. Anlauf M, Perren A, Kloppel G. Endocrine precursor lesions and microadenomas of the duodenum and pancreas with and without MEN1: criteria, molecular concepts and clinical significance. Pathobiology 2007;74(5): 279–84.

116. Imamura M. Treatment for pancreatic endocrine tumors with or without multiple endocrine neoplasia type 1. Nihon Geka Gakkai Zasshi 2005;106(8):472–8 [in Japanese].

117. Imamura M, Komoto I, Ota S, et al. Biochemically curative surgery for gastrinoma in multiple endocrine neoplasia type 1 patients. World J Gastroenterol 2011;17(10):1343–53.

118. Norton JA, Jensen RT. Current surgical management of Zollinger-Ellison syndrome (ZES) in patients without multiple endocrine neoplasia-type 1 (MEN1). Surg Oncol 2003;12(2):145–51.

119. O'Riordain DS, O'Brien T, van Heerden JA, et al. Surgical management of insulinoma associated with multiple endocrine neoplasia type I. World J Surg 1994; 18(4):488–93 [discussion: 493–4].

120. Grama D, Skogseid B, Wilander E, et al. Pancreatic tumors in multiple endocrine neoplasia type 1: clinical presentation and surgical treatment. World J Surg 1992;16(4):611–8 [discussion: 618–9].

121. Mignon M, Ruszniewski P, Podevin P, et al. Current approach to the management of gastrinoma and insulinoma in adults with multiple endocrine neoplasia type I. World J Surg 1993;17(4):489–97.

122. Thompson NW. Management of pancreatic endocrine tumors in patients with multiple endocrine neoplasia type 1. Surg Oncol Clin N Am 1998; 7(4):881–91.

123. Gauger PG, Thompson NW. Early surgical intervention and strategy in patients with multiple endocrine neoplasia type 1. Best Pract Res Clin Endocrinol Metab 2001;15(2):213–23.

124. Bartsch DK, Langer P, Wild A, et al. Pancreaticoduodenal endocrine tumors in multiple endocrine neoplasia type 1: surgery or surveillance? Surgery 2000; 128(6):958–66.

125. Kulke MH, Anthony LB, Bushnell DL, et al. NANETS treatment guidelines: well-differentiated neuroendocrine tumors of the stomach and pancreas. Pancreas 2010;39(6):735–52.
126. Krampitz GW, Norton JA, Poultsides GA, et al. Lymph nodes and survival in pancreatic neuroendocrine tumors. Arch Surg 2012;147(9):820–7.
127. Bartsch DK, Fendrich V, Boninsegna L, et al. Impact of lymphadenectomy on survival after surgery for sporadic gastrinoma. Br J Surg 2012;99:1234–40.
128. Hashim YM, Linehan DC, Strasberg SS, et al. Regional lymphadenectomy is indicated in the surgical treatment of pancreatic neuroendocrine tumors (PNETS). Ann Surg 2014;259:197–203.
129. Norton JA, KG, Zemek A, et al. Surgical perspectives: changing causes of death in patients with MEN-1. Ann Surg, in press.
130. Kunz PL, Reidy-Lagunes D, Anthony LB, et al. Consensus guidelines for the management and treatment of neuroendocrine tumors. Pancreas 2013;42(4): 557–77.
131. Thakker RV. Multiple endocrine neoplasia type 1. Endocrinol Metab Clin North Am 2000;29(3):541–67.
132. Goudet P, Murat A, Binquet C, et al. Risk factors and causes of death in MEN1 disease. A GTE cohort study among 758 patients. World J Surg 2010;34: 249–55.
133. Bartsch DK, Knoop R, Kann PH, et al. Enucleation and limited pancreatic resection provide long-term cure for insulinoma in multiple endocrine neoplasia type 1. Neuroendocrinology 2014;98(4):290–8.
134. Tonelli F, Fratini G, Nesi G, et al. Pancreatectomy in multiple endocrine neoplasia type 1-related gastrinomas and pancreatic endocrine neoplasias. Ann Surg 2006;244(1):61–70.
135. Sakurai A, Yamazaki M, Suzuki S, et al. Clinical features of insulinoma in patients with multiple endocrine neoplasia type 1: analysis of the database of the MEN Consortium of Japan. Endocr J 2012;59(10):859–66.
136. Cougard P, Goudet P, Peix JL, et al. Insulinomas in multiple endocrine neoplasia type 1. Report of a series of 44 cases by the multiple endocrine neoplasia study group. Ann Chir 2000;125(2):118–23 [in French].
137. Hiramoto JS, Feldstein VA, LaBerge JM, et al. Intraoperative ultrasound and preoperative localization detects all occult insulinomas; discussion 1025-6. Arch Surg 2001;136(9):1020–5.
138. Doppman JL, Miller DL, Chang R, et al. Gastrinomas: localization by means of selective intraarterial injection of secretin. Radiology 1990;174:25–9.
139. Vezzosi D, Cardot-Bauters C, Bouscaren N, et al. Long-term results of the surgical management of insulinoma patients with MEN1: a Groupe d'étude des Tumeurs Endocrines (GTE) retrospective study. Eur J Endocrinol 2015;172: 309–19.
140. Pipeleers-Marichal M, Donow C, Heitz PU, et al. Pathologic aspects of gastrinomas in patients with Zollinger-Ellison syndrome with and without multiple endocrine neoplasia type I. World J Surg 1993;17(4):481–8.
141. Bartsch DK, Langer P, Rothmund M. Surgical aspects of gastrinoma in multiple endocrine neoplasia type 1. Wien Klin Wochenschr 2007;119(19–20):602–8.
142. Skogseid B, Oberg K, Eriksson B, et al. Surgery for asymptomatic pancreatic lesion in multiple endocrine neoplasia type I. World J Surg 1996;20(7):872–6 [discussion: 877].
143. Kann PH, Balakina E, Ivan D, et al. Natural course of small, asymptomatic neuroendocrine pancreatic tumours in multiple endocrine neoplasia

type 1: an endoscopic ultrasound imaging study. Endocr Relat Cancer 2006; 13(4):1195–202.

144. Kann PH, Kann B, Fassbender WJ, et al. Small neuroendocrine pancreatic tumors in multiple endocrine neoplasia type 1 (MEN1): least significant change of tumor diameter as determined by endoscopic ultrasound (EUS) imaging. Exp Clin Endocrinol Diabetes 2006;114(7):361–5.

145. D'souza SL, Elmunzer BJ, Scheiman JM. Long-term follow-up of asymptomatic pancreatic neuroendocrine tumors in multiple endocrine neoplasia type I syndrome. J Clin Gastroenterol 2014;48:458–61.

146. Tonelli F. How to follow-up and when to operate asymptomatic pancreatic neuroendocrine tumors in multiple endocrine neoplasia type 1. J Clin Gastroenterol 2014;48:387–9.

147. Gauger PG, Scheiman JM, Wamsteker EJ, et al. Role of endoscopic ultrasonography in screening and treatment of pancreatic endocrine tumours in asymptomatic patients with multiple endocrine neoplasia type 1. Br J Surg 2003; 90(6):748–54.

148. Froeling V, Elgeti F, Maurer MH, et al. Impact of Ga-68 DOTATOC PET/CT on the diagnosis and treatment of patients with multiple endocrine neoplasia. Ann Nucl Med 2012;26(9):738–43.

149. Sabet A, Nagarajah J, Dogan AS, et al. Does PRRT with standard activities of 177Lu-octreotate really achieve relevant somatostatin receptor saturation in target tumor lesions?: insights from intra-therapeutic receptor imaging in patients with metastatic gastroenteropancreatic neuroendocrine tumors. EJNMMI Res 2013;3(1):82.

150. Stoeltzing O, Loss M, Huber E, et al. Staged surgery with neoadjuvant 90Y-DOTATOC therapy for down-sizing synchronous bilobular hepatic metastases from a neuroendocrine pancreatic tumor. Langenbecks Arch Surg 2010;395(2): 185–92.

151. Levy-Bohbot N, Merle C, Goudet P, et al, Groupe des Tumeurs Endocrines. Prevalence, characteristics and prognosis of MEN 1-associated glucagonomas, VIPomas, and somatostatinomas: study from the GTE (Groupe des Tumeurs Endocrines) registry. Gastroenterol Clin Biol 2004;28(11):1075–81.

152. Gatta-Cherifi B, Murat A, Niccoli P, et al. Adrenal involvement in MEN1. Analysis of 715 cases from the Groupe d'etude des tumeurs endocrines database. Eur J Endocrinol 2012;166:269–72.

153. Sachithanandan N, Harle RA, Burgess JR. Bronchopulmonary carcinoid in multiple endocrine neoplasia type 1. Cancer 2005;103(3):509–15.

154. Teh BT, McArdle J, Chan SP, et al. Clinicopathologic studies of thymic carcinoids in multiple endocrine neoplasia type 1. Medicine (Baltimore) 1997;76(1):21–9.

155. Scherubl H, Cadiot G, Jensen RT, et al. Neuroendocrine tumors of the stomach (gastric carcinoids) are on the rise: small tumors, small problems? Endoscopy 2010;42(8):664–71.

156. Debelenko LV, Emmert-Buck MR, Zhuang Z, et al. The multiple endocrine neoplasia type I gene locus is involved in the pathogenesis of type II gastric carcinoids. Gastroenterology 1997;113(3):773–81.

157. Fossmark R, Sørdal Ø, Jianu CS, et al. Treatment of gastric carcinoids type 1 with the gastrin receptor antagonist netazepide (YF476) results in regression of tumours and normalisation of serum chromogranin A. Aliment Pharmacol Ther 2012;36(11–12):1067–75.

158. Manfredi S, Pagenault M, de Lajarte-Thirouard AS, et al. Type 1 and 2 gastric carcinoid tumors: long-term follow-up of the efficacy of treatment with a

slow-release somatostatin analogue. Eur J Gastroenterol Hepatol 2007;19(11): 1021–5.

159. Williams ED, Pollock DJ. Multiple mucosal neuromata with endocrine tumours: a syndrome allied to von Recklinghausen's disease. J Pathol Bacteriol 1966;91(1): 71–80.

160. Bordi C, Falchetti A, Azzoni C, et al. Aggressive forms of gastric neuroendocrine tumors in multiple endocrine neoplasia type I. Am J Surg Pathol 1997;21(9): 1075–82.

161. Grieco A, Bianco A, Alfei B, et al. Liver metastases of endocrine tumour associated with multiple endocrine neoplasia type 1: a sustained response to interferon therapy or a peculiar benign course? Hepatogastroenterology 2000; 47(35):1269–72.

162. Belizzi AM. Assigning site of origin in metastatic neuroendocrine neoplasms: a clinically significant application of diagnostic immunohistochemistry. Adv Anat Pathol 2013;20(5):285–314.

163. Ito T, Igarashi H, Jensen RT. Therapy of metastatic pancreatic neuroendocrine tumors (pNETs): recent insights and advances. J Gastroenterol 2012;47(9):941–60.

164. Pavel M, Baudin E, Couvelard A, et al. ENETS consensus guidelines for the management of patients with liver and other distant metastases from neuroendocrine neoplasms of foregut, midgut, hindgut, and unknown primary. Neuroendocrinology 2012;95(2):157–76.

165. Yao JC, Shah MH, Ito T, et al. Everolimus for advanced pancreatic neuroendocrine tumors. N Engl J Med 2011;364(6):514–23.

166. Raymond E, Dahan L, Raoul JL, et al. Sunitinib malate for the treatment of pancreatic neuroendocrine tumors. N Engl J Med 2011;364(6):501–13.

167. Rinke A, Müller HH, Schade-Brittinger C, et al. Placebo-controlled, double-blind, prospective, randomized study on the effect of octreotide LAR in the control of tumor growth in patients with metastatic neuroendocrine midgut tumors: a report from the PROMID Study Group. J Clin Oncol 2009;27(28):4656–63.

168. Blumberg J, CM, The UK and Ireland NET Society/NETS. The CLARINET study-assessing the effect of Lantreotide Autogel on tumor progression-free survival in patients with non-functioning gastroenteropancreatic neuroendocrine tumors (GEP-NETS). AGA; 2012. p. C4.

169. Bergsma H, van Vliet EI, Teunissen JJ, et al. Peptide receptor radionuclide therapy (PRRT) for GEP-NETs. Best Pract Res Clin Gastroenterol 2012;26(6): 867–81.

170. Lee M, Pellegata NS. Multiple endocrine neoplasia type 4. Front Horm Res 2013; 41:63–78.

171. Thakker RV. Multiple endocrine neoplasia type 1 (MEN1) and type 4 (MEN4). Mol Cell Endocrinol 2014;386:2–15.

172. Tham E, Grandell U, Lindgren E, et al. Clinical testing for mutations in the MEN1 gene in Sweden: a report on 200 unrelated cases. J Clin Endocrinol Metab 2007;92:3389–95.

173. Pellegata NS, Quintanilla-Martinez L, Siggelkow H, et al. Germ-line mutations in p27Kip1 cause a multiple endocrine neoplasia syndrome in rats and humans. Proc Natl Acad Sci U S A 2006;103:15558–63.

174. Pardi E, Mariotti S, Pellegata NS, et al. Functional characterization of a CDKN1B mutation in a Sardinian kindred with multiple endocrine neoplasia type 4 (MEN4). Endocr Connect 2014. [Epub ahead of print].

175. Marinoni I, Pellegata NS. p27kip1: a new multiple endocrine neoplasia gene? Neuroendocrinology 2011;93:19–28.

176. Agarwal SK, Mateo CM, Marx SJ. Rare germline mutations in cyclin-dependent kinase inhibitor genes in multiple endocrine neoplasia type 1 and related states. J Clin Endocrinol Metab 2009;94(5):1826–34.

177. Norton JA, Kunz P. Multiple endocrine neoplasias. cancer: principles and practice of oncology. 10th edition. Wolters Kluwer 2015.

178. Moline J, Eng C. Multiple endocrine neoplasia type 2: an overview. Genet Med 2011;13:755–64.

179. Sizemore GW, Health H 3rd, Carney JA. Multiple endocrine neoplasia type 2. Clin Endocrinol Metab 1980;9(2):299–315.

180. Howe JR, Norton JA, Wells SA Jr. Prevalence of pheochromocytoma and hyperparathyroidism in multiple endocrine neoplasia type 2A: results of long-term follow-up. Surgery 1993;114(6):1070–7.

181. Norton JA, Froome LC, Farrell RE, et al. Multiple endocrine neoplasia type IIb: the most aggressive form of medullary thyroid carcinoma. Surg Clin North Am 1979;59(1):109–18.

182. Carney JA, Go VL, Sizemore GW, et al. Alimentary-tract ganglioneuromatosis. A major component of the syndrome of multiple endocrine neoplasia, type 2b. N Engl J Med 1976;295(23):1287–91.

183. Farndon JR, Leight GS, Dilley WG, et al. Familial medullary thyroid carcinoma without associated endocrinopathies: a distinct clinical entity. Br J Surg 1986; 73(4):278–81.

184. Sipple J. The association of pheochromocytoma with carcinoma of the thyroid gland. Am J Med 1961;31(1):163–6.

185. Steiner AL, Goodman AD, Powers SR. Study of a kindred with pheochromocytoma, medullary thyroid carcinoma, hyperparathyroidism and Cushing's disease: multiple endocrine neoplasia, type 2. Medicine (Baltimore) 1968;47(5):371–409.

186. Schimke RN, Hartmann WH, Prout TE, et al. Syndrome of bilateral pheochromocytoma, medullary thyroid carcinoma and multiple neuromas. A possible regulatory defect in the differentiation of chromaffin tissue. N Engl J Med 1968; 279(1):1–7.

187. Raue F, Frank-Raue K. Update multiple endocrine neoplasia type 2. Fam Cancer 2010;9(3):449–57.

188. Durbec P, Marcos-Gutierrez CV, Kilkenny C, et al. GDNF signalling through the Ret receptor tyrosine kinase. Nature 1996;381(6585):789–93.

189. Robertson K, Mason I. The GDNF-RET signalling partnership. Trends Genet 1997;13(1):1–3.

190. Nosrat CA, Tomac A, Hoffer BJ, et al. Cellular and developmental patterns of expression of Ret and glial cell line-derived neurotrophic factor receptor alpha mRNAs. Exp Brain Res 1997;115(3):410–22.

191. Trupp M, Arenas E, Fainzilber M, et al. Functional receptor for GDNF encoded by the c-ret proto-oncogene. Nature 1996;381(6585):785–9.

192. Wells SA Jr, Santoro M. Targeting the RET pathway in thyroid cancer. Clin Cancer Res 2009;15(23):7119–23.

193. Jing S, Wen D, Yu Y, et al. GDNF-induced activation of the ret protein tyrosine kinase is mediated by GDNFR-alpha, a novel receptor for GDNF. Cell 1996; 85(7):1113–24.

194. Golden JP, Hoshi M, Nassar MA, et al. RET signaling is required for survival and normal function of nonpeptidergic nociceptors. J Neurosci 2010;30(11):3983–94.

195. Tee JB, Choi Y, Shah MM, et al. Protein kinase A regulates GDNF/RET-dependent but not GDNF/Ret-independent ureteric bud outgrowth from the Wolffian duct. Dev Biol 2010;347(2):337–47.

196. Ryu H, Jeon GS, Cashman NR, et al. Differential expression of c-Ret in motor neurons versus non-neuronal cells is linked to the pathogenesis of ALS. Lab Invest 2011;91(3):342–52.

197. Ohgami N, Ida-Eto M, Sakashita N, et al. Partial impairment of c-Ret at tyrosine 1062 accelerates age-related hearing loss in mice. Neurobiol Aging 2012;33(3): 626.e25–34.

198. Pachnis V, Mankoo B, Costantini F. Expression of the c-ret proto-oncogene during mouse embryogenesis. Development 1993;119(4):1005–17.

199. Moore SW, Zaahl MG. Multiple endocrine neoplasia syndromes, children, Hirschsprung's disease and RET. Pediatr Surg Int 2008;24(5):521–30.

200. Reginensi A, Clarkson M, Neirijnck Y, et al. SOX9 controls epithelial branching by activating RET effector genes during kidney development. Hum Mol Genet 2011;20(6):1143–53.

201. Brantley MA Jr, Jain S, Barr EE, et al. Neurturin-mediated ret activation is required for retinal function. J Neurosci 2008;28(16):4123–35.

202. Schuchardt A, D'Agati V, Larsson-Blomberg L, et al. Defects in the kidney and enteric nervous system of mice lacking the tyrosine kinase receptor Ret. Nature 1994;367(6461):380–3.

203. Schuchardt A, D'Agati V, Larsson-Blomberg L, et al. RET-deficient mice: an animal model for Hirschsprung's disease and renal agenesis. J Intern Med 1995; 238(4):327–32.

204. Rungby J. RET, a gene responsible for familial endocrine neoplasias and Hirschsprung disease. Ugeskr Laeger 1994;156(21):3194 [in Danish].

205. Lyonnet S, Edery P, Mulligan LM, et al. Mutations of RET proto-oncogene in Hirschsprung disease. C R Acad Sci III 1994;317(4):358–62 [in French].

206. Edery P, Lyonnet S, Mulligan LM, et al. Mutations of the RET proto-oncogene in Hirschsprung's disease. Nature 1994;367(6461):378–80.

207. Romeo G, Ronchetto P, Luo Y, et al. Point mutations affecting the tyrosine kinase domain of the RET proto-oncogene in Hirschsprung's disease. Nature 1994; 367(6461):377–8.

208. Smith DP, Eng C, Ponder BA. Mutations of the RET proto-oncogene in the multiple endocrine neoplasia type 2 syndromes and Hirschsprung disease. J Cell Sci Suppl 1994;18:43–9.

209. Attie T, Edery P, Lyonnet S, et al. Identification of mutation of RET proto-oncogene in Hirschsprung disease. C R Seances Soc Biol Fil 1994;188(5–6): 499–504 [in French].

210. Jeanpierre C, Mace G, Parisot M, et al. RET and GDNF mutations are rare in fetuses with renal agenesis or other severe kidney development defects. J Med Genet 2011;48(7):497–504.

211. Jain S. The many faces of RET dysfunction in kidney. Organogenesis 2009;5(4): 177–90.

212. Skinner MA, Safford SD, Reeves JG, et al. Renal aplasia in humans is associated with RET mutations. Am J Hum Genet 2008;82(2):344–51.

213. Gestblom C, Sweetser DA, Doggett B, et al. Sympathoadrenal hyperplasia causes renal malformations in Ret(MEN2B)-transgenic mice. Am J Pathol 1999;155(6):2167–79.

214. Schuchardt A, D'Agati V, Pachnis V, et al. Renal agenesis and hypodysplasia in ret-k- mutant mice result from defects in ureteric bud development. Development 1996;122(6):1919–29.

215. Mathew CG, Chin KS, Easton DF, et al. A linked genetic marker for multiple endocrine neoplasia type 2A on chromosome 10. Nature 1987;328(6130):527–8.

216. Simpson NE, Kidd KK, Goodfellow PJ, et al. Assignment of multiple endocrine neoplasia type 2A to chromosome 10 by linkage. Nature 1987;328(6130): 528–30.
217. Donis-Keller H, Dou S, Chi D, et al. Mutations in the RET proto-oncogene are associated with MEN 2A and FMTC. Hum Mol Genet 1993;2(7):851–6.
218. Mulligan LM, Kwok JB, Healey CS, et al. Germ-line mutations of the RET proto-oncogene in multiple endocrine neoplasia type 2A. Nature 1993;363(6428): 458–60.
219. Hofstra RM, Landsvater RM, Ceccherini I, et al. A mutation in the RET proto-oncogene associated with multiple endocrine neoplasia type 2B and sporadic medullary thyroid carcinoma. Nature 1994;367(6461):375–6.
220. Santoro M, Carlomagno F, Romano A, et al. Activation of RET as a dominant transforming gene by germline mutations of MEN2A and MEN2B. Science 1995;267(5196):381–3.
221. Unger K, Malisch E, Thomas G, et al. Array CGH demonstrates characteristic aberration signatures in human papillary thyroid carcinomas governed by RET/PTC. Oncogene 2008;27(33):4592–602.
222. Xue F, Yu H, Maurer LH, et al. Germline RET mutations in MEN 2A and FMTC and their detection by simple DNA diagnostic tests. Hum Mol Genet 1994;3(4):635–8.
223. Chi DD, Toshima K, Donis-Keller H, et al. Predictive testing for multiple endocrine neoplasia type 2A (MEN 2A) based on the detection of mutations in the RET protooncogene. Surgery 1994;116(2):124–32 [discussion: 132–3].
224. Pazaitou-Panayiotou K, Kaprara A, Sarika L, et al. Efficient testing of the RET gene by DHPLC analysis for MEN 2 syndrome in a cohort of patients. Anticancer Res 2005;25(3B):2091–5.
225. Brandi ML, Gagel RF, Angeli A, et al. Guidelines for diagnosis and therapy of MEN type 1 and type 2. J Clin Endocrinol Metab 2001;86(12):5658–71.
226. Kloos RT, Eng C, Evans DB, et al. Medullary thyroid cancer: management guidelines of the American Thyroid Association. Thyroid 2009;19(6):565–612.
227. Frank-Raue K, Rondot S, Schulze E, et al. Change in the spectrum of RET mutations diagnosed between 1994 and 2006. Clin Lab 2007;53(5–6):273–82.
228. Jasim S, Ying AK, Waguespack SG, et al. Multiple endocrine neoplasia type 2B with a RET proto-oncogene A883F mutation displays a more indolent form of medullary thyroid carcinoma compared with a RET M918T mutation. Thyroid 2011;21(2):189–92.
229. Siqueira DR, Romitti M, da Rocha AP, et al. The RET polymorphic allele S836S is associated with early metastatic disease in patients with hereditary or sporadic medullary thyroid carcinoma. Endocr Relat Cancer 2010;17(4):953–63.
230. Wells SA Jr, Chi DD, Toshima K, et al. Predictive DNA testing and prophylactic thyroidectomy in patients at risk for multiple endocrine neoplasia type 2A. Ann Surg 1994;220(3):237–47 [discussion: 247–50].
231. Scholten A, Valk GD, Ulfman D, et al. Unilateral adrenalectomy for pheochromocytoma in multiple endocrine neoplasia type 2 patients. Ann Surg 2011;254: 1022–7.
232. Lamers CB. Familial multiple endocrine neoplasia type I (Wermer's syndrome). Neth J Med 1978;21(6):270–4.
233. Doherty GM, Olson JA, Frisella MM, et al. Lethality of multiple endocrine neoplasia type I. World J Surg 1998;22(6):581–6 [discussion:586–7].
234. Geerdink EA, Van der Luijt RB, Lips CJ. Do patients with multiple endocrine neoplasia syndrome type 1 benefit from periodical screening? Eur J Endocrinol 2003;149(6):577–82.

Sequence Variants of Uncertain Significance

What to Do When Genetic Test Results Are Not Definitive

Marc S. Greenblatt, MD

KEYWORDS

- Cancer • Genetic testing • Variants of uncertain significance (VUS) • Gene panels
- Pathogenic variant • Hereditary cancer syndrome

KEY POINTS

- Variants of uncertain significance (VUS) comprise a significant and growing number of results from germline testing associated with many hereditary cancer syndromes.
- The biological interpretation and clinical significance of VUS are complex and challenging.
- Unlike pathogenic germline DNA variants, VUS are generally not useful for clinical management; however, the goal of the genetics community is to gather different types of evidence that will eventually lead to the classification of all VUS as either pathogenic or neutral.
- It is important for clinicians, and surgical oncologists in particular, to understand that they can contribute to VUS classification efforts by documenting clinicopathologic data, referring patients and their families to genetic counselors, and encouraging patients to share data and participate in cancer genetics research studies.
- Management of patients at increased cancer risk, and evaluation of difficult genetic variants and their cancer risks, are both complex tasks that rely on combining multiple lines of evidence.

TERMINOLOGY AND DEFINITIONS IN CANCER GENETICS

Clinicians in the coming era will need to be familiar with the basics of genetic terminology and principles, so this article reviews some terms and principles that apply to DNA variations.[1] Some of the nomenclature of DNA variant interpretation is new and confusing to clinicians, and often to researchers as well. Ongoing international efforts

Disclosure: The author has nothing to disclose.
University of Vermont College of Medicine, Given E214, 89 Beaumont Ave, Burlington, VT 05405, USA
E-mail address: marc.greenblatt@uvmhealth.org

Surg Oncol Clin N Am 24 (2015) 833–846
http://dx.doi.org/10.1016/j.soc.2015.06.009
1055-3207/15/$ – see front matter © 2015 Elsevier Inc. All rights reserved.

exist to standardize genetic and phenotypic terminology so that the field is more accessible to researchers, clinicians, and patients.[2]

Basic Genetics

Only about 2% of human DNA codes for genes that produce proteins. Much of the remaining 98% of the genome's noncoding DNA is now known to have regulatory functions that are incompletely understood but are the subject of intense study.[3] Current genetic testing for cancer susceptibility generally deals almost exclusively with protein-coding genes. However, it is anticipated that in the future more regulatory regions will be associated with hereditary diseases, including cancer susceptibility syndromes.

A gene is composed of DNA sequences that usually span thousands of base pairs (adenine [A] pairing with thymine [T], guanine [G] pairing with cytosine [C]). The cell reads the DNA code of genes, first producing a complementary strand of messenger RNA (mRNA), by the process of gene transcription. mRNA is then converted into a chain of amino acids that forms a cellular protein by the process of translation using the triplet nucleotide code (3 nucleotide bases translate into 1 amino acid). Genes contain several regions with different functions. In the coding sequences, called exons, the genetic code is read by cellular machinery and converted into a protein. Coding exons are short stretches of DNA separated by sequences called introns, which are stretches of DNA ranging from dozens to thousands of DNA bases that do not code for protein. They are transcribed into mRNA, but are spliced out before mRNA is translated. In addition, there are regulatory sequences that indicate the beginning and end of a gene, and others that code for whether the cell should produce the protein and in what amounts. The consensus normal sequence of a gene and protein is called the wild type. DNA can be altered (mutated) in any gene region,[4,5] and any of these alterations may result in (1) abnormal protein structure, function, and/or expression, causing increased disease susceptibility; or (2) protein structure, function, and expression that is not significantly changed from the normal sequence and does not cause disease.

Clinicians interpret the effects of a DNA change based on knowledge of genetic principles and on observed effects in vivo and in vitro. Reports from clinical genetic testing may indicate abnormalities caused by changes in amino acid, truncation of protein length, abnormal splicing, large gene deletion, and other mechanisms. Interpretation may be uncertain regarding any of these mechanisms. The different types of variants that are seen are:

Missense
Change from one amino acid to another without changing protein length.

Nonsense
Creation of a premature stop codon, coding for a shortened protein that may or may not be transcribed by the cell.

Frameshift
Deletion or insertion of a few DNA nucleotides, not in multiples of 3, that changes the reading frame of the mRNA message. This variant almost always results in a few new incorrect amino acids followed by a premature stop codon.

Insertion or deletion
Insertion or deletions (indels) can be large or small. Small indels are deletions or insertions of a few DNA nucleotides in multiples of 3, which result in the addition or

subtraction of 1 or a few amino acids from the protein chain. Large deletions can involve many thousands of DNA nucleotides, resulting in the loss of large regions or an entire protein.

Splicing
Splicing is deletion of a full exon or exons, resulting in a deletion of a segment of the protein, and possibly also a frameshift.

Regulatory
Change in a DNA nucleotide in a region that controls whether a gene is successfully translated into a protein by the cell.

Silent
A change in DNA nucleotide that results in a different DNA code for the same amino acid. Silent mutations sometimes affect splicing or regulatory functions.

Genetic Variation Nomenclature

Clinical reports from genetic testing can be confusing. In the past, a genetic change that was seen commonly in populations and presumed to be benign was called a polymorphism, and one that was thought to cause disease was called a mutation. The term variant is now often used to refer to any DNA change. With the recognition of many variants of uncertain significance (VUS), the term mutation has become ambiguous and cannot be assumed to mean that the change is associated with disease. The clearest terminology is now to refer to all DNA changes as variants, and to classify them as pathogenic (disease causing) or neutral (benign) when the association with disease has been assessed. Other terms have been borrowed from different areas of variant science. Important examples that are seen and are related to, but not identical to, pathogenic or neutral include damaging, which is the preferred way to refer to a change that alters a protein's function versus mutation; and deleterious, referring to a change that is harmful to an organism and therefore is not seen in any species through evolution.[6] Both of these terms apply to specific types of nonclinical evidence, and do not reflect clinical interpretation.

CLASSIFYING VARIANTS

Until the last few years, there were no standard systems for reporting the classification of genetic variants. Variants were generally reported in 3 categories: (1) pathogenic mutations that cause disease; (2) benign or neutral, and (3) VUS. Genetic testing laboratories tend to be conservative in classifying variants, wanting to avoid errors because of the important decisions that result from these conclusions. There has been considerable variation among researchers and laboratories regarding how much evidence should be required in order to classify a given variant. National and international organizations are attempting to develop standardized systems for interpreting and reporting such results.[2,7,8]

A 5-tiered classification system that can be used to define clinical management of variants in hereditary cancer genes was proposed by the International Association for Research on Cancer (IARC) Working Group on Unclassified Genetic Variants,[7] and has been applied to several syndromes in clinical cancer genetics (hereditary breast and ovarian cancer [HBOC], Lynch syndrome [LS], familial melanoma).[9–11] When possible, each class is associated with a probability that a variant is pathogenic, derived from statistical studies[7] that incorporate data from various independent sources that are important to disease pathology (**Table 1**). The American College of Medical Genetics

Table 1				
IARC 5-class system				
Class	Quantitative or Qualitative Probability of Pathogenicity	Clinical Testing of Relatives	Surveillance for Relatives	Research Testing
5	>0.99	Yes	Yes: high risk	No
4	0.95–0.99	Yes	Yes: high risk	Yes
3	0.05–0.949	No	Based on family history and so forth	Yes
2	0.001–0.049	No	Treat as no mutation detected	Yes
1	<0.001	No	Treat as no mutation detected	No

Five classes of variants linked to clinical recommendations. Based on probability of pathogenicity.

Adapted from Plon SE, Eccles DM, Easton D, et al. Sequence variant classification and reporting: recommendations for improving the interpretation of cancer susceptibility genetic test results. Hum Mutat 2008;29(11):1287; with permission.

and Genomics (ACMG) and the Association for Molecular Pathology have jointly recommended guidelines that closely parallel the IARC scheme.[12] Both systems include 5 classes of variants, and the IARC system links these to probabilities of pathogenicity (class 5, pathogenic, >99%; class 4, likely pathogenic, 95%–99%; class 3, uncertain, 5%–95%; class 2, likely neutral, 0.1%–5%; and class 1, neutral, <0.1%) and recommendations for management of HBOC and LS.[7] It is hoped that the presence of guidelines from these major organizations will lead to standardization of the terminology and processes, which will assist in both clinical management and further research.

VARIANTS IN COMMON AND RARE HEREDITARY CANCER SYNDROMES

When interpreting genetic testing results, cancer geneticists must consider typical versus atypical presentations of the clinical syndrome in question. Atypical presentations could represent a variant of the common syndrome or a different condition that mimics the classic syndrome. The most commonly seen hereditary cancer syndromes are HBOC and LS; more than 50 other syndromes have been described. Genetic testing in these syndromes can be difficult to interpret because many cancers are commonly seen as sporadic cases, and it may not even be clear whether a hereditary syndrome is present in a family. New genetic technologies will identify many new genes that rarely cause a hereditary cancer syndrome, and many that confer intermediate (not high) risk for cancer, leading to new layers of uncertainty in variant interpretation.[5,13,14] LS usually results from mutation to one of the 4 mismatch repair (MMR) genes, but can also be caused by an inherited deletion of the end of the EPCAM gene, just upstream of the MSH2 gene, which changes regulation of MSH2 and results in loss of MSH2 protein.[15] The identification of other unusual examples of genetic mechanisms of pathogenicity is anticipated.

Definitive proof of hereditary cancer syndromes is sought in the DNA from normal cells, usually peripheral blood lymphocytes, looking for an inherited pathogenic mutation in a relevant gene. DNA changes that are inherited are present in every somatic cell of the body. For cancer to develop, the inherited gene mutation is followed by a second mutation in the copy of the gene in a relevant somatic cell (eg, colon, breast, ovary). In this clone of cells, both copies of the gene (eg, BRCA, MMR) are thus mutated. As a result, no normal proteins that the gene encodes are produced. The second abnormality abrogates the physiologic process that these proteins perform (eg, DNA MMR in LS, homologous recombination repair in HBOC). Evidence of these abnormal processes can sometimes be found in cells or tissues of patients.

VUS have been a large part of genetic testing since its inception in the 1990s. Their frequency varies by gene and syndrome. For HBOC, the fraction of BRCA1 and BRCA2 variants that are VUS has steadily decreased in recent years, but new, rare VUS in these genes are still identified with significant frequency.[16] However, the frequency of VUS in intermediate-risk breast cancer genes is high. The database of MMR gene variants associated with LS includes more than 2000 VUS, about 20% to 30% of variants[4] (http://insight-group.org/variants/database/).

INTERPRETING GENETIC TESTING RESULTS

Some changes found in germline DNA almost certainly affect protein or cellular function; others almost certainly do not. Interpreting genetic testing results can be complicated, and potential results are not limited to positive or negative. In general, genetic testing can result in one of 3 possible interpretations of the molecular findings. These molecular interpretations must then be applied by clinicians to manage patients and their families properly.

Potential interpretations of molecular genetic testing for cancer predisposition syndromes are:

Pathogenic Variant Detected

There is an increased hereditary predisposition to cancer because of the DNA variant that can be clearly classified as pathogenic. A classification of pathogenic may mean that the variant has been seen before and is clearly associated with the corresponding condition. Some uncommon variants are easy for the laboratory to recognize as a mutation that disrupts the gene's normal function. The most common types of variants for which pathogenicity is implied by the type of mutation involve a change in the DNA code that is predicted to result in the production of no protein or a very abnormal protein. These variants include (1) a nonsense mutation resulting in a stop codon; (2) a large deletion or insertion; (3) a frameshift deletion or insertion of a small number of nucleotides not divisible by 3; (4) some changes in which exons and introns meet and mRNA splicing is almost certainly altered, leading to an aberrant protein missing 1 or more of its critical parts. If any of these types of mutations are detected in a patient, the laboratory report will state that an inherited pathogenic mutation has been identified. Management of the patient can be planned accordingly, and testing of the patient's relatives becomes an option.

Pathogenic DNA Variant Not Detected

The important caveat for this result is that it applies only to the genes examined, based on the specific technology applied. If only a variant that is known to be neutral is identified, this is considered a negative result. If no pathogenic variant is identified, this result must be interpreted cautiously; it does not automatically mean that there is no hereditary cancer risk present. Factors that affect interpretation of negative results are:

Who was tested?

Did the tested individual have cancer, and, if so, how likely is it that this individual carries the hereditary syndrome that was tested? If an unaffected relative was tested, then it is not possible to be certain that there is no pathogenic mutation present in others in the family. It is possible that no pathogenic mutation exists in the family, but it is also possible that other relatives carry a pathogenic mutation but this individual does not. Even if the tested individual has had cancer, the full personal and family history must be carefully evaluated. It is possible that the tested individual had a sporadic cancer but other relatives had a hereditary cancer (especially in the case of common cancers such as breast and colon). Several models have been developed to predict the likelihood of mutations in MMR or BRCA genes, but all of them have limitations. Each model represents a single tool that may or may not assist the surgical oncologist to navigate a difficult clinical scenario.[17,18]

What test was done?

Which gene or genes was tested? It is possible that a mutation exists in a gene that was not tested. It is possible that not every relevant known gene was tested, and it is possible that a pathogenic mutation exists in a gene that is not yet known to be associated with hereditary cancer. Which parts of the gene were studied? It is possible that a variant exists in a regulatory region that was not tested. Some genetic technologies can miss large deletions. In addition, sometimes even the full coding region of a gene is not checked. For example, if a specific variant is known to be carried by a family, this specific variant can be sought at low cost without studying the rest of the gene. However, personal and family histories are critical in order to properly interpret the results of such site-specific testing.

Identification of a Variant of Uncertain Significance

This result usually means that further work is required by the clinical and/or research laboratories before the result can be used clinically. VUS can be in either regulatory or coding regions of the gene. A large body of scientific literature exists regarding how to interpret VUS, mostly on missense variants but also on some regulatory variants. Clinicians are not expected to perform these interpretations, but they should be aware of the principles regarding underlying variant analysis, and how clinicians can help advance the field for the benefit of patients and their families.

SEEKING EVIDENCE FOR PATHOGENICITY IN ASSESSING VARIANTS OF UNCERTAIN SIGNIFICANCE

The consensus of experts in classifying variants is that multiple lines of evidence should be used, and no single piece of evidence by itself is conclusive.[7] Presently, there is no simple way to instantly and with certainty clinically classify many missense and regulatory region mutations. Instead, many points of evidence for or against pathogenicity are collected for each missense mutation. In general, 2 types of evidence should be obtained: (1) evidence that associates the variant with the clinical syndrome, and (2) evidence that associates the variant with abnormal biological function. Several research efforts are ongoing to establish criteria for classifying variants, and multidisciplinary teams of experts have been addressing the problem for HBOC and LS (http://insight-group.org/variants/classifications/, http://enigmaconsortium.org/).[10,19,20] Clinicians can be important contributors to this process by recognizing that a report of a VUS requires further study, and helping to refer individuals in these families to cancer genetics programs in which they can be enrolled in research studies to advance variant interpretation. This process can take years before clinically useful conclusions can be drawn, but the effort and results can pay off for the families that carry the VUS.

Several good technical reviews on this process have been published.[14,21–24] This article discusses the evidence in less technical terms. This evidence includes clinicopathologic and epidemiologic studies that are familiar to clinicians but also in vivo or in vitro functional assays, and computational (in silico) analyses, which are less familiar to clinicians.[6,23,25]

ASSOCIATION, OR LACK OF ASSOCIATION, OF THE VARIANT WITH HEREDITARY CANCER

Segregation: Finding the Variant in Multiple Affected Family Members

If a variant causes a hereditary cancer syndrome in a family, then all of the relatives clinically affected with the syndrome should carry that variant. Geneticists use the term segregation when they study this co-occurrence. Relatives close to each other in a pedigree are likely to share a random gene variant simply by chance. The more distant relatives are from each other, the more likely it is that sharing both the hereditary condition and the variant is not coincidental. Each pair of first-degree relatives has a 50% chance of sharing a given variant. Calculations of the probability of a variant being shared by chance are based on exponents of 2 (1 in 2, 1 in 4, 1 in 8, 1 in 16 chance, and so forth). A large family with many affected individuals can provide strong evidence that co-occurrence of a variant is not likely to be caused by chance. However, large families with DNA and clinical information about many of the relatives for segregation studies are rare.

Even if there is a large family with many affected relatives who share the variant, can clinicians then conclude this variant to be the cause of the syndrome? This evidence is strong, but not conclusive. It is possible that the variant is harmless but is physically close on its chromosome to a different, undetected pathogenic variant that is the real cause of the syndrome in that family. If there is a strong segregation in a family then geneticists might still consider the variant to be a good genetic marker for cancer risk and use it for presymptomatic DNA testing in that family. There are good documented examples of this for both common and uncommon cancer predisposition syndromes. For example, a missense mutation changing the 29th amino acid of the MLH1 protein from alanine to serine (p.Ala29Ser) was observed in several families with colorectal cancer (CRC) and segregated with affected individuals within each of the families. However, functional studies suggested that the altered protein had the same function as wild-type MLH1.[26] Therefore, for 7 years, this result was not used in managing unaffected family members. In some affected families, sequencing included the regions slightly upstream of the coding exons, and a second variant in this regulatory region (c.-27C>A) was found to be linked to the original missense variant in all of the affected families studied worldwide. Functional studies of the upstream regulatory variant showed that it was the cause of decreased MLH1 production and resulting LS phenotype.[27,28] With this information, the c.-27C>A variant can now be used for predictive testing.

Population Frequency

With the many recent projects that have determined the DNA sequence of many individuals worldwide, one of the first things to look for is whether the variant has appeared in normal populations, and its frequency. If it is a common variant then it is unlikely to be a cause for hereditary cancer risk. Databases include dbSNP (www.ncbi.nlm.nih.gov/projects/SNP/), the 1000 Genomes Project,[29] and others. Some studies of hereditary cancer in the scientific literature also contain data on genetic variants in control populations.[30] If a variant has been reported in control populations with sufficient frequency (usually >1%), then this is evidence that it is not pathogenic. If a variant has not been reported, clinicians must take into account the ethnicity and geographic location of the reported populations. If a variant is absent in a population, but the reported populations do not match the ethnicity of your patient, then the fact that the variant has not been reported before does not rule out a harmless variant (referred to in the past as a polymorphism) that is specific to that ethnicity.

Occurrence of the Variant in Other Families with Hereditary Cancer

If a variant has not been observed in appropriate control populations for a patient, but instead has been observed in patients affected with cancer from different families, this favors pathogenicity. However, the caveats mentioned earlier regarding specifics of the family history apply here. Statistical methods can sometimes be applied to try to quantify the likelihood of pathogenicity. If the family history of patients with identified clearly pathogenic variants can be shown to be significantly different from the histories of patients with negative test results, then this can be used to help calculate the likelihood that a VUS is pathogenic. This approach has been used in BRCA1 and BRCA2 VUS analysis but has not yet been fully developed for other syndromes.[24,31]

Tumor Characteristics

Sometimes, specific histologic features suggest that a cancer arose from a specific hereditary syndrome. This association can apply to both common and uncommon hereditary cancer syndromes. The presence or absence of specific tumor attributes offers one line of evidence in favor of pathogenicity or neutrality of a VUS. For example, in HBOC, breast cancers are much more likely to be estrogen receptor negative, progesterone receptor negative, and HER2/neu negative (ie, triple negative[19]). Ovarian cancers in BRCA1 and BRCA2 mutation carriers are more likely to be invasive serous adenocarcinomas and unlikely to be borderline or mucinous tumors.[32]

CRCs that develop in the setting of LS may show characteristic histologic features: tumor-infiltrating lymphocytes, a Crohn-like lymphocytic response, an excess of mucin, or signet-ring cells with poor differentiation.[33] They usually show evidence of faulty MMR in the tumor, which can be detected as abnormalities of either protein or DNA. The most commonly performed abnormal tumor pathology test is immunohistochemistry (IHC), which shows loss of staining for 1 or more of the MMR proteins in the cancer, with normal staining in the surrounding normal tissue. Abnormal IHC is found in ~90% of LS-associated CRCs.[33] However, observed staining for an MMR protein is only proof of the presence of that protein, not of its normal function. Missense mutations may give rise to proteins that are less functional than their normal counterpart but still contain those regions that are bound by the IHC antibodies. For this reason, the possibility of a VUS being pathogenic if the corresponding protein is detected in the tumor cannot be discarded.

The resulting pattern of DNA damage from failure to fix DNA mismatches can be detected by measuring the lengths of repeated DNA bases known as microsatellites (eg, ACACACAC). These segments are prone to lengthening or shortening in cells with faulty MMR. This phenomenon is known as microsatellite instability (MSI). MSI also is found in ~85% to 90% of LS-associated CRCs.[33,34] Absence of MSI in CRC in a VUS carrier argues against LS and pathogenicity of the VUS.[3] IHC and MSI abnormalities are seen less frequently in non-CRC LS-associated cancers and are therefore more difficult to interpret.[35]

These findings can be used as another line of evidence to support the molecular diagnosis of LS, although alone they are not conclusive to classify a given VUS as pathogenic. Inactivation of MMR in a cell can be noninherited. MSI occurs in 15% to 20% of sporadic CRC because of somatic, noninherited suppression of MLH1 protein caused by methylation of the MLH1 promoter region, which controls protein expression. Other tests must be done to follow up this finding. Observing MLH1 promoter hypermethylation strongly suggests a noninherited cause of observed MSI and loss of MLH1 staining. Finding a V600E noninherited mutation of the *BRAF* gene in a colorectal tumor indicates sporadic tumors with MSI, although it is present in only 50% to 70% of such cases.[34]

Other characteristic histologic tumor features that suggest inherited cancer syndromes include papillary kidney cancers (associated with germline mutations in the c-met and fumarate hydratase genes [hereditary leiomyomatosis and kidney cell cancer]), chromophobe and oncocytic kidney cancers associated with Birt-Hogg-Dube syndrome,[36] and sebaceous adenocarcinomas of the skin associated with the Muir-Torre variant of LS.[33]

Co-occurrence of Variants of Uncertain Significance with a Known Inherited Pathogenic Variant of the Gene

Sometimes a VUS is detected in the presence of a second, clearly pathogenic, variant in the other copy of the same gene (sometimes this must be sorted out by testing for the variants in the patient's parents or other relatives). Inheriting 2 mutated copies of a gene sometimes is not compatible with life (eg, BRCA1),[37] and other times causes a different distinctive condition. For example, inheriting 2 pathogenic BRCA2 mutations causes Fanconi anemia type D1,[38] and inheriting 2 pathogenic MMR gene mutations causes a condition referred to as constitutional mismatch repair deficiency syndrome, with childhood or young adult onset featuring café-au-lait skin spots, gastrointestinal tumors, leukemia, lymphomas, and brain tumors.[39] Therefore, detecting a VUS in the presence of a clearly pathogenic mutation in the other copy of the gene in question suggests that the VUS is pathogenic if the patient has the features of the special syndrome, and is strong evidence that the VUS is neutral if seen in a gene that causes embryonic lethality or if the syndrome that corresponds with 2 pathogenic variants is not present.

ASSOCIATION OF A VARIANT WITH ABNORMAL PROTEIN STRUCTURE, FUNCTION, OR EXPRESSION
Functional Analysis

Many laboratory tests have been developed to test the various functional aspects of protein variants, comparing them with normal protein. Human and nonhuman cell-based assays as well as in vitro biochemical assays are used in functional analysis, which have been performed for BRCA, MMR, and other genes.[11,21,22,25,40–42] These tests are a promising mechanism to assign pathogenicity. However, they are difficult to interpret, differ from syndrome to syndrome, and do not necessarily reflect the action of variant MMR protein in its normal human environment and its relation to clinical disease. Often, different tests suggest different levels of function for the same variant. However, observed consistent loss of normal protein functions in these assays generally does suggest pathogenicity. Normal function in test environments does not necessarily imply that a VUS is neutral, because other explanations for pathogenicity may exist (eg, abnormal protein expression or splicing,[43] or unrealistic assay conditions). No consensus on the type of testing best suited for a diagnostic setting has been reached yet, and tests still need to be validated for this purpose before they can move out of the research laboratories and into the clinic.

Computational (in Silico) Analysis of Gene and Protein

Missense mutations in the DNA sequence change the predicted protein sequence. Software tools have been developed that consider the biophysical properties and evolutionary conservation of the variant protein and its underlying genetic code to help predict whether or not the protein function will be disrupted. Such analysis is referred to as in silico (reviewed in Ref.[6]).

These analyses may compare the biophysical properties of the old and new amino acid, such as changes in polarity and volume. Other tools check for evolutionary conservation. In this approach, the amino acid composition of the proteins and their underlying DNA sequences are carefully compared among multiple species. Parts of the sequences and their corresponding protein parts that have shown little or no change during the evolution of lower and higher organisms are considered to be of crucial importance to the protein function. Variants that affect these amino acids are more likely to alter a key function, because no living organisms contain them, and are therefore predicted to be pathogenic. In silico prediction of the effects of variants on RNA splicing is another important area of variant analysis.[41] Recent versions of tools to predict the pathogenicity of missense variants correlate well with other methods of assessing pathogenicity in the MMR and BRCA genes, if the analyses are performed carefully. For BRCA and MMR variants, they perform as well as predictive tools as many commonly used clinical tests, and can be safely used for pathogenicity prediction.[34,44] These results should be confirmed in other syndromes before they are used as clinical tools.

CLASSIFYING VARIANTS BY COMBINING EVIDENCE

Pulling all these lines of evidence together to reach a verdict on pathogenicity is a challenge. Mutation databases frequently contain conflicting interpretations of variants.[4,45] Current research aims to develop clinically validated algorithms that integrate results from all lines of evidence into a final classification, ideally with an objectively calculated probability in favor of pathogenicity.[9,21,23,34]

Initial efforts to create standardized systems to integrate data and classify variants have been made by several international groups. The IARC working group developed a matrix to support this type of translation[7] (see **Table 1** for a version adapted for LS). The Variant Interpretation Committee of the International Society for Hereditary Gastrointestinal Tumors (InSiGHT, www.insight-group.org) has used the Plon matrix to develop a set of qualitative rules to classify MMR gene missense variants.[34] The committee has reached consensus on what combination of features corresponds with 99%, 95%, less than 5%, and less than 0.1% probability of pathogenicity, and has used these criteria to classify the missense variants in the InSiGHT database (N>2000). These variants can now be used to develop quantitative statistics for the types of evidence described earlier, so that they can be integrated using objective evidence rather than expert opinion. The ENIGMA (Evidence-based Network for the Interpretation of Germline Mutant Alleles) consortium is tackling the same issues for the BRCA1/BRCA2 genes.[46] Initial progress has been made on quantitative models to calculate the likelihood of pathogenicity based on objective data,[9,23] and standards are evolving.

SUMMARY: TRANSLATION INTO CLINICAL MANAGEMENT

Ultimately, a VUS result from clinical genetic testing cannot be used for management; it must be regarded as a finding of no pathogenic mutation at the present time. When clinicians receive a result of a VUS from genetic testing, subsequent management decisions must be made based on the clinical scenario, considering both personal and family histories. Cancer genetics clinicians recommend clinical surveillance and management based on the patient's cancer risk status as determined from all of these data.

An Example of a Challenging Variant of Uncertain Significance Scenario

A 32-year-old woman without evidence of breast disease presents to a clinician's office to inquire about prophylactic mastectomy. Her sister was recently diagnosed with *invasive breast cancer at age 33 years, and underwent genetic testing. A variant in BRCA1 was found. The patient was also recently tested and was found to carry the same BRCA1 variant identified in her sister. The testing company has stated the variant is a VUS and there are no clinical recommendations related to the finding at this time. However, the patient and her surgeon have reviewed the literature and found a report of the variant affecting some aspect of cell function, creating the suspicion that the variant might be deleterious, and increasing anxieties in both patient and surgeon.*

At first reading of this scenario, a clinician might respond that, if the woman accepts the clinical risks of the requested surgery despite genetic risk uncertainty but recognizing some degree of increased risk based on her known family history, then what harm is done? In reality, the decision making in such a situation is complex. Important considerations include (1) lifetime risk of breast cancer, given this family history, but no definitive evidence of a pathologic mutation. Several models estimate our patient's lifetime risk of breast cancer at approximately 25%, assuming no other cases of breast cancer in the family. This risk could be 40% or more if there are additional cases of breast or ovarian cancer, especially at early ages. Regardless of genetic testing results, correct management of this patient involves the physician and patient understanding her true cancer risk and how comfortable they are with different clinical strategies to manage that risk, be they increased screening with mammography or MRI, prophylactic surgery, or other plans. (2) Risk that a pathologic mutation does exists in the family despite the initial VUS finding. Given only the patient's history, the risk that a BRCA1 or BRCA2 mutation exists in this family is less than 10% and possibly not more than 5%. Again, additional cases of breast or ovarian cancer could increase this risk, possibly to 50% or more (depending on number of cases, ages of onset, and ethnicity). Knowing that a single hereditary cancer mutation in BRCA1 or BRCA2 is likely versus not likely might lead to different key clinical decisions. (3) The status of other, syndrome-related organs. Again, additional family history can play a major role in establishing whether the patient needs to worry about ovarian or other cancers as well. A single prophylactic surgery may not fully eliminate the patient's increased risk and need for concern, and could provide false reassurance. (4) The risk that a mutation exists in another separate gene that has not, to date, been tested.

Taking all of this into consideration, a dangerous potential scenario for this patient would be to assume that no other organs are at risk and no further genetic evaluation is needed after prophylactic breast surgery. It is important for the surgical oncologist to be reassured that an appropriate cancer genetics consultation in a case such as this can be extremely helpful. Such consultation includes diligent assessment of the likelihood of the relevant cancer syndromes, such as HBOC. However, VUS in BRCA are frequently reclassified as neutral.[9] Further testing could be indicated, for conditions such as Li-Fraumeni syndrome (predisposing to many cancers, including breast cancer), hereditary diffuse gastric cancer syndrome (lobular breast and diffuse gastric cancer), or LS (colon, endometrial, and many other cancers). In addition, a comprehensive cancer genetics evaluation can help address the patient's anxiety and help facilitate a plan that may or may not include a recommendation for prophylactic mastectomy.

It is also important for practicing clinicians to know they can play a major role in future research that will help decipher genetic variation for the benefit of patients and families, by: (1) referring patients and families to cancer genetics programs, in which the subtle details can be elicited that can help with variant interpretation, and patients can be referred to appropriate research studies.[47] The National Society of Genetic Counselors Web site (http://www.nsgc.org/) is also an excellent resource for identifying counselors across North America. (2) Recording and reporting phenotype data in as much detail as possible. (3) Encouraging and facilitating patients' participation in research studies that will help to interpret genetic variation. Clinicians, diagnostic tests, and researchers working together on an international scale provide the best chance to bring the data together for continued advances in definitive clarification of the clinical significance of VUS.

REFERENCES

1. Lindor NM, Goldgar DE, Tavtigian SV, et al. BRCA1/2 sequence variants of uncertain significance: a primer for providers to assist in discussions and in medical management. Oncologist 2013;18(5):518–24.
2. Howard HJ, Horaitis O, Cotton RG, et al. The Human Variome Project (HVP) 2009 Forum "Towards Establishing Standards". Hum Mutat 2010;31(3):366–7.
3. Sijmons RH, Greenblatt MS, Genuardi M. Gene variants of unknown clinical significance in Lynch syndrome. An introduction for clinicians. Fam Cancer 2013; 12(2):181–7.
4. Plazzer JP, Sijmons RH, Woods MO, et al. The InSiGHT database: utilizing 100 years of insights into Lynch syndrome. Fam Cancer 2013;12(2):175–80.
5. Easton DF, Pharoah PD, Antoniou AC, et al. Gene-panel sequencing and the prediction of breast-cancer risk. N Engl J Med 2015;372(23):2243–57.
6. Tavtigian SV, Greenblatt MS, Goldgar DE, et al, for the IARC Unclassified Genetic Variants Working Group. Overview of results from the IARC Unclassified Genetic Variants Working Group. Hum Mutat 2008;29:1261–4.
7. Plon SE, Eccles DM, Easton D, et al, IARC Unclassified Genetic Variants Working Group. Sequence variant classification and reporting: recommendations for improving the interpretation of cancer susceptibility genetic test results. Hum Mutat 2008;29(11):1282–91.
8. Richards S, Aziz N, Bale S, et al. Standards and guidelines for the interpretation of sequence variants: a joint consensus recommendation of the American College of Medical Genetics and Genomics and the Association for Molecular Pathology. ACMG Laboratory Quality Assurance Committee. Genet Med 2015; 17(5):405–24.
9. Vallée MP, Francy TC, Judkins MK, et al. Classification of missense substitutions in the BRCA genes: a database dedicated to ex-UVs. Hum Mutat 2012;33(1):22–8.
10. Thompson BA, Spurdle AB, Plazzer JP, et al. Application of a 5-tiered scheme for standardized classification of 2,360 unique mismatch repair gene variants in the InSiGHT locus-specific database. Nat Genet 2014;46(2):107–15.
11. Miller PJ, Duraisamy S, Newell JA, et al. Classifying variants of CDKN2A using computational and laboratory studies. Hum Mutat 2011;32:900–11.
12. Richards S, Aziz N, Bale S, et al. Standards and guidelines for the interpretation of sequence variants: a joint consensus recommendation of the American College of Medical Genetics and Genomics and the Association for Molecular Pathology. Genet Med 2015;17(5):405–23.
13. Yurgelun MB, Allen B, Kaldate RR, et al. Identification of a variety of mutations in cancer predisposition genes in patients with suspected Lynch syndrome. Gastroenterology 2015. [Epub ahead of print].
14. Tavtigian SV, Chenevix-Trench G. Growing recognition of the role for rare missense substitutions in breast cancer susceptibility. Biomark Med 2014;8(4): 589–603.
15. Ligtenberg MJ, Kuiper RP, Chan TL, et al. Heritable somatic methylation and inactivation of MSH2 in families with Lynch syndrome due to deletion of the 3' exons of TACSTD1. Nat Genet 2009;41(1):112–7.

16. Lindor NM, Goldgar DE, Tavtigian SV, et al. BRCA1/2 sequence variants of uncertain significance: a primer for providers to assist in discussions and in medical management. Oncologist 2013;18(5):518–24.

17. Win AK, Macinnis RJ, Dowty JG, et al. Criteria and prediction models for mismatch repair gene mutations: a review. J Med Genet 2013;50(12):785–93.

18. Parmigiani G, Chen S, Iversen ES Jr, et al. Validity of models for predicting BRCA1 and BRCA2 mutations. Ann Intern Med 2007;147(7):441–50.

19. Spurdle AB, Couch FJ, Parsons MT, et al. Refined histopathological predictors of BRCA1 and BRCA2 mutation status: a large-scale analysis of breast cancer characteristics from the BCAC, CIMBA, and ENIGMA consortia. Breast Cancer Res 2014;16(6):3419.

20. Rehm HL, Berg JS, Brooks LD, et al. ClinGen–the Clinical Genome Resource. N Engl J Med 2015;372(23):2235–42.

21. Rasmussen LJ, Heinen CD, Royer-Pokora B, et al. Pathological assessment of mismatch repair gene variants in Lynch syndrome: past, present, and future. Hum Mutat 2012;33(12):1617–25.

22. Heinen CD, Juel Rasmussen L. Determining the functional significance of mismatch repair gene missense variants using biochemical and cellular assays. Hered Cancer Clin Pract 2012;10(1):9.

23. Thompson BA, Greenblatt MS, Vallee MP, et al. Calibration of multiple in silico tools for predicting pathogenicity of mismatch repair gene missense substitutions. Hum Mutat 2013;34:255–65.

24. Goldgar DE, Easton DF, Byrnes GB, et al, IARC Unclassified Genetic Variants Working Group. Genetic evidence and integration of various data sources for classifying uncertain variants into a single model. Hum Mutat 2008;29(11): 1265–72.

25. Couch FJ, Rasmussen LJ, Hofstra R, et al. For the IARC Unclassified Genetic Variants Working Group, Assessment of Functional Effects of Unclassified Genetic Variants. Human Mutation 2008;29:1314–26.

26. Raevaara TE, Korhonen MK, Lohi H, et al. Functional significance and clinical phenotype of nontruncating mismatch repair variants of MLH1. Gastroenterology 2005;129(2):537–49.

27. Hitchins MP, Rapkins RW, Kwok CT, et al. Dominantly inherited constitutional epigenetic silencing of MLH1 in a cancer-affected family is linked to a single nucleotide variant within the 5'UTR. Cancer Cell 2011;20(2):200–13.

28. Kwok C-T, Vogelaar IP, van Zelst-Stams WA, et al. The MLH1 c.-27C>A and c.85G>T variants are borne on a European ancestral haplotype which underlies a dominantly inherited form of MLH1 epimutation. Eur J Hum Genet 2014;22(5): 617–24.

29. 1000 Genomes Project Consortium, Abecasis GR, Altshuler D, Auton A, et al. A map of human genome variation from population-scale sequencing. Nature 2010;467(7319):1061–73.

30. Barnetson RA, Cartwright N, van Vliet A, et al. Classification of ambiguous mutations in DNA mismatch repair genes identified in a population-based study of colorectal cancer. Hum Mutat 2008;29(3):367–74.

31. Easton DF, Deffenbaugh AM, Pruss D, et al. A systematic genetic assessment of 1,433 sequence variants of unknown clinical significance in the BRCA1 and BRCA2 breast cancer-predisposition genes. Am J Hum Genet 2007;81(5): 873–83.

32. Lakhani SR, Manek S, Penault-Llorca F, et al. Pathology of ovarian cancers in BRCA1 and BRCA2 carriers. Clin Cancer Res 2004;10(7):2473–81.

33. Lynch HT, Lynch PM, Lanspa SJ, et al. Review of the Lynch syndrome: history, molecular genetics, screening, differential diagnosis, and medicolegal ramifications. Clin Genet 2009;76(1):1–18.

34. Thompson BA, Goldgar DE, Paterson C, et al, Colon Cancer Family Registry. A multifactorial likelihood model for MMR gene variant classification incorporating probabilities based on sequence bioinformatics and tumor characteristics: a report from the Colon Cancer Family Registry. Hum Mutat 2013;34:200–9.

35. Gylling AH, Nieminen TT, Abdel-Rahman WM, et al. Differential cancer predisposition in Lynch syndrome: insights from molecular analysis of brain and urinary tract tumors. Carcinogenesis 2008;29(7):1351–9.

36. Haas NB, Nathanson KL. Hereditary kidney cancer syndromes. Adv Chronic Kidney Dis 2014;21(1):81–90.

37. Gowen LC, Johnson BL, Latour AM, et al. Brca1 deficiency results in early embryonic lethality characterized by neuroepithelial abnormalities. Nat Genet 1996;12(2):191–4.

38. D'Andrea AD. Susceptibility pathways in Fanconi's anemia and breast cancer. N Engl J Med 2010;362(20):1909–19.

39. Wimmer K, Kratz CP, Vasen HF, et al, EU-Consortium Care for CMMRD (C4CMMRD). Diagnostic criteria for constitutional mismatch repair deficiency syndrome: suggestions of the European consortium 'care for CMMRD' (C4CMMRD). J Med Genet 2014;51(6):355–65.

40. Drost M, Zonneveld JB, van Dijk L, et al. A cell-free assay for the functional analysis of variants of the mismatch repair protein MLH1. Hum Mutat 2010;31(3):247–53.

41. Spurdle AB, Couch FJ, Hogervorst FB, et al, IARC Unclassified Genetic Variants Working Group. Prediction and assessment of splicing alterations: implications for clinical testing. Hum Mutat 2008;29(11):1304–13.

42. Loke J, Pearlman A, Upadhyay K, et al. Functional variant analyses (FVAs) predict pathogenicity in the BRCA1 DNA double-strand break repair pathway. Hum Mol Genet 2015;24(11):3030–7.

43. Tournier I, Vezain M, Martins A, et al. A large fraction of unclassified variants of the mismatch repair genes MLH1 and MSH2 is associated with splicing defects. Hum Mutat 2008;29(12):1412–24.

44. Moghadasi S, Hofland N, Wouts JN, et al. Variants of uncertain significance in BRCA1 and BRCA2 assessment of in silico analysis and a proposal for communication in genetic counseling. J Med Genet 2013;50(2):74–9.

45. Landrum MJ, Lee JM, Riley GR, et al. ClinVar: public archive of relationships among sequence variation and human phenotype. Nucleic Acids Res 2014;42(Database issue):D980–5.

46. Spurdle AB, Healey S, Devereau A, et al. ENIGMA–evidence-based network for the interpretation of germline mutant alleles: an international initiative to evaluate risk and clinical significance associated with sequence variation in BRCA1 and BRCA2 genes. Hum Mutat 2012;33(1):2–7.

47. Catts ZA, Hampel H. Certified Genetic Counselors: A Crucial Clinical Resource in the Management of Patients with Suspected Hereditary Cancer Syndromes. Surg Oncol Clin N Am, in press.

United States Postal Service

Statement of Ownership, Management, and Circulation
(All Periodicals Publications Except Requester Publications)

1. Publication Title	2. Publication Number	3. Filing Date
Surgical Oncology Clinics of North America	0 1 2 - 5 6 5	9/18/15

4. Issue Frequency	5. Number of Issues Published Annually	6. Annual Subscription Price
Jan, Apr, Jul, Oct	4	$290.00

7. Complete Mailing Address of Known Office of Publication (Not printer) (Street, city, county, state, and ZIP+4®)

Elsevier Inc.
360 Park Avenue South
New York, NY 10010-1710

Contact Person
Stephen R. Bushing

Telephone (Include area code)
215-239-3688

8. Complete Mailing Address of Headquarters or General Business Office of Publisher (Not printer)

Elsevier Inc., 360 Park Avenue South, New York, NY 10010-1710

9. Full Names and Complete Mailing Addresses of Publisher, Editor, and Managing Editor (Do not leave blank)

Publisher (Name and complete mailing address)

Linda Belfus, Elsevier Inc., 1600 John F. Kennedy Blvd., Suite 1800, Philadelphia, PA 19103

Editor (Name and complete mailing address)

John Vassallo, Elsevier Inc., 1600 John F. Kennedy Blvd., Suite 1800, Philadelphia, PA 19103-2899

Managing Editor (Name and complete mailing address)

Adrianne Brigido, Elsevier Inc., 1600 John F. Kennedy Blvd., Suite 1800, Philadelphia, PA 19103-2899

10. Owner (Do not leave blank. If the publication is owned by a corporation, give the name and address of the corporation immediately followed by the names and addresses of all stockholders owning or holding 1 percent or more of the total amount of stock. If not owned by a corporation, give the names and addresses of the individual owners. If owned by a partnership or other unincorporated firm, give its name and address as well as those of each individual owner. If the publication is published by a nonprofit organization, give its name and address.)

Full Name	Complete Mailing Address
Wholly owned subsidiary of	1600 John F. Kennedy Blvd, Ste. 1800
Reed/Elsevier, US holdings	Philadelphia, PA 19103-2899

11. Known Bondholders, Mortgagees, and Other Security Holders Owning or Holding 1 Percent or More of Total Amount of Bonds, Mortgages, or Other Securities. If none, check box ☐ None

Full Name	Complete Mailing Address
N/A	

12. Tax Status (For completion by nonprofit organizations authorized to mail at nonprofit rates) (Check one)
The purpose, function, and nonprofit status of this organization and the exempt status for federal income tax purposes:
☐ Has Not Changed During Preceding 12 Months
☐ Has Changed During Preceding 12 Months (Publisher must submit explanation of change with this statement)

13. Publication Title	14. Issue Date for Circulation Data Below
Surgical Oncology Clinics of North America	July 2015

PS Form 3526, July 2014 (Page 1 of 3 (Instructions Page 3)) PSN 7530-01-000-9931 PRIVACY NOTICE: See our Privacy policy in www.usps.com

15. Extent and Nature of Circulation			Average No. Copies Each Issue During Preceding 12 Months	No. Copies of Single Issue Published Nearest to Filing Date
a. Total Number of Copies (Net press run)			440	389
b. Legitimate Paid and/or Requested Distribution (By Mail and Outside the Mail)	(1)	Mailed Outside-County Paid/Requested Mail Subscriptions stated on PS Form 3541. (Include paid distribution above nominal rate, advertiser's proof copies and exchange copies)	171	152
	(2)	Mailed In-County Paid/Requested Mail Subscriptions stated on PS Form 3541. (Include paid distribution above nominal rate, advertiser's proof copies and exchange copies)		
	(3)	Paid Distribution Outside the Mails Including Sales Through Dealers And Carriers, Street Vendors, Counter Sales, and Other Paid Distribution Outside USPS®	67	65
	(4)	Paid Distribution by Other Classes of Mail Through the USPS (e.g. First-Class Mail®)		
c. Total Paid and/or Requested Circulation (Sum of 15b (1), (2), (3), and (4))		▲	238	217
d. Free or Nominal Rate Distribution (By Mail and Outside the Mail)	(1)	Free or Nominal Rate Outside-County Copies included on PS Form 3541	21	24
	(2)	Free or Nominal Rate In-County Copies included on PS Form 3541		
	(3)	Free or Nominal Rate Copies mailed at Other classes Through the USPS (e.g. First-Class Mail®)		
	(4)	Free or Nominal Rate Distribution Outside the Mail (Carriers or Other means)		
e. Total Nonrequested Distribution (Sum of 15d (1), (2), (3) and (4))		▲	21	24
f. Total Distribution (Sum of 15c and 15e)			259	241
g. Copies not Distributed (See instructions to publishers #4 (page #3))		▲	181	148
h. Total (Sum of 15f and g)		▲	440	389
i. Percent Paid and/or Requested Circulation (15c divided by 15f times 100)		▲	91.89%	90.04%

* If you are claiming electronic copies go to line 16 on page 3. If you are not claiming Electronic copies, skip to line 17 on page 3.

16. Electronic Copy Circulation	Average No. Copies Each Issue During Preceding 12 Months	No. Copies of Single Issue Published Nearest to Filing Date
a. Paid Electronic Copies		
b. Total paid Print Copies (Line 15c) + Paid Electronic copies (Line 16a)		
c. Total Print Distribution (Line 15f) + Paid Electronic Copies (Line 16a)		
d. Percent Paid (Both Print & Electronic copies) (16b divided by 16c X 100)		

☐ I certify that 50% of all my distributed copies (electronic and print) are paid above a nominal price

17. Publication of Statement of Ownership
If the publication is a general publication, publication of this statement is required. Will be printed in the _October 2015_ issue of this publication.

18. Signature and Title of Editor, Publisher, Business Manager, or Owner

Stephen R. Bushing – Inventory Distribution Coordinator

Date
September 18, 2015

I certify that all information furnished on this form is true and complete. I understand that anyone who furnishes false or misleading information on this form or who omits material or information requested on the form may be subject to criminal sanctions (including fines and imprisonment) and/or civil sanctions (including civil penalties).

PS Form 3526, July 2014 (Page 3 of 3)

Moving?

Make sure your subscription moves with you!

To notify us of your new address, find your **Clinics Account Number** (located on your mailing label above your name), and contact customer service at:

Email: journalscustomerservice-usa@elsevier.com

800-654-2452 (subscribers in the U.S. & Canada)
314-447-8871 (subscribers outside of the U.S. & Canada)

Fax number: 314-447-8029

Elsevier Health Sciences Division
Subscription Customer Service
3251 Riverport Lane
Maryland Heights, MO 63043

*To ensure uninterrupted delivery of your subscription, please notify us at least 4 weeks in advance of move.

Printed and bound by CPI Group (UK) Ltd, Croydon, CR0 4YY

07/10/2024

01040498-0004